—

MEDICAL EVALUATION OF CHILD SEXUAL ABUSE

A Practical Guide

3rd Edition

Edited by

Martin A. Finkel, DO, FACOP, FAAP
Child Abuse Research Education & Service Institute
School of Osteopathic Medicine
University of Medicine and Dentistry
of New Jersey

Angelo P. Giardino, MD, PhD, MPH, FAAP
Texas Children's Health Plan
and
Baylor College of Medicine

American Academy of Pediatrics
141 Northwest Point Blvd
Elk Grove Village, IL 60007-1098

AAP Department of Marketing and Publications

Maureen DeRosa, MPA, Director, Department of Marketing and Publications
Mark Grimes, Director, Division of Product Development
Diane Lundquist, Senior Product Development Editor
Sandi King, MS, Director, Division of Publishing and Production Services
Kate Larson, Manager, Editorial Services
Theresa Wiener, Manager, Editorial Production
Linda Diamond, Manager, Art Direction and Production
Jill Ferguson, Director, Division of Marketing
Linda Smessaert, Manager, Clinical and Professional Publications Marketing
Robert Herling, Director, Division of Sales

Library of Congress Control Number: 2008938292
ISBN: 978-1-58110-320-5
MA0463

The recommendations in this publication do not indicate an exclusive course of treatment or serve as a standard of care. Variations, taking into account individual circumstances, may be appropriate.

Brand names are furnished for identification purposes only. No endorsement of the manufacturers or products mentioned is implied.

9-204/1208

Last digit is the print number: 9 8 7 6 5 4 3 2 1

About the Editors

Martin A. Finkel, DO, FACOP, FAAP

Dr Finkel is a professor of pediatrics and the medical director and cofounder of the Child Abuse Research Education & Service (CARES) Institute at the University of Medicine and Dentistry of New Jersey's School of Osteopathic Medicine. The CARES Institute is a statewide resource to inform best practices in the delivery of medical and mental health diagnostic and treatment services. Dr Finkel is an internationally recognized authority on the medical evaluation and treatment of the child alleged to have been sexually abused. Dr Finkel has been instrumental in developing New Jersey's statewide network of regional child abuse diagnostic and treatment centers. These centers of excellence provide services for sexually and physically abused children and educate professionals within the medical, child protection, law enforcement, and mental health communities on the evaluation of the child victim. He has been a pioneer in the use of videocolposcopy for the assessment and documentation of residua to sexual abuse. He is the author of the first scientific paper published in the medical literature on the healing and interpretation of acute genital and anal trauma and the first paper in the literature on signs and symptoms associated with genital contact in girls. He has published numerous articles, authored chapters, and coedited 2 previous editions of this textbook on the medical evaluation of the sexually abused child.

Dr Finkel was appointed by 6 governors to cochair, with the commissioner of the Department of Children and Families, New Jersey's Task Force on Child Abuse and Neglect and 2 Governor's Blue Ribbon Panels to review child protection practices. He is a founding commissioner of New Jersey's Children's Trust Fund to prevent child abuse. Dr Finkel has been on the national board of the American Professional Society on the Abuse of Children, where he had oversight for the development of national standards regarding medical terminology and the interpretation of medical findings. He is a founding member of the Ray E. Helfer Society, the American Academy of Pediatrics Section on Child Abuse and Neglect, and the American Professional Society on the Abuse of Children. He served a 6-year term on the National Board of Prevent Child Abuse America. He is former president of the American College of Osteopathic Pediatricians.

Angelo P. Giardino, MD, PhD, MPH, FAAP

Dr Giardino is the medical director of Texas Children's Health Plan, a clinical associate professor of pediatrics at Baylor College of Medicine, and an attending physician on both the Texas Children's Hospital Child Protection Team and the forensic pediatrics service at the Children's Assessment Center in Houston, TX. In addition, Dr Giardino serves as the physician advisor to the Texas Children's Hospital Center for Childhood Injury Prevention. Dr Giardino earned his doctor of medicine and doctor of philosophy degrees at the University of Pennsylvania and his master of public health from the University of Massachusetts. Dr Giardino completed his pediatric residency and child maltreatment fellowship training at The Children's Hospital of Philadelphia (CHOP) and also completed training in secondary data analysis related to child maltreatment from the National Data Archive on Child Abuse and Neglect's Summer Research Institute at Cornell University.

Dr Giardino's clinical work focuses on child maltreatment, and in 1995 he collaborated with a multidisciplinary team to develop and lead the Abuse Referral Center for Children with Special Health Care Needs at the Children's Seashore House, which was funded by a 3-year grant from a local philanthropy in Philadelphia. This program was designed to provide medical evaluations to children with developmental disabilities who were suspected of having been abused or neglected. In 1998 he was appointed associate chair for clinical operations in the department of pediatrics at CHOP and also served on the hospital's child abuse evaluation service. In 2002 Dr Giardino joined the department of pediatrics at Drexel College of Medicine as the associate chair for clinical affairs and was appointed associate physician in chief at St Christopher's Hospital for Children, where he also served as the medical director for the hospital's Suspected Child Abuse and Neglect Program. This program collaborated with the Institute for Safe Families and Lutheran Settlement House to secure a Pennsylvania Children's Trust Fund grant, which supported a community-based Intimate Partner Violence Screening program at St Christopher's aimed at identifying at-risk families and working to prevent child maltreatment. Additionally, while at St Christopher's, Dr Giardino collaborated with colleagues at the Drexel University School of Public Health to launch the Philadelphia Grow Project, which provided clinical care to children with the diagnosis of failure to thrive and also conducted policy research on the issues surrounding food insecurity and childhood hunger. Dr Giardino is board certified in pediatrics, is a fellow of the American Academy of Pediatrics and a member of both the Texas Pediatric Society and the Harris County Medical Society. He is a member of the Helfer Society, the American College of Physician Executives, and the American College of Medical Quality. Dr Giardino is a certified physician executive and is also certified in medical quality. Prior to relocating to Houston, Dr Giardino served as chair of the Philadelphia Branch Board of the Southeastern Chapter of the American Red Cross; president of the board for Bethany Christian Services in Fort Washington, PA; and a 2-term member of the board for the Support Center for Child Advocates, where he was named a 2005 Champion for Children. His academic accomplishments include published articles and textbooks on child abuse and neglect, contributions to several national curricula on the evaluation of child maltreatment, presentations on a variety of pediatric topics at both national and regional conferences and, most recently, completion of a 3-year term on the National Review Board (NRB) for the US Conference of Catholic Bishops, providing advice on how best to protect children from sexual abuse. While on the NRB, Dr Giardino served as the chair for its Research Committee. Currently, Dr Giardino serves on the national board of directors for Justice for Children (an advocacy organization providing assistance for children and families involved with the court system around issues related to child abuse and neglect), the national advisory board for the Institute for Safe Families (an advocacy organization that seeks to train professionals in screening and prevention around issues related to intimate partner violence), and the national board of directors for Prevent Child Abuse America.

About the Contributors

Faye A. Blair, RN, PhD

Dr Faye Blair is an associate clinical professor in the College of Nursing at Texas Women's University in Houston, TX. Dr Blair received her bachelor of nursing degree from the University of Texas Medical Branch and her master of science and post-master's certificate as an emergency nurse practitioner at the School of Nursing at the University of Texas Health Sciences at Houston. She completed her doctoral program at Texas Women's University. Dr Blair has coordinated and lead several Sexual Assault Nurse Examiner (SANE) programs in Houston and is a frequent lecturer on the evaluation of children and adolescents for possible sexual abuse and sexual assault. An emergency nurse for many years, Dr Blair has served as a nursing leader in several emergency departments and is an active member of the Emergency Nurses Association (ENA), having served 2 terms as the president of the Houston Chapter of the ENA. Additionally, she serves on Houston's Regional Advisory Council on Trauma and completed 4 years as a member of its Board of Managers. Her academic work includes teaching about emergency care, trauma services, and the evaluation of suspected abuse and neglect as well as participating as a coinvestigator on several projects exploring the utility of a comprehensive database related to child sexual abuse quality assurance.

Ann S. Botash, MD, FAAP

Dr Botash is professor of pediatrics at the State University of New York Upstate Medical University and vice chair for educational affairs at the SUNY Upstate Department of Pediatrics. She is director of the University Hospital's Child Abuse Referral and Evaluation (CARE) program in Syracuse, NY, and is one of the founders of the McMahon/Ryan Child Advocacy site as well as medical director of the site.

To better serve all children and adolescents in New York State, Dr Botash created and is director of the Child Abuse Medical Provider (CHAMP) Network to educate health care professionals in the identification and management of child sexual abuse cases. Dr Botash has written a primer for medical providers, *Evaluating Child Sexual Abuse: Education Manual for Medical Professionals* (Johns Hopkins Press; 2000) and many research articles and chapters.

Dr Botash is a recipient of the Ambulatory Pediatric Association's Award for Public Policy and Advocacy (2005).

Cindy W. Christian, MD, FAAP

Dr Christian holds The Children's Hospital of Philadelphia Chair in the Prevention of Child Abuse and Neglect. She is codirector of Safe Place: The Center for Child Protection and Health at The Children's Hospital of Philadelphia and associate professor of pediatrics at the University of Pennsylvania School of Medicine. Dr Christian devotes much of her clinical and academic work to the care of abused children. She is a faculty director of the Field Center for Children's Policy, Practice and Research at the University of Pennsylvania. Dr Christian presently serves on the Committee on Child Abuse and Neglect for the American Academy of Pediatrics and is a founding member of the Ray E. Helfer Society. Dr Christian's research and educational efforts are related to the medical evaluation and care of abused children.

Sharon W. Cooper, MD, FAAP

Dr Cooper is chief executive officer of Developmental and Forensic Pediatrics, a consulting firm that provides medical care, training, and expert witness experience in child maltreatment cases, as well as medical care for children with disabilities. She works regularly with numerous national and international investigative agencies on Internet crimes against children cases. Dr Cooper spent 21 years in the armed forces, retiring as a colonel, and has for the past several years worked in both the civilian and military arenas in child abuse and developmental pediatrics. She holds a faculty position at the University of North Carolina Chapel Hill School of Medicine and the Uniformed Services University of Health Sciences in Bethesda, MD. She is an instructor at the Army Medical Education Department Center and School at Fort Sam Houston, San Antonio, TX, where she provides multidisciplinary training in all forms of child maltreatment to health care providers, law enforce-ment, attorneys, judges, therapists, chaplains, and social workers. For the past several years, Dr Cooper has served as an instructor at the National Center for Missing & Exploited Children, where she teaches about the victim aspects of Internet crimes against children and the sexual exploitation through prostitution of children and youths. She has published chapters in texts and is the lead author of the first comprehensive text on the medical, legal, and social science aspects of child sexual exploitation and Internet crimes against children.

Esther Deblinger, PhD

Dr Deblinger is cofounder and codirector of the New Jersey Child Abuse Research Education & Service (CARES) Institute and professor of clinical psychiatry at the University of Medicine and Dentistry of New Jersey (UMDNJ) School of Osteopathic Medicine. In collaboration with her colleagues at the institute, Dr Deblinger has conducted cutting-edge research, funded by the Foundation of UMDNJ, the National Center on Child Abuse and Neglect, and the National Institute of Mental Health, examining the impact of child sexual abuse and the treatment of post-traumatic stress disorder and related difficulties. As a result of this work, Dr Deblinger and her colleagues developed a cognitive-behavioral therapy program that was recognized for its effectiveness in treating child sexual abuse with a 2001 Exemplary Program Award, presented by the US Department of Health and Human Services, Substance Abuse and Mental Health Services Administration. Dr Deblinger served 2 terms on the board of the American Professional Society on the Abuse of Children and she is a member of the National Child Traumatic Stress Network. In addition to publishing numerous journal articles, Dr Deblinger is the coauthor of the professional books *Treating Trauma and Traumatic Grief in Children and Adolescents* (2007) and *Treating Sexually Abused Children and Their Nonoffending Parents: A Cognitive Behavioral Approach* (1996), as well as the children's book *Let's Talk About Taking Care of You: An Educational Book About Body Safety* (2003).

Lori D. Frasier, MD, FAAP

Dr Frasier attended the University of Utah College of Medicine and completed a pediatric residency at the University of Washington. She was fellow at the Harborview Sexual Assault Center under Dr Carole Jenny from 1988 to 1990. Dr Frasier was on faculty of the department of pediatrics at the University of Iowa from 1990 to 1995, establishing the sexual abuse evaluation clinic there and participating in evaluations of physical abuse and neglect. From 1995 to 2002 Dr Frasier was on the faculty of the department of child health at the University of Missouri-Columbia, director of the child protection program there, and from 1994 to 2002 was the medical director of the Missouri SAFE-CARE Network, a network of medical providers trained to provide medical evaluations to abused and neglected children. She is currently the medical director of the Medical Assessment Team at the Center for Safe and Healthy Families, Primary Children's Medical Center, Salt Lake City, UT, and a professor in the department of pediatrics at the University of Utah School of Medicine. She has published many articles and chapters in the field of child abuse and has lectured locally and nationally. She is the immediate past chair of the executive committee for the Section on Child Abuse and Neglect of the American Academy of Pediatrics and on the board of directors of the American Professional Society on the Abuse of Children. Dr Frasier has been appointed to the American Board of Pediatrics first sub-board in child abuse pediatrics.

Eileen R. Giardino, RN, PhD, CRNP, FNP-BC

Dr Giardino is an associate professor at the School of Nursing at the University of Texas Health Science Center (UTHSC) at Houston. Dr Giardino received her bachelor of science in nursing and doctor of philosophy degrees from the University of Pennsylvania, her master of science in nursing from Widener University, and her nurse practitioner certification in adult and family from LaSalle University. Clinically, Dr Giardino works as a nurse practitioner at a university student health service. Her academic accomplishments include coediting several textbooks in the areas of child maltreatment and intimate partner violence and presenting at professional meetings on issues related to physical assessment and conducting a differential diagnosis. Prior to moving to

Houston, Dr Giardino served on the board of directors for Bethany Christian Services in Fort Washington, PA; was on the advisory board for the LaSalle University Nursing Center in Philadelphia; and completed 2 terms on the board of directors for the Philadelphia Children's Alliance, where she also chaired the program evaluation committee. Finally, Dr Giardino teaches on a variety of topics in the adult and family nurse practitioner tracks at UTHSC at Houston and is involved in supervising a number of clinical preceptorships within the nurse practitioner training program.

Julie Lippmann, PsyD

Dr Lippmann is director of Evaluation Services at the Child Abuse Research Education & Service (CARES) Institute and assistant professor of clinical psychiatry at the University of Medicine and Dentistry of New Jersey School of Osteopathic Medicine. She has served as the senior supervising psychologist at the institute since its inception, conducting specialized evaluations and psychotherapy with children alleged to have been sexually abused, and with their nonoffending parents, for the past 20 years. She participates in federally funded research, expert legal testimony, and teaching and training statewide. Her publications focus on results of treatment outcome research and mental health evaluation.

Michelle A. Lyn, MD, FAAP

Dr Lyn is an associate professor of pediatrics at Baylor College of Medicine, chief of the Child Protection Section of Emergency Medicine at Texas Children's Hospital, and medical director of The Children's Assessment Center. Dr Lyn earned her doctor of medicine degree from State University of New York at Buffalo School of Medicine; completed her residency in pediatrics at Albert Einstein College of Medicine-Montefiore Medical Center in Bronx, NY, where she served as the pediatric chief resident; and completed a fellowship in pediatric emergency medicine at Baylor College of Medicine in Houston, TX. Her academic, clinical, research, and community outreach work focuses largely on children in crisis. She teaches medical students, interns, residents, and fellows of emergency medicine and family practice about child maltreatment and she educates community medical professionals, teachers, law enforcement officers, military personnel, and first responders through the SCAN (Suspect Child Abuse & Neglect) community outreach program. Dr Lyn is a board-certified pediatrician who is also certified in pediatric emergency medicine. She is a fellow of the American Academy of Pediatrics. Her community board memberships include St Luke's Episcopal Health Charities and Healthy Family Initiatives, both in Houston, TX. She has presented numerous lectures and made many television and radio appearances speaking on topics of pediatric and adolescent physical and sexual abuse. Dr Lyn's work to help children in crisis and to teach medical professionals about the field of child maltreatment and pediatric emergency medicine has been recognized by her receiving Baylor College of Medicine's (BCM) Department of Pediatrics Award of General Excellence in Teaching as well as the BCM Fulbright and Jaworski Excellence Teaching Award. Additionally, community recognition has manifested itself as the Texas Executive Women's Women on the Move honoree, Martin Luther King Foundation's Keeping the Dream Alive recipient, and the Wesleyan College Alumni Recognition Award. Prior to leading the Child Protection Team at Texas Children's Hospital, Dr Lyn served as the medical director for pediatric emergency medicine at Ben Taub General Hospital in Houston, which is dedicated to serving the underinsured and uninsured population in Harris County Texas.

John E. B. Myers, JD

John E.B. Myers, JD, is distinguished professor and scholar at the University of the Pacific-McGeorge School of Law in Sacramento, CA. Professor Myers has authored numerous books, chapters, and articles on legal issues in child abuse. His writing has been cited by more than 140 courts, including the US Supreme Court. He is a frequent speaker at child abuse conferences, having made more than 400 presentations across America and abroad.

Vincent J. Palusci, MD, MS, FAAP

Dr Palusci graduated with honors in chemistry from the University of Pennsylvania. He received his medical degree from the University of Medicine and Dentistry of New Jersey and completed his internship and residency in pediatrics at New York University/Bellevue Hospital Center in New York. He entered private practice and later joined the faculty of the College of Human Medicine at Michigan State University, where he was also a TRECOS scholar and earned a master of science degree in epidemiology. He recently returned to NYU School of Medicine and Bellevue Hospital's Frances L. Loeb Child Protection and Development Center. Dr Palusci's work has focused on epidemiologic and health services issues for child abuse victims and the educational needs of general and specialist pediatricians. He received the Ray E. Helfer Award for child abuse prevention in 2004. He has edited *Shaken Baby Syndrome: A Multidisciplinary Response* with Dr Steven Lazoritz and *A Colour Atlas of Child Abuse and Neglect*, due out in 2009.

Lawrence R. Ricci, MD, FAAP

Dr Ricci is a clinical associate professor of pediatrics at the University of Vermont College of Medicine and is director of the Spurwink Child Abuse Program, a statewide referral center for Maine children, located in Portland, ME. He has been a full-time child abuse pediatrician specializing in the evaluation and treatment of abused children for the past 20 years. Dr Ricci has served on a number of state and national child abuse committees, including former chair of the Section on Child Abuse of the American Academy of Pediatrics (1990–1994) and former president of the Ray Helfer Society, an honorary society of physicians specializing in the care of abused children (2002–2004). He has presented numerous child abuse workshops throughout Maine and around the country to social workers, mental heath professionals, legal professionals, and medical professionals and has published approximately 25 articles and book chapters in the field of child abuse evaluation and treatment.

Melissa K. Runyon, PhD

Dr Runyon is director of treatment services at the Child Abuse Research Education & Service (CARES) Institute and associate professor of psychiatry at the University of Medicine and Dentistry of New Jersey School of Osteopathic Medicine. Through federally funded grants, she and her colleagues have developed evidence-based practices for children and families at risk for child physical abuse: combined parent-child cognitive behavioral therapy (CPC-CBT). Dr Runyon also serves as a supervisor and coinvestigator on federally funded research grants examining the effectiveness of trauma-focused cognitive behavioral therapy for children who have experienced sexual abuse. She has provided training and ongoing consultation in the implementation of CPC-CBT for children and parents at risk for child physical abuse on a local, national, and international basis. She has several publications in the area of child maltreatment and is an author of the therapeutic children's book, *Helping Families Heal: A Story of Child Physical Abuse*.

Philip V. Scribano, DO, MSCE, FAAP

Dr Scribano graduated from Rutgers University and The University of Medicine and Dentistry of New Jersey School of Osteopathic Medicine. He also received a master of science degree in clinical epidemiology at the University of Pennsylvania.

He is the medical director of the Center for Child and Family Advocacy at Nationwide Children's Hospital, chief of the division of child and family advocacy, and associate professor of clinical pediatrics at the Ohio State University College of Medicine. He is the recipient of multiple research and program grants including awards from the Administration on Children and Families, Agency for Healthcare Research and Quality, and the Centers for Disease Control and Prevention.

Dr Scribano is active with the American Academy of Pediatrics (AAP) and is chair of the Ohio AAP Committee on Child Abuse and Neglect. He is a board member of the Academy on Violence and Abuse and cochair of the Helfer Society's Program Directors Committee.

Deborah C. Stewart, MD

Dr Stewart is the medical director of the University of California Davis Child and Adolescent Abuse Resource and Evaluation Diagnostic and Treatment Center. She is a professor of pediatrics at the University of California Davis. Her clinical and research interests involve sexually transmitted infections in sexually abused children, medical issues in child neglect, and medical issues in drug-endangered children, as well as other youth violence issues.

She is past president of Chapter V, District IX of the American Academy of Pediatrics and prior recipient of multiple grants including Healthy Tomorrows Preventing Teen Violence 8% Early Intervention Program and the National Institutes of Health/National Institute on Drug Abuse Optimizing Toxicologic Screening in Drug Endangered Children.

Thank you...

To the children, parents, and professionals
who have entrusted me to help.

To my colleagues with whom shared insights
have helped build the foundation of our understanding
of meeting the medical needs
of children suspected of being sexually abused.

To my child protection, mental health,
and legal colleagues
for teaching me how the system can
and must work to help children.

To the staff of the Child Abuse Research Education
& Service Institute
for their tireless dedication and professionalism.

To the administration of the School of Osteopathic Medicine
at the University of Medicine & Dentistry of New Jersey
for providing the environment and tools to succeed.

To my wife Bonnie and my children Benjamin and Julia
for their encouragement, understanding, and support.

Martin A. Finkel, DO

To the following colleagues, who over the past 2 decades
have graciously shared
their teaching materials and wise counsel:

Carol D. Berkowitz, MD

Allan R. DeJong, MD

Robert M. Reece, MD

Lawrence R. Ricci, MD

Angelo P. Giardino, MD, PhD, MPH

Contents

Foreword

This book, now in its third edition, continues to provide a valuable resource to clinicians and child advocates on the front line who are directly serving children and families affected by suspicions of child sexual abuse. It is over 30 years since the pioneering reports on the medical findings of child sexual abuse surfaced in the pediatric literature. Over the past 3 decades our professional understanding of normal and posttraumatic prepubertal and pubertal anatomy has increased, and has become even more refined. The emerging evidence base that professionals now use on a daily basis to conduct and interpret the health care evaluation findings in children who are assessed for suspicions of possible sexual abuse is clearly evident in the book's ensuing chapters written by an illustrious array of child sexual abuse experts. Professionals who confront the challenges inherent in evaluating children suspected of having been sexually abused will find coherent and readily applied information that will assist them in conducting a thorough health care evaluation. Additionally, to its credit this third edition taken as a whole also reflects a profound respect for the multidisciplinary approach to child sexual abuse investigations, and the chapter on multidisciplinary teams serves as a primer on effective team functioning, which is so essential for our collective work on behalf of the children and families we as health care providers and child advocates seek to serve. And yet as our knowledge increases around ideal ways to evaluate child abuse allegations in the health care setting, new dangers continue to emerge that confront our children, including the Internet with exposure to pornography and enticement into sexual encounters and interactions with experienced predators. The chapter on exploitation provides a framework from which to view this growing risk to children as well.

With the benefit of more than 3 decades of professional attention, we can now look back and see where we have been as a group of professionals and child advocates. Amazingly, recent epidemiological data suggest that the prevalence as well as the incidence of child sexual abuse may be declining in our US society in recent years. The reason for such a downward trend is unclear, however. In the early 1980s there was an explosion of reported cases of child sexual abuse. In Los Angeles County alone, about 25% of reported cases of child abuse were for child sexual abuse. After the furor of the preschool allegations and multiple victim cases, the reported statistics settled to about 8% of all cases of maltreatment were for child sexual abuse, and the figure remains at that lower value even today at this writing. Optimistically, data also suggest that the total numbers of cases of physical child maltreatment are also declining. Are we better at early detection and intervention, and reducing the rates of recidivism and repeat abuse? After the upsurge of cases in the 1980s, I had assumed that we had perhaps caught up with a backlog of affected children who previously might not have been believed or seen by a medical examiner. Studies suggested that the time lapse between onset of abuse and disclosure was about 8 years. Clinical care keeps us grounded, and I recently encountered a 3-year-old who on returning from a 4-day trip with extended family members told her mother that Uncle Don (a boyfriend of an aunt) had touched her "little butt" (genital area). Her mother immediately brought her to our pediatric emergency department for an assessment. In the past we might not have encountered such a child because children were frequently not believed, and their claims about inappropriate touching by family members were discounted. ("Uncle Don would never had done that. Just stay away from Uncle Don.") The time interval has significantly shortened, and I would speculate that the backlog of cases has been addressed and that children are more likely to be heard and believed.

Effective advocacy builds on what we know about the risks facing children and families, so what are the remaining issues and challenges in the arena of child sexual abuse? Finkelhor, an early and consistent contributor to the field, suggests 2 issues that should form the basis of future research efforts: (1) defining the specifics that ensure the accurate assessment of whether or not an individual was sexually abused and (2) defining the factors that minimize the long-term consequences of such abuse. The latter is a question that is frequently posed when Dr Vincent Felitti presents data from the Adverse Childhood Experiences (ACE) studies. Dr Felitti has clearly identified how multiple factors related to abuse and dysfunctional family issues increase the likelihood of a child experiencing health issues as an adult. But does intervention change these risks? Does stopping the abuse and providing a child with therapy alter the outcome? What impact does placement in foster care or parental incarceration have on adult well-being? I am reminded of the scenario in which a town adjacent to a river is confronted by cries of help coming from the water. The townspeople run to the river's edge and see a man struggling in the river. They hurriedly grab a rowboat and row out to the man, saving him from drowning. Several days later they are confronted by a similar scenario and again they are successful in the rescue. They decide to meet and discuss ways to improve their rescue operations. They then leave a rowboat near the point in the river closest to where the men were retrieved. They develop a roster of citizens to serve on rescue duty. The town receives an award for their heroism and rescue protocol. But no one ever goes upstream to see why people are falling into the river. Prevention is not even on the town's radar. So, are we only rescuing or are we also preventing? And is there any way to prevent child sexual abuse—not just repeat episodes of abuse, but even the initial event?

This is truly a challenging question. In the field of pediatric medicine, we have seen the success of newly created vaccines—the virtual elimination of invasive *Haemophilus influenzae* type b disease, and the marked reduction in both invasive and noninvasive pneumococcal disease and the human papillomavirus vaccine, which holds the promise of reducing cases of cervical cancer in future generations of women. Unfortunately, immunizing against child maltreatment does not seem a likely possibility. Yet, we have been able to develop strategies for minimizing the risk of injuries associated with events such as motor vehicle crashes and falls from bicycles. We have crafted playground equipment to also safeguard against injuries from the falls that naturally occur during play. And we have taught parents to place their infants on their backs when they go to sleep, cutting the rate of sudden infant death syndrome by about two-thirds. So, we have to continue to push forward with searching out ways to reduce the risk to children of child sexual abuse—it may be difficult, but it is a goal that we must redouble our efforts toward achieving. Now that we have refined our diagnostic acumen and learned about the value of working in multidisciplinary teams, we need to focus more attention on prevention. We have seen the documented success in efforts related to preparing a new parent to handle infant crying and the subsequent reduction in the incidence of shaken baby syndrome. But whom to teach? Teaching children to stand up to a molester is both naïve and destructive. How can a 45-pound 6-year-old ward off a 175-pound 25-year-old (especially when the older individual is a trusted family member or friend)? Teaching parents how to open dialogues with their children is, however, an important path to early detection and interruption. The prevention gauntlet is down, and it is time to move to the next level and intervene so the numbers of children who are victims of child sexual abuse will continue to fall both in the United States and abroad. Perhaps we can look forward to a time when child sexual abuse will be a condition of historic interest only, rather like polio.

So, in summary, we have our work as health care professionals and child advocates cut out for us. When we are faced with children who may have been sexually abused, we can use this third edition of the Drs Finkel and Giardino book to guide a thorough health care evaluation and collaborate with other disciplines in conducting a complete investigation into the allegation. However, we seek ultimately to find ways to keep children safe and mitigate the risk of exposure to sexually abusive or exploitive criminal behavior. Our clinical work, our policy work, and our prevention efforts need to be informed by evidence and rigorous research and, fortunately, this book collects a lot of that evidence in a useful, straightforward manner that clinicians and child advocates can begin using today. As we use this information to guide our professional work, let us all unite in the collective effort to fashion a world that allows fewer and fewer of cases of sexual abuse to ever occur and need an evaluation to begin with!

Carol D. Berkowitz, MD

Preface

We are very pleased to offer this revised and expanded third edition of *Medical Evaluation of Child Sexual Abuse: A Practical Guide*. We are honored to have this book published by the American Academy of Pediatrics (AAP). It has been 16 years since the publication of the first edition. During this intervening time, our collective understanding of the sexual victimization of children has increased dramatically. The impact of our increasing evidence base and professional skill development has dramatically improved our diagnostic acumen, improved protection and prevention of child sexual abuse, and refined our therapeutic intervention. It is truly heartening to see the systems designed to recognize sexual abuse and investigate allegations in a manner that is informed and sensitive to victims' special needs becoming steadily more accessible throughout the United States, and beyond. As the field of child maltreatment has matured, pediatricians continue to play a leading role in defining and meeting the specialized medical needs of sexually abused children, and soon board certification will be available in child abuse pediatrics. The multidisciplinary landscape has continued to change over time as well, a spectrum of strategies has evolved to coordinate investigations, collect forensic evidence, and meet the medical and mental health needs of sexually abused children. With all of these changes and the difficulty in meeting the clinical demands for medical services, pediatricians in the vanguard along with the AAP remain very important members of the multidisciplinary expertise necessary to meet all the needs of child victims. We believe that when children enter a system designed to assess and then protect, if needed, those children should have access to the most knowledgeable, skilled, and sensitive clinicians. This book brings together the collective expertise of skilled clinicians whose vast experience in addressing the needs of sexually abused children is shared in a manner that we hope clinicians will find practical and easily applied.

This edition reflects continued refinement of our knowledge of the scientific foundation of the medical diagnosis of child sexual abuse and our roles as medical professionals in diagnosing and treating children who have suffered sexual abuse. Medical professionals, whether physicians or nurses, are on the front lines, and their clinical expertise is critical to addressing residua to sexual contact. The medical professional's opinion is one of the many important pieces of the diagnostic puzzle that leads ultimately to a fuller understanding of what a child may have experienced. A well-documented medical diagnosis and opinion often contribute to the substantiation of allegations, protection from further abuse, and referral for treatment of the psychological sequelae. There are few aspects of medical practice that require a multidisciplinary approach and cooperation with other disciplines more than the field of maltreatment. Throughout this text, the important contributions of the many disciplines that comprise the child protection system are emphasized.

This text is written not only for medical professionals but also as a reference for child protection workers, mental health clinicians, investigators, and the courts. It is incumbent on professionals in each of the disciplines to understand what a complete and comprehensive medical evaluation entails, when to seek an examination, the importance of a medical history, how discrepancies between a child's history and physical findings can be explained, how the medical record should be structured, what types of documentation should be expected, and how a medical diagnosis is formulated.

This latest edition includes new chapters on the burgeoning problem of child pornography and the risks of the Internet. Because the primary impact of any form of sexual victimization is psychological, a new chapter has been added to complement the chapter on psychological evaluation to help the pediatrician understand the spectrum of mental health therapy choices as well as the latest on the prevention of sexual abuse. We hope that readers will find this third edition to be practical, providing both the knowledge and skills necessary to readily translate new information into clinical practice.

The contributors hope that this text will enhance professionals' working knowledge of how to make the diagnosis of child sexual abuse, resulting in objective, balanced, and defensible medical diagnoses. We salute professionals who select this very rewarding field and hope that each of our authors' contributions to this text will assist you in providing the best of care. Children will be the beneficiaries of all of our efforts.

Martin A. Finkel, DO   Angelo P. Giardino, MD, PhD, MPH

Chapter 1

The Problem

Angelo P. Giardino
Michelle A. Lyn

Introduction

Sexual abuse is a complex medical and social problem that manifests itself in a variety of ways and is best defined by an early synthesis of several definitions that go beyond the typically narrow legal definition found in various state criminal codes.[1-3] *Sexual abuse, sexual maltreatment, sexual misuse, sexual molestation,* and *sexual exploitation* are all related terms referring to the involvement in sexual activities by a dominant or more powerful person of a dependent, developmentally immature child or adolescent for that dominant person's own sexual stimulation, or for the gratification of other persons, as in child pornography or prostitution. The activities defined by sexual abuse of a child by a more powerful person or adult include exhibitionism; inappropriate viewing of the child; allowing the child to view inappropriate sexual material; taking sexually related photographs of the child; sexualized

kissing; fondling; masturbation; digital or object penetration of the vagina or anus; and oral-genital, genital-genital, and anal-genital contact. These sexual activities are by their very nature imposed on a child or an adolescent because the child cannot provide informed consent because of his or her age or developmental stage.[1,2] The essential components of the definition of sexual abuse involve the child's developmental immaturity and inability to consent, and the perpetrator's betrayal of the child's trust. The perpetrator in cases of sexual abuse has authority and power over the child ascribed by his or her age or position, and is thus able, either directly or indirectly, to coerce the child into sexual compliance. In intrafamilial sexual abuse, the involvement of the child in sexual activities violates the social taboos of family roles.[1,4] Terms associated with sexual abuse include *intrafamilial abuse, pedophilia,* and *rape.* Intrafamilial abuse (referred to as *incest* in older literature) is sexual activity between individuals who are not permitted to marry, including step-relatives.[5] In the cases involving step-family relationships, the presence or absence of blood relationship is not as important as the kinship role the abuser has in relation to the child.[6] Pedophilia is defined as the preference of an adult for sexual contact with children.[7] Pedophiles are typically skilled at ingratiating themselves with children and are likely to target the most vulnerable among them for sexual contact. Finally, *rape* is a legal term defined by various statutes, typically seen as a violent act that includes some form or variant of forcible sexual intercourse. Rape includes actual or threatened physical force sufficient to coerce the victim.[8]

In recent years, with the ever-increasing availability of computers and access to the World Wide Web, Internet sexual solicitation and exploitation have emerged as a risk to children and adolescents. Reporting on this growing risk were the 2 Youth Internet Safety Surveys (YISS-1 and YISS-2), which were conducted on 2 different nationally representative samples of children and teens between the ages of 10 and 17 years who used the Internet regularly. The YISS-1 was published in 2001 and then repeated 5 years later as the YISS-2 and published in 2006.[9,10] Between the 2 surveys, each looking at a 1-year period, 19% of children and 13% of teens received unwanted sexual solicitations. An increased proportion of children and teens encountered unwanted exposures

to sexual material (25% and 34%, respectively) as well as increased online harassment (6% and 9%, respectively). The increased exposure to unwanted sexually oriented material occurred despite increased use of filtering, blocking, and monitoring software between the periods separating the YISS-1 and YISS-2 (33% and 55%, respectively).

Paradigms

Health care professionals must be careful about making generalizations because each case of sexual abuse is unique. Various paradigms provide useful frameworks from which to gain understanding of the clinical information that is collected during the medical evaluation of child and adolescent sexual abuse.

In a now classic publication, Sgroi and colleagues[11] articulated a longitudinal model of the sexual abuse phenomenon that describes how child sexual abuse may occur in a fairly predictable fashion over a given period. Child sexual abuse may occur as an isolated event or it may, more commonly, consist of repeated episodes of an increasingly invasive nature and happening over an extended period. Finkelhor[12] looked at a set of circumstances, which he termed *preconditions,* that are consistently present in cases of sexual abuse and that help explain how situations arise that may place a child at risk for sexual abuse. Additionally, Finkelhor and Browne[13] proposed a traumagenic model of sexual abuse that describes how 4 dynamics come together to uniquely harm the child exposed to sexual abuse.

No model or set of typical characteristics can be offered regarding perpetrators other than the information contained in Finkelhor's set of preconditions because it does not exist.[14] Convicted sexual abuse perpetrators, however, characteristically are (1) known to their child victims and (2) commonly abuse more than one child with one report showing that about 30% of perpetrators admit to abusing more than one child.[15] Sex offenders in general are 7.5 times more likely to be rearrested for a new sexual offense compared with those convicted of other offenses.[15]

Longitudinal Progression of Child Sexual Abuse

Sgroi et al[11] described a pattern of ongoing sexual abuse that is characterized by a staged increase in contact between the perpetrator and the child victim. These researchers describe a spectrum of age-inappropriate activities that constitute sexually abusive behavior. The spectrum includes nudity, disrobing, genital exposure, observation of the child, kissing, fondling, masturbation, fellatio, cunnilingus, digital or object penetration of the anus, digital or object penetration of the vagina, vulvar coitus, intragluteal coitus, penile penetration of the vagina, and penile penetration of the anus.

Sgroi and colleagues[11] suggested a 5-stage sequence that may characterize child sexual abuse: engagement, sexual interaction, secrecy, disclosure, and suppression. These phases constitute a model for the longitudinal progression of sexual abuse.

Engagement

The perpetrator engages the child around nonsexual issues and becomes a friend or a person who provides material rewards and meets psychological needs. The perpetrator acquires access to the child and develops a relationship with him or her. The characteristics of this phase include access to the child and the development of a relationship with the child. The child may be sensitive to the threat of losing a relationship that provides attention and perceived affection.

Sexual Interaction

In the sexual interaction phase, the perpetrator engages the child in age-inappropriate sexual contact. The perpetrator manipulates the relationship developed in the engagement phase to include sexual contact. The sexual contact may progress from exhibitionism and inappropriate kissing to fondling and ultimately to oral-genital, genital-genital, or anal-genital contact. Even if sexual interaction does not progress to fondling and genital contact, the child is still a victim of age-inappropriate sexual activity.

Secrecy

The objectives of the perpetrator are to ensure access to the child and to facilitate a continuation of sexual contact. Maintaining secrecy is essential to the perpetrator's continued access to the child. Secrecy is maintained through direct or indirect coercion. The perpetrator may use bribes or threats. The threats may be as subtle as the perpetrator stating that he or she will disapprove of the child if the child does not comply or as explicit as threats of harm to the child or loved ones. From the perpetrator's perspective secrecy removes accountability.

Disclosure

The disclosure of sexual abuse by a child victim may occur in a variety of ways.[16] Sgroi and colleagues originally characterized disclosure as occurring in 2 broad categories described below, namely accidental and purposeful. Some have suggested adding a third disclosure category, which may occur after a precipitating event such as after the child attends a program discussing child sexual abuse or hears a news cast about sexual molestation, which then prompts, or elicits, the child to disclose additional information after this precipitating event.[17]

- *Accidental.* Accidental disclosure occurs in a variety of ways because of external circumstances: (a) a third party observes the participants and tells someone else; (b) signs of physical injury draw outside attention to the sexual behavior; (c) diagnosis of a sexually transmitted infection or, more rarely, an injury in the genital or anal area is discovered; (d) pregnancy occurs; and (e) nonspecific behavior changes take place, including sexually stylized behavior that is developmentally inappropriate. In accidental disclosure a crisis may occur, because neither participant decided to reveal the secret.
- *Purposeful.* The child consciously reveals the abusive activity. A variety of reasons exist for the child to disclose, and they may vary with the developmental level of the child.

Suppression

Once disclosure takes place, the case may enter a suppression phase with the primary task of the perpetrator shifting to undermining the credibility of the child. Caregivers may not want to deal with the reality of the disclosure because of denial, guilt, or fear of family disruption. The perpetrator, caregivers, or relatives may exert pressure on the child to retract his or her account of the abusive events. The child's history may be characterized as fabrication or dismissed as fantasy.

Preconditions for Child Sexual Abuse:

Finkelhor[12] characterized 4 preconditions that are typically present when sexual abuse occurs: motivation of the perpetrator, overcoming internal inhibitions, overcoming external inhibitions, and overcoming a child's resistance.

Motivation of the Perpetrator

The first precondition is that of the motivation on the part of the perpetrator. The offender experiences emotional congruence with the concept of sexual arousal related to children. Congruence may arise from prior sexual abuse of the perpetrator during his or her own childhood, from a lack of availability of alternative sources of gratification, or from the perpetrator's perception that the alternative sources are less gratifying. Motivational factors set the stage for subsequent abusive behavior if other preconditions are met.

Overcoming Internal Inhibitions

The second precondition involves the perpetrator's ability to overcome his or her internal inhibitions against committing a sexually abusive act. Although normal adults may at times become sexually aroused by children, internal codes of behavior, morals, or superego prevent them from acting on these feelings. Sexual abusers, however, overcome their normal internal inhibitions. In some cases, perpetrators may suffer from substance addictions or other forms of mental illness or instability. Such conditions may be factors in their decision to abuse children.

Overcoming External Inhibitions

The third precondition to sexual abuse is a perpetrator's ability to overcome the external inhibitors of sexually abusive behavior. The protective environment of a family setting usually serves as a check to the victimization of a child. Abuse may occur when there is physical or emotional absence of a parent.

Overcoming a Child's Resistance

Finally, the fourth precondition for sexual abuse is the persistence of the abuser in overcoming the child's resistance to abusive acts. The abuser may use either implicit or direct coercion to impose age-inappropriate sexual contact on the psychologically immature child. The abuser may manipulate the child and offer attention to ensure participation.

Traumagenic Dynamics Model

Finkelhor and Browne[13] developed a framework that systematically explains the psychological injury inflicted on a child who is sexually abused. The framework in this model is based on 4 traumagenic dynamics that are at the core of the injury: traumatic sexualization, betrayal, powerlessness, and stigmatization. These dynamics come together, and in a unique manner, alter the children's cognitive and emotional orientation to the world and distort their self-concept, worldview, and capacity to give and receive affection.

Traumatic Sexualization

Traumatic sexualization is a process in which the child's sexual feelings and attitudes are shaped in a developmentally inappropriate and interpersonally dysfunctional manner. The child learns that sexual behavior may lead to rewards, attention, or privileges. It may also occur when the child's sexual anatomy is given distorted importance and meaning and, in some cases, it may occur when sexual activity becomes associated with frightening memories in the child's mind. The observed effects of traumatic sexualization may be seen in the sexual preoccupation and repetitive sexual behavior displayed by some children. Additionally, the developmentally inappropriate knowledge of sexual activity, often in extensive detail, is a hallmark of traumatic sexualization and may be associated with misconception about sex and healthy sexual relationships as a result of the perpetrator's actions with the child.

Betrayal

Betrayal is a process in which the child learns that a trusted individual has caused them harm, misrepresented moral standards, or failed to protect them properly. In this process the betrayal can be by the perpetrator or by the family and other adults when the child realizes that they did not receive what they needed by way of protection and support, especially after the disclosure occurs. The child may be observed to be having a grief reaction or depression over the loss of a trusted figure. They may display disappointment and disillusionment as well as an intense desire to reestablish trusting relationships. This desire to have trusting relationships may place the child in a vulnerable position post-abuse if their judgment is impaired as they assess future relationships with peers and adults.

Powerlessness

Powerlessness is a process of disempowerment in which the child's sense of self-efficacy and will are consistently thwarted by the perpetrator's actions with the child. The child is coerced and manipulated by the perpetrator, and their personal space and body are violated by the abusive activity. The child may manifest symptoms of fear and anxiety and may demonstrate impaired coping strategies as a result of the powerlessness. Symptoms associated with fear and anxiety may include nightmares, phobias, hypervigilance, clinging behavior, and various somatic complaints. The symptoms associated with impaired coping may include despair, depression, learning problems, running away, and school activity/ employment difficulties.

Stigmatization

Stigmatization is a process whereby the child's self-image becomes incorporated with the negative connotation of the words used to communicate about the sexual abuse, including such words as *bad, awful, shameful,* and *guilty.* The negativity may be communicated directly by the perpetrator or those around the child in describing the activity, or it may be indirectly understood by the child from what he or she hears from those in the family or community as they discuss the abuse. This is consistent with the "damaged goods" mentality originally described by Sgroi[2] in which the child feels deviant and not as whole as they did prior to the abuse. The child may be observed to feel isolated as a result of the stigmatization. Some stigmatized children may gravitate toward other stigmatized individuals or groups and become involved with drugs, alcohol, or other criminal types of activity. Some others may feel isolated and become depressed, attempt suicide, or engage in self-destructive behavior. Many victims of sexual abuse experience high degrees of guilt and shame and manifest a low self-esteem.

Scope of the Problem: The Numbers

In attempting to study the magnitude of child sexual abuse in the population, essentially 2 approaches are possible: those focusing on the incidence and those focusing on the prevalence.

Incidence studies look at the number of new cases of sexual abuse that occur in a given period, typically a year's time, while prevalence studies look at the proportion of the population that has been sexually abused during childhood.

Incidence

In the last years of the 20th century national compilations of state reported incidence data consistently found that approximately 3 million reports of suspected child maltreatment were made to child protective services (CPS) agencies for investigation and that ultimately after processing and investigation, approximately 900,000 to 1 million children were estimated to have been maltreated. The breakdown showed that more than one-half were neglected, approximately one-fifth to one-quarter were physically abused, and nearly 10% were sexually abused, with the others

representing a variety of other forms of maltreatment.[18] The overall rates for various forms of child maltreatment varied over the years of the 1990s and mid-2000s as demonstrated in Figure 1.1. The graph shows that the rate per 10,000 for neglect declined by 6% between 1992 and 2004 and the rate per 10,000 for physical abuse declined by 43% during that period. This favorable declining trend was also seen when examining the rates for child sexual abuse between 1990 and 2004, during which a decrease in incidence of 49% was observed.

Looking specifically at 2006 data,[18] the following observations may be made:

Maltreatment Overall
- Approximately 905,000 children were known by CPS to have been victims of maltreatment.
- 64.2% experienced neglect.
- 16.0% experienced physical abuse.

FIGURE 1.1
US Maltreatment trends, 2004 update.

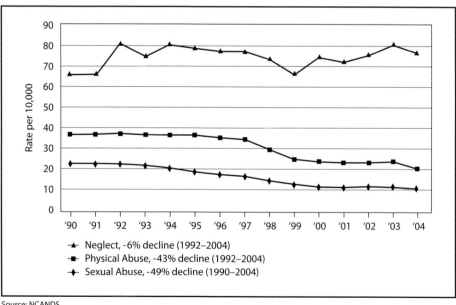

Source: NCANDS

- 8.8% experienced sexual abuse.
- 6.6% experienced emotional/psychological abuse.
- Overall the victimization rate was 12.1 per 1,000 children in the US population.

Sexual Abuse

- 8.8% or an estimated 79,640 children were known by CPS to have been sexually abused.
- The sexual abuse victimization rate was approximately 1.1 per 1,000 children.

Age

(for the slightly >78,000 children for whom age data were available)

- 6% or approximately 5,000 were younger than 4 years.
- 22% or approximately 17,500 were 4 through 7 years old.
- 23% or approximately 18,300 were 8 through 11 years old.
- 47% or nearly 37,000 were 12 years old or older.

Gender

- *Child Maltreatment 2006* does not report a gender breakdown for sexual abuse cases; however, Douglas and Finkelhor[14] note that incidence studies routinely confirm that girls are more often reported to be sexually abused than are boys. They conclude that all reliable studies conclude that girls experience more sexual abuse than boys and that the percentage of victims who are female ranges from 78% to 89%.

Incidence studies rely on data reported to county, state, and national authorities, such as seen with the National Child

Abuse and Neglect Data System (NCANDS) data reported previously, and are recognized as deficient because of the suspected large amount of under-reporting to professionals of sexual abuse. Early on in the professional study of child sexual abuse, Finkelhor[19] observed that yearly occurrence rates for maltreatment substantially underes-timated its incidence primarily because the identification and reporting of sex-ual abuse was discouraged due to the nature of sexual abuse, its secrecy and shame, the criminal sanctions against it, and the young age of its victims. In addition, because varying levels of professional education and public awareness affect the frequency of case detection, it was difficult to judge the true scope of the problem accurately. Most authorities agree that published incidence figures dealing with the occurrence of child sexual abuse are in reality underestimates of the actual incidence in sexual maltreatment.

Beginning in 2001 Finkelhor and Jones[20] reported marked declines in rates of child sexual abuse during the 1990s (see Figure 1.1). In their report it was noted that the number of substantiated cases of child sexual abuse from 1992 to 1998 had declined by 31%, from an all-time high of 149,800 in 1992 to 103,600 in 1998.[20] At that time they offered several possible explanations, including a true decline in the incidence of child sexual abuse cases and/or changes in attitudes, policies, or standards that resulted in fewer substantiated cases (Figure 1.2). In 2004 Finkelhor and Jones again looked at the data and concluded that the decline continued into the early

FIGURE 1.2
Possible factors influencing the decline in substantiated cases of child sexual abuse.[20]

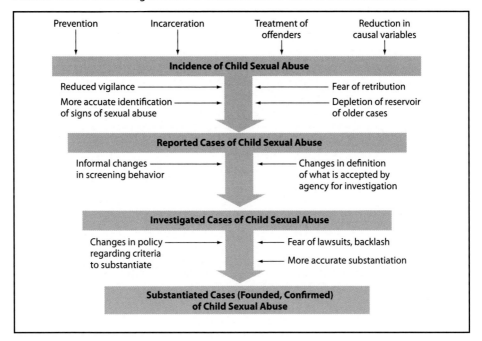

2000s.[21] Information from NCANDS for 1990 through 2004 revealed that the rate of substantiated cases of sexual abuse had declined by 49% during that 14-year period[22] (Figure 1.3). Sexual assault of teenagers, juvenile victim homicides, and other crimes involving juveniles had also seen similar declines.[22]

There is general agreement that a decline in substantiated cases of child sexual abuse has occurred over the past decade. However, there is no consensus on the specific reasons for this dramatic occurrence. Finkelhor and Jones[22] concluded that factors such as economic prosperity, increasing number of agents of social intervention, and the availability of more sophisticated psychiatric pharmacologic treatments were likely to have had a role in reducing the incidence rates but that these areas need

further investigation. Ultimately the overall decline seems to be multifactorial, and further investigation into the significance of each potential reason is crucial to continue to sustain a further decline in child victimization seen during the 1990s and early 2000s.

Prevalence

Prevalence studies, on the other hand, rely on victim and offender self-reports. Because it is believed that most sexual abuse goes unreported, studies that rely on large survey data from a variety of potential victim populations may more accurately reflect the scope of the problem. Prevalence surveys, however, may suffer from several problems including (1) differences in definitions of sexual abuse, some including noncontact sexual abuse exposure, inappropriate

FIGURE 1.3
Juvenile victimization trends, 1993–2004 (NCVS).

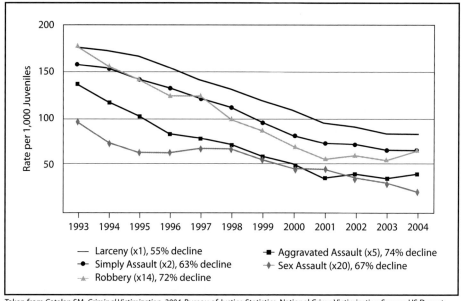

Taken from Catalan SM. *Criminal Victimization, 2004.* Bureau of Justice Statistics. National Crime Victimization Survey. US Department of Justice, Office of Justice Programs, September 2005 (www.ojp.usdoj.gov/bjs/pub/pdf/cv04.pdf).

comments or requests for sex, others might be more restrictive to contact forms of sexual abuse, and others may include incidents involving peers as perpetrators or specific age differences between perpetrator and victim (eg, greater than 5 years difference whereas others might exclude peers or include any perpetrator/victim age difference); (2) differences in group studies with sample characteristics differing in age, education level, and ethnicity of subjects as well as variation in region of the country surveyed, which calls into question the comparability and generalizability of the findings; and (3) differing methodological characteristics of studies around sampling and questioning techniques. The sampling techniques may vary around random versus nonrandom techniques (eg, random

dialing telephone surveys vs nonrandom surveys of undergraduates taking an introductory psychology course[19]), and questioning techniques may vary around face-to-face interviews, self-administered questionnaires, and phone call surveys.[23]

In a comprehensive review of 16 survey type prevalence studies of nonclinical, North American samples that were performed over a 3-decade period, Gorey and Leslie[24] attempted to adjust or correct the reported prevalence figures for females and males who had experienced sexual abuse in their childhood. The adjustments were done to account for as much variation as possible that may be attributed to differences in each study's response rate and the definitions of abuse used. The authors explained that the corrections were necessary because adults who are aware that they experienced sexual abuse in their childhood are more likely to respond to surveys addressing the issue, so a high response rate is necessary to balance this out. Additionally, the definition adjustment was necessary because how the survey questions are asked is central to how the respondents answer the questions. The unadjusted prevalence rates for having experienced childhood sexual abuse were 22.3% for women and 8.5% for men. When adjustments were made in the calculation for a survey response rate of 60% or more (considered a good survey), the prevalence rates were 16.8% for women and 7.9% for men. Additionally, when rates were calculated excluding the broadest, noncontact form of sexual abuse (exhibitionism) from the comparisons, the prevalence figures were 14.5% for women and 7.2% for men. Using these adjustments, the authors argued that the prevalence rates during the 3 decades in which the studies were done did not change significantly.

Professionals in the child abuse field have conservatively used Finkelhor's[25] prevalence estimates of 20% for women and 5% to 10% for men. The careful analysis by Gorey and Leslie[24] suggest that prevalence figures should, at their upper end, be set at about 17% for women and 8% for men.[26] Both Runyan[27] and Leventhal[26] individually call for rigorous epidemiologically sound future studies that limit bias and that are longitudinal in design and focused on the clinically relevant areas of risk and prognosis.

Children With Special Needs

Since the early study of child abuse and neglect, children with special needs were thought to be at potentially higher risk for victimization.[28] A number of clinical reports support this view.[29,30] Several reasons have been identified to explain why children with a variety of developmental disabilities may be at increased risk for sexual maltreatment and they include (1) cognitive impairments and limited capacity for judgment that may place the child with special needs in situations that are high risk for inappropriate sexual activities; (2) limited language and verbal abilities that may make disclosure more difficult; (3) likelihood to have multiple caregivers throughout the day between home, school, and health care setting, and transportation required to get to these settings; (4) possibility of residing in an institutional setting; (5) high degree of dependency around typically private behaviors such as bathing and toileting; and (6) physical impairments that may prevent escape from sexually inappropriate situations.[31,32] In 1993, in response to a Congressional mandate, the National Center on Child Abuse and Neglect issued a report that presented data showing that children with a variety of special needs were at approximately 2 times the risk for child maltreatment compared with children who did not have disabilities.[33] The incidence of child sexual abuse among children with special needs was 3.5 per 1,000 children compared with an incidence rate of 2.1 per 1,000 for all children, and an incidence of 2.0 per 1,000 for children without special needs. This study, using a nationally representative sample of children, validated what had long been a clinical observation: Children with disabilities are at increased risk for child abuse and neglect, specifically sexual abuse.[31,34–36] Sullivan and Knutson[36] subsequently conducted 2 population-based studies that built on this early epidemiological study. In one using a hospital-based epidemiological approach, they provided further evidence that a disability rate among maltreated children was approximately twice the disability rate among non-maltreated children.[37] In a subsequent study using a school-based population approach, they reported that children with disabilities were 3.4 times more likely to be maltreated than their non-disabled peers.[37]

Performing the medical evaluation of children with special needs presents a number of unique challenges to the health care provider related to both the interview and the physical examination that require extra attention and additional training.[38]

Consequences

There is no recognized universal set of responses nor a uniform impact from the experience of child or adolescent sexual abuse.[39,40] Individual differences in response to the trauma of childhood abusive events have been attributed to the nature of the abuse experience and individual psychological adaptation.[41] The impact of sexual abuse can be seen in both physical and mental health areas.

The impact on physical health from child sexual abuse is often limited in nature and once identified is treated

with standard medical therapies.[42] Berkowitz[43] has summarized the more commonly recognized medical sequelae of child sexual abuse using an organ systems approach. In addition to the immediate injuries and possible sexually transmitted infections that may be identified during the initial medical evaluation, the possible physical effects that can be credibly attributed to the impact of sexual abuse include

- Gastrointestinal (GI) disorders: Considered to be secondary to association of GI symptoms and stressful events related to effects on acid secretion and intestinal motility. Disorders associated with sequelae from sexual abuse tend to show no structural, infectious, or metabolic basis and as such are called *functional.* Include irritable bowel syndrome, non-ulcer dyspepsia, and chronic abdominal pain.
- Gynecologic disorders: Considered related to the inappropriate focus on the child's genital region that may occur in the context of sexual activity. In general, those with long-term gynecologic symptomatology associated with child sexual abuse tend to have no organic etiology identified. Include chronic pelvic pain, dysmenorrhea, and menstrual irregularities.
- Somatization: Considered associated with a preoccupation with bodily processes. Conflicting research in this area makes definitive statements difficult, but some clinical population studies suggest that somatization may account for the reported increased complaints of chronic headache and backache as well as other functional neurologic complaints in children

and adults who report having been sexually abused.

At the core of the mental health impact is the fundamental harm inflicted on the child by the imposition of developmentally inappropriate sexual behavior that is by definition nonconsensual.[44] The psychological foundation of the child's sense of self-worth, normal development, and adjustment are all placed at risk by the perpetrator's actions around sexual abuse. In considering the likely mental health impacts that may be seen in child sexual abuse, one can examine them in terms of several continua of symptoms including (1) a severity continuum ranging from mild to severe; (2) along a time course ranging from relatively short-term effects to those that are long term, sometimes even lifelong; and (3) from an internalizing versus externalizing type of symptom pattern ranging from children who internalize and respond to the stress by withdrawing and becoming depressed to those children who externalize and who become aggressive and disruptive in response to the trauma.

Keeping in mind that each child comes to the experience with their own set of coping behaviors and environmental realities that may modulate the severity, acuity, and expression of their response to the sexual abuse, a number of possible mental health effects have been described that include[44]

- Behavioral problems: Clinically significant increases in problematic behavioral problems have been identified when children who have been abused are compared with non-abused comparison groups. This includes generic behavioral problems as well as increased sexual behaviors.
- Post-traumatic stress disorder (PTSD) symptoms: Related to the child's response to the anxiety around the sexual abuse. Although many children do not meet the full criteria for a formal PTSD diagnosis, many demonstrate symptoms characteristically associated with PTSD.
- Interpersonal difficulties: Associated with the child's view of themselves after the abuse and their ability to establish trusting relationships.
- Cognitive and emotional distortions: Conflicting evidence makes clear statements difficult in this realm, but complex and multi-determined symptom patterns have been observed clinically. School performance and emotional functioning seem most at risk.

Paolucci et al[40] conducted a meta-analysis of published research on the effects of child sexual abuse and identified 37 studies published between 1981 and 1995 that collectively contained 25,367 people. The analysis found clear evidence of a link between child sexual abuse and a set of multifaceted negative short-term and long-term consequences to development, including PTSD, depression, suicide, sexual promiscuity, victim-perpetrator cycle, and poor academic performance. Like other studies before it, this meta-analysis did not find evidence to support a specific child sexual abuse syndrome, but it did find support for a multifaceted model of traumatization after child sexual abuse that had potential for significant negative consequences for the victimized child.

The adult survivor of sexual abuse is often used to describe persons who as adults have problems in functioning that are related to early damaging sexual experiences.[45] Some researchers have described a link between sexual abuse and a host of emotional and behavioral dysfunctions. Among them are depression, low self-esteem, suicide attempts, multiple personality disorder, school failure, regressive behavior, PTSD, drug and alcohol abuse, running away, sexual promiscuity, prostitution, and delinquent behavior.[46–48]

During the 1980s and early 1990s public health information about risk factors for disease were widely researched and used in public education and prevention programs. It became clear that risk factors such as smoking, alcohol abuse, and risky sexual behaviors were not randomly distributed in the population. Surprisingly, what emerged from further study was that risk factors for many chronic diseases in adulthood tended to be associated with a number of adverse childhood experiences such as exposure to domestic violence in the home and sexual victimization as a child. A series of studies were conducted using a large database from the Kaiser-Permanente health system called the Adverse Childhood Experiences (ACE) studies[49] that provided sound epidemiological evidence to support this association of poorer adult health being associated with a variety of adverse childhood experiences. The ACE Pyramid (Figure 1.4) represents the conceptual model that underlies the process by which negative health outcomes occur well into adulthood.

Continued study is needed to further elucidate the connection between adverse events in childhood and later health and disease in adulthood, but the ACE studies[47] have broken new ground and have challenged health care providers to think broadly about the potential impact of victimization on children and adult survivors.

Practical Implications for the Health Care Professional

Very early in the professional response to child sexual abuse, Sgroi[6] pointed out that a prerequisite for the diagnosis of sexual abuse is the willingness of the health care professional to consider the possibility that such abuse may occur. Since the publication of this seminal work, the number of reported cases of sexual abuse of children has dramatically increased, as has our collective understanding of the magnitude that this child health problem poses to children and families today. Sexual abuse can be conceptualized as an abuse of power and authority over a child to engage them in inappropriate sexual activities for which they cannot consent. When children are abused by someone they know and trust they feel betrayed. As a result children may have difficulty developing trusting relationships. The medical evaluation of children and adolescents who have been sexually victimized must not then become one more instance in which powerful adults impose their authority on the child's body and remove the child's control of events in his or her life. One way of educating children that they have choices and the power to decide for themselves is to provide them with choices throughout the medical history and examination. If the medical history and examination are not conducted in a knowledgeable and sensitive manner, the process itself may be perceived as invasive and threatening. Therefore, the health care professional and team can optimize this experience for the child or adolescent by conveying a gentle, concerned manner and by explaining to the child or adolescent what to expect during the evaluation. A calm, gentle, and unhurried approach will go a long way toward making the examination part of the recovery process rather than an instance of another form of assault. Awareness of the circumstances that these children and adolescents may have experienced, along with anticipating and addressing their fears, can help make them more secure throughout the examination process and will enhance their cooperativeness. When a child is uncooperative, the health care provider should not resort to force to complete the examination, but rather should address the underlying concerns of the child. This, coupled with efforts to demystify what the child will experience, will increase the chances of successfully completing an examination. The approach of the examining health care professional and the entire multidisciplinary team should be to complete the necessary medical evaluation in as nonthreatening and therapeutic a manner as possible.

Looking Toward the Future

Sound medical practice is based on evidence generated in well-designed clinical studies. Research in the field of child abuse and neglect has been likened to "walking up a mountain with many false summits" in that the further we go, the more progress we make, the more

FIGURE 1.4
ACE pyramid.[a]

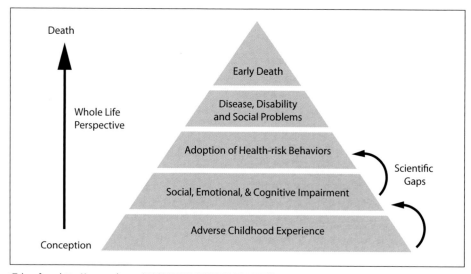

[a]Taken from http://www.cdc.gov/NCCDPHP/ACE/PYRAMID.HTM.[47]

we see, the more we realize how far we have to go to reach the summit and substantially understand child abuse and neglect.[50] There is a long-standing recognition that rigorous research in the area of child sexual abuse is necessary but full of challenges. Finkelhor[51] criticized the current research efforts as being "confined to increasingly redundant, retrospective case-control studies that attempt to confirm…associations between sexual abuse and later…outcomes." He goes on to comment that although these studies were important when the field was just starting, they are now of marginal significance. Thus it is important to move on and push the field and its research base toward more rigor and utility. Finkelhor[51] states that 2 far-ranging questions should be placed at the top of the child sexual abuse research agenda, namely: (1) Which investigative policies, procedures, and standards (medical, legal, child welfare) maximize the likelihood for accurate and efficient confirmation or dismissal of allegations of sexual abuse? and (2) Which investigative, therapeutic, criminal justice, and case management procedures of confirmed cases maximize the security, mental health, and sense of justice for victims and their families and the rest of the community? Putnam[52] has called for large-scale effectiveness research trials with longitudinal follow-up to test treatment models. He also calls for resources to be directed toward the development of the necessary research infrastructure for large-scale studies to be possible. As we await the design, implementation, and publication of this high-quality research, clinicians must of necessity continue

to serve children and families affected by child sexual abuse with care that is as evidenced-based as possible and when short on evidence, with care that is firmly rooted in best practice and sound pediatric principles. In the chapters that follow, an approach to the medical evaluation of children suspected of having been sexually abused is presented that is based on available evidence, consensus opinions of seasoned clinicians, and many years of combined experience serving children and families struggling to deal with the possibility of child sexual abuse and its consequences.

References

1. Kempe CH. Sexual abuse, another hidden pediatric problem: the 1977 C. Anderson Aldrich Lecture. *Pediatrics.* 1978;62:382–389

2. Sgroi SM, ed. *Handbook of Clinical Intervention in Child Sexual Abuse.* Lexington, MA: Lexington; 1982

3. Sedlak AJ, Broadhurst DD. *Third National Incidence Study of Child Abuse and Neglect (NIS-3 Final Report).* Washington, DC: US Department of Health and Human Services (Contract #105-94-1840); 1996

4. Faller KC. *Child Sexual Abuse: An Interdisciplinary Manual for Diagnosis, Case Management, and Treatment.* New York, NY: Columbia University Press; 1988

5. Kempe CH. Incest and other forms of sexual abuse. In: Kempe CH, Helfer RE, eds. *The Battered Child.* 3rd ed. Chicago, IL: University of Chicago Press; 1980:1198–1214

6. Sgroi SM. Sexual molestation of children: the last frontier in child abuse. *Child Today.* 1975;4:18–21, 44

7. American Psychiatric Association. *Diagnostic and Statistical Manual of Mental Disorders.* 4th ed. Text revision. Washington, DC: American Psychiatric Association; 2000

8. Sexual Assault. ACOG Technical Bulletin Number 172—September 1992. *Int J Gynaecol Obstet.* 1993;42:67–72

9. Mitchell KJ, Finkelhor D, Wolak J. Risk factors for and impact of online sexual solicitation of youth. *JAMA.* 2001;285:3011–3014

10. Wolak L, Mitchell K, Finkelhor D. *Online Victimization of Youth: Five Years Later.* Alexandria, VA: National Center for Missing & Exploited Children; 2006

11. Sgroi SM, Blick LC, Porter FS. A conceptual framework for child sexual abuse. In: Sgroi SM, ed. *Handbook of Clinical Intervention in Child Sexual Abuse.* Lexington, MA: Lexington; 1982:9–37

12. Finkelhor D. *Child Sexual Abuse: New Theory and Research.* New York, NY: Free Press; 1984

13. Finkelhor D, Browne A. The traumatic impact of child sexual abuse: a conceptualization. *Am J Orthopsychiatry.* 1985;55(4):530–541

14. Douglas EM, Finkelhor D. Child sexual abuse fact sheet. Durham, NH: Crimes against Children Research Center, Family Research Laboratory, University of New Hampshire; 2005. http://www. unh.edu/ccrc/factsheet/pdf/CSA-FS20. pdf. Accessed September 2007

15. Prevent Abuse Now Sexual Abuse Statistics. 2000. Prevent abuse now. http:// www.prevent-abuse-now.com/stats2. htm. Accessed September 21, 2000

16. Nagel DE, Putnam FW, Noll JG, Trickett PK. Disclosure patterns of sexual abuse and psychological functioning at a 1-year follow-up. *Child Abuse Negl.* 1997;21(2):137–147

17. Campis LB, Hebden-Curtis J, Demaso DR. Developmental differences in detection and disclosure of sexual abuse. *J Am Acad Child Adolesc Psychiatry.* 1993;3:920–924

18. US Department of Health and Human Services, Administration on Children, Youth and Families. *Child Maltreatment 2006.* Washington, DC: US Government Printing Office; 2008

19. Finkelhor D. *A Sourcebook on Child Sexual Abuse.* Beverly Hills, CA: Sage Publications; 1986

20. Jones L, Finkelhor D. The Decline in Child Sexual Abuse Cases. Bulletin. Washington, DC: US Department of Justice, Office of Justice Programs, Office of Juvenile Justice and Delinquency Prevention; 2001. http:// www.ncjrs.gov/pdffiles1/ojjdp/184741. pdf. Accessed October 14, 2008

21. Finkelhor D, Jones LM. Explanations for the Decline in Child Sexual Abuse Cases. Washington, DC: US Department of Justice, Office of Justice Programs, Office of Juvenile Justice Delinquency; 2004. http://www. nchrs.gov/pdffiles1/ojjdp/199298. pdf. Accessed October 14, 2008

22. Finkelhor D, Jones L. Why have child maltreatment and child victimization declined? *J Soc Issues.* 2006;62:685–716

23. Wyatt GE, Peters SD. Methodological consideration in research on the prevalence of child sexual abuse. *Child Abuse Negl.* 1986;10:241–251

24. Gorey KM, Leslie DR. The prevalence of child sexual abuse: integrative review adjustment for potential response and measurement biases. *Child Abuse Negl.* 1997;21(4):391–398

25. Finkelhor D. Current information on the scope and nature of child sexual abuse. *Future Child.* 1994;4:31–53

26. Leventhal JM. Epidemiology of sexual abuse of children: old problems, new directions. *Child Abuse Negl.* 1998;22(6):481–491

27. Runyan DK. Prevalence, risk, sensitivity, and specificity: a commentary on the epidemiology of child sexual abuse and the development of a research agenda. *Child Abuse Negl.* 1998:22(6):493–498

28. Gil DG. *Violence Against Children: Physical Child Abuse in the United States.* Cambridge, MA: Harvard University Press; 1970

29. Valentine DP. Double jeopardy: child maltreatment and mental retardation. *Child Adolesc Social Work J.* 1990;7:487–499

30. Zirpoli TJ. Characteristics of persons with mental retardation who have been abused by caregivers. *J Spec Educ.* 1987;21:31–41

31. Garbarino J, Brookhouser P, eds. *Special Children, Special Risks: The Maltreatment of Children with Disabilities.* New York, NY: Aldine; 1987

32. Sullivan PM, Brookhouser PE, Scanlan JM, Knutson JF, Schulte LE. Patterns of physical and sexual abuse of communicatively handicapped children. *Ann Otol Rhinol Laryngol.* 1991;100:188–194

33. US Department of Health and Human Services. *A Report on the Maltreatment of Children with Disabilities.* Washington, DC: Westat, Inc; 1993. No. 105-89-16300/

34. Elvik SL, Berkowitz C. Sexual abuse in the developmentally disabled: dilemmas of diagnosis. *Child Abuse Negl.* 1990; 14:497–502

35. Baladerian N. Sexual abuse of people with developmental disabilities. *Sex Disabil.* 1991;9:323–335

36. Sullivan PM, Knutson JF. The association between child maltreatment and disabilities in a hospital-based epidemiological study. *Child Abuse Negl.* 1998;22(4):271–288

37. Sullivan PM, Knutson JF. Maltreatment and disabilities: a population-based epidemiological study. *Child Abuse Negl.* 2000;24(10):1257–1273

38. Hudson KM, Giardino AP. Child abuse and neglect. In: Kurtz LA, Dowrick PW, Levy SE, Batshaw ML, eds. *Handbook of Developmental Disabilities.* Gaithersburg, MD: Aspen Publishers, Inc.; 1996:542–554

39. Kendall-Tackett K, Williams L, Finkelhor D. Impact of sexual abuse on children: a review and synthesis of recent empirical studies. *Psychol Bull.* 1993;113:164–180

40. Paolucci EO, Genuis ML, Violato C. A meta-analysis of the published research on the effects of child sexual abuse. *J Psychol.* 2001;135:17–36

41. McCann J, Pearlman LA, Sakheim DK, Abrahamson DJ. Assessment and treatment of the adult survivor of childhood sexual abuse within a schema framework. In: Sgroi SM, ed. *Vulnerable Populations.* Lexington, MA: Lexington; 1988:77–101

42. Jenny C. Medical issues in sexual abuse. In: Briere J, Berliner L, Bulkley JA, Jenny C, Reid T, eds. *The APSAC Handbook on Child Maltreatment.* Thousand Oaks, CA: Sage Publications; 1996

43. Berkowitz CD. Medical consequences of child sexual abuse. *Child Abuse Negl.* 1998;22:541–554

44. Berliner L, Elliott DM. Sexual abuse of children. In: Briere J, Berliner L, Bulkley JA, Jenny C, Reid T, eds. *The APSAC Handbook on Child Maltreatment.* Thousand Oaks, CA: Sage Publications; 1996

45. Sgroi SM, Bunk BS. A clinical approach to adult survivors of child sexual abuse. In: Sgroi SM, ed. *Vulnerable Populations.* Lexington, MA: Lexington; 1988:137–186

46. Bachmann GA, Moeller TP, Benett J. Childhood sexual abuse and the consequences in adult women. *Obstet Gynecol.* 1988;71:631–642

47. Jenny C, Sutherland SE, Sandahl BB. Developmental approach to preventing the sexual abuse of children. *Pediatrics.* 1986;78:1034–1038

48. Whitman BY, Munkel W. Multiple personality disorder: a risk indicator, diagnostic marker and psychiatric outcome for severe child abuse. *Clin Pediatr.* 1991;30:422–428

49. Felitti VJ, Anda RF, Nordenberg D, et al. Relationship of childhood abuse and household dysfunction to many of the leading causes of death in adults. *Am J Prev Med.* 1998;14:245–258

50. Gough D, Lynch MA. Taking child abuse research seriously. *Child Abuse Rev.* 2000;9:1–5

51. Finkelhor D. Improving research, policy, and practice to understand child sexual abuse. *JAMA.* 1998;280:1864–1865

52. Putnam FW. Ten-year research update review: child sexual abuse. *J Am Acad Child Adolesc Psychiatry.* 2003;42:269–278

Chapter 2

The Evaluation

Martin A. Finkel

The fruit of healing grows on the tree of understanding. Without diagnosis, there is no rational treatment. Examination comes first, then judgment, and then one can give help.

— Carl Gerhardt, 1873

The medical examination of the child suspected of being sexually abused is conducted to diagnose and treat any residua to sexual contact, should there be such. Residua to sexually inappropriate interactions might include acute or chronic signs of injury; sexually transmitted infections (STIs); or evidence of sexual contact, as in trace materials, seminal products, or expressed worries regarding body intactness. When evaluating any patient suspected of being abused, the clinician must conduct a comprehensive evaluation that includes a complete medical history, review of systems, history of alleged events from the child, physical examination, and pertinent laboratory studies and/or procedures. In cases of suspected child sexual abuse, the medical history obtained from the child is of paramount importance. Thus the time-honored practice of clinicians obtaining a medical history and formulating a diagnostic impression prior to conducting a physical examination applies to the medical evaluation of the child alleged to have been sexually abused as it would to any other medical diagnostic con-dition. This chapter serves as an introduction to many of the key concepts important to the medical evaluation of the child suspected of being sexually abused, and these concepts are developed further in subsequent chapters.

Making the Diagnosis: The Medical Model

Throughout medical training, physicians learn about the pathophysiology and clinical expression of diseases, and we ultimately develop the skills necessary to obtain a medical history from the patient before us. The medical history is the foundation on which we formulate our diagnostic impression prior to conducting a physical examination. Ultimately, the ability to diagnosis any clinical condition requires knowledge of the "disease" that we are trying to diagnose.[1-3] Making the diagnosis of sexual abuse requires the following basic skills and tasks:

1. Having an in-depth understanding of the "disease" known as *sexual victimization*
2. Obtaining a medical history of the child's experience in a nonjudgmental, facilitating, and empathetic manner
3. Documenting historical details in an accurate and meticulous manner
4. Conducting a detailed anogenital and extragenital examination to diagnose acute and chronic residua to trauma and STIs, and to collect forensic evidence
5. Considering a differential diagnosis of behavioral complaints and anogenital signs that may mimic sexual abuse
6. Obtaining photographic/video documentation of all diagnostic findings interpreted to be residual to abuse
7. Formulating a complete and detailed medical report with diagnostic and treatment recommendations
8. Participating in a peer review process
9. Testifying in court when required

Obtaining a Medical History

The clinician will need to obtain historical details from a variety of sources to understand the concerns surrounding the alleged victimization of the child to be evaluated. Historical details will be obtained from the caretaker and potentially a child

protective services (CPS) worker and/or law enforcement professionals. Each of those histories will be afforded its own weight. The most critical history will be the medical history obtained from the child. The caretaker's history provides information regarding the child's medical history, the caretaker's understanding of the chronology of events leading up to the disclosure/suspicion of sexual abuse, and an opportunity to address any worries or concerns the caretaker might have.

The emotionally charged nature of child sexual abuse requires that clinicians maintain an objective demeanor throughout their interactions with the child; caretakers; CPS/law enforcement; and the court, if challenged. The ability to modulate one's visceral response to highly charged issues is not intuitive and is a learned/modeled skill that develops with time. The most challenging skill to develop is the ability to obtain the medical history in a non-leading and non-suggestive manner that is appropriate for the child's developmental, cognitive, and linguistic capabilities.

It is important not only to be able to obtain the medical history of the child's experience but also to document the historian's questions and record the history as asked and the child's verbatim response. An easy way to document the child's complete medical history while enhancing one's skills in history taking is to use a handheld tape recorder to record the medical history.

The tape recorder is introduced to the child as a way to assist the doctor in carefully listening to what the child has to say. The statement to the child should be simple, such as the following:

> *Everything you have to say is important to me. I would like to be able to listen carefully as we talk. So I don't have to write while we talk, I would like to use this tape recorder. Is that OK with you? Would you like to hear your voice in the recorder?*

The physician then asks the child to speak into the recorder, and then replays the child's name for the child before setting the recorder aside to obtain the history. When fully engaged in conversation, most children will not be distracted by the presence of the recorder. After completing the medical history, and prior to formulating a report, the clinician should review the history and transcribe verbatim the questions asked and the child'sresponse. This approach offers an unparalleled opportunity to both critique the manner in which one asks questions and further analyze the child's responses. With time, the clinician's self-review of medical histories will result in improved formulation of developmentally appropriate questions that are increasingly less leading/suggestive and comfortable for the child to answer. Once a level of skill and comfort in medical history taking has been achieved, the use of a recorder should be unnecessary and future medical histories are simply recorded as a verbatim written record that then is dictated into the consultative report. The physicians handwritten notes serve to refresh any recollection

of the medical history obtained when preparing the consultative report.

In the case of suspected sexual abuse, the historical details provided by the child allow the greatest insight into what a child experienced and the potential for residua to the alleged contact. When the anogenital examination is conducted because of a suspicion of sexual abuse, it must occur only within the context of a head-to-toe examination. By conducting the anogenital examination in the context of a complete examination the clinician provides an important message to the child that all body parts are important.

Unfortunately, too few primary health care providers—whether pediatricians, family physicians, or nurse practitioners—feel comfortable with evaluating children suspected of sexual abuse and are thus ill prepared for the responsibility of providing the diagnostic and treatment services that these children require. All clinicians need to enhance their professional awareness of the problem of sexual abuse and the issues surrounding its identification, evaluation, and management.[4-7] Clinicians who decide not to provide medical care to these children must be aware of their responsibility to report, as well as the available resources to which to refer children suspected of experiencing sexual abuse within their community.

Clinician Preparedness for Conducting Examinations

Medical school and residency training programs provide only sparse instruction concerning the fundamentals of child maltreatment, including sexual abuse evaluation.[8-10] This is especially true regarding the prepubertal genital examination.[5,11]

In 1986 Ladson et al[5] surveyed 123 pediatricians and family and emergency department (ED) physicians to determine their knowledge and biases regarding child sexual abuse. Ten years later, Lentsch and Johnson[4] repeated the initial survey by Ladson et al, to which 166 physicians responded. In both studies, physicians were asked to identify normal genital structures, indicate the frequency with which they routinely conduct genital examinations, and indicate whether they believed there was an association between sociological factors and vulnerability for child sexual abuse. Although the 1996 survey shows that physicians in general have become more knowledgeable about the socioeconomic and behavioral aspects of child sexual abuse, they continue to have difficulty with the physical examination (ie, identifying normal genital structures) and with reporting suspected sexual abuse.[4]

In 1986, 77% of the physicians included the genital examination as a part of their complete physical examination more than 50% of the time, whereas in 1996 the percentage dropped to 72%. All respondents were provided a photograph of the genitalia of a 6-year-old child and asked to identify normal genital structures. In 1986 genital anatomy was correctly identified as follows: hymen, 59.1%; labia minora, 76.4%; and urethra, 78.4%. In 1996 the

percentages changed as follows: hymen, 61.5% ($P < .05$); labia minora, 83%; and urethra, 72.4%.

One possible explanation for the difficulty in correctly identifying genital anatomy is physicians' discomfort with and lack of experience in examining the genitalia. Any discomfort with the genital examination should be overcome over time by routinely incorporating the anogenital examination into the annual physical examination. Within the context of preparing the child for the anogenital component of the well-child examination, the clinician is also afforded an opportunity to provide anticipatory guidance regarding OK and not OK touching and teach the child the appropriate names for private parts, providing the language to communicate should anything inappropriate happen.

A more difficult issue to overcome may be the anxieties and fears that physicians may have when confronted with the need to address the possibility of sexual abuse. Box 2.1 expresses some of the perceived fears of a family physician. The fears expressed may be more universal than we might like to acknowledge. However, when we understand our fears and anxieties, we can confront them. The Ladson et al[5] and Lentsch and Johnson[4] surveys addressed the examination of prepubertal children, but physicians may have a similar level of discomfort when examining pubertal children.

Inexperience with the examination of children's genitalia leads to unfamiliarity with the broad range of

BOX 2.1
Another Dilemma for the Family Physician

I.   As a family physician, I become concerned regarding the possibility of child sexual abuse based on historical/behavioral factors.

II. Do I perform a genital examination? If I do (which I should)

A.   Mom will become alarmed. (What if she is aware of the abuse?)

B.   What will my examination show? (I probably will not know, because there are too many variables; also, I have seen so few normal preadolescent genitalia.) Besides, even in abuse situations, by virtue of time delay, any trauma may have already completely healed.

C.   Mom will want to know what I have found. If I say everything is OK, I may give a false sense of security. But if I give a false-negative, I may further hurt or frustrate the child emotionally.

1.   If I say that problems exist, I have created a whirlwind of difficulties.

2.   Mom will accuse someone as the perpetrator.

3.   That someone may come and challenge me.

4.   I must report alleged (or suspected) abuse to authorities.

5.   I have to deal with attorneys, police, courts, and depositions.

6.   I will probably lose the family as patients.

7.   If the courts do not convict, the family/alleged perpetrator can bring a countersuit. I will have a damaged reputation and many sleepless nights.

III. If my diagnosis/suspicion is not confirmed (yet is true), a child continues to be hurt psychologically, emotionally, and physically

IV. If my suspicions are false, I may be sued. I may be shot or beaten up. My practice will suffer through whisper campaigns.

V.   But if I am not vigilant and decisive, children may continue to be destroyed.

Perhaps the only solution is specially trained community teams, including doctors to whom suspected cases must be referred.

normal anatomical variants.[12,13] Whatever the reason for uneasiness when called on to complete a genital examination, the health care professional who is uncomfortable will undoubtedly convey this discomfort to the patient. The examining health care professional has a responsibility to develop confidence in his or her ability to complete the anogenital examination of both prepubertal and pubertal children. Strategies to overcome skill limitations in practicing physicians will be different from those used with residents in training. Program directors need to provide residents with the opportunity to gain experience in preparing children for and conducting anogenital examinations. While residents are in training, exposure to the spectrum of normal and abnormal findings, as well as participation in the assessment of children alleged to have been sexually abused, will help physicians develop good skills and prepare them for the challenges of clinical practice. Only with experience can the spectrum of normal variants of anogenital anatomy and the healed residua to trauma be recognized.

Each year more physicians are specializing in the discipline of the medical diagnosis and treatment of children suspected of being abused, but the number remains small relative to the need. With the advent of board certification in child abuse pediatrics, more communities will have access to pediatricians with specialized training in child abuse.[14] Because experienced child abuse pediatricians (whether that expertise developed from years of clinical care or formal fellowship training) are limited throughout the country, most communities will rely on local physicians for recognition and care of children suspected of being abused.[15] Children's hospitals are increasingly recognizing the importance of dedicating resources to provide communities with the specialized services of a child abuse team.[16]

Although it is not necessary to be a specialist in sexual abuse, the health care professional should be familiar with the basic aspects of a sexual abuse evaluation to make the necessary decisions for initial intervention, reporting, and/or referral: (a) conducting a medical history directed at uncovering the details of the experience interpreted to be sexually inappropriate,

(b) performing a physical examination that includes a careful inspection of the genitalia and anus of the child, (c) collecting and preserving laboratory and forensic specimens, (d) considering a differential diagnosis of behavioral complaints and anogenital signs that may suggest sexual abuse, (e) describing and documenting diagnostic findings observed during the examination, and (f) providing treatment and follow-up when appropriate.

These skills are important for all clinicians to have because cases of suspected sexual abuse can be discovered not only by primary care practitioners but also by ED physicians at general and community hospitals, urgent care centers, and clinics. Familiarity with the components of the evaluation and the requirements for mandated reporting of cases of suspected sexual abuse are essential skills for all health care providers.

Presenting Signs and Symptoms

The child suspected of being sexually abused may present to the health care professional with diverse behavioral and/or physical complaints. The parent or another caregiver frequently observes behavioral changes in the child, overhears a child say something that includes sexually explicit content, or responds to a physical complaint from the child. Some children will deliberately disclose their inappropriate experiences, or the disclosure may stem from a direct observation of sexual interactions.

The health care professional begins the assessment of the presenting concerns by taking a complete medical history. He or she then determines any immediate risk to the child and sets the stage to both report the suspected abuse and pursue a more formal evaluation. A CPS worker or a law enforcement officer may accompany the child for a sexual abuse evaluation following the child's disclosure. If this is the case, an investigation presumably has begun, and the issues of continued risk and protection should have been addressed. Regardless of how a child presents to the physician, the physician's role and responsibility is to obtain a detailed medical history of alleged victimization, identify any residua from the alleged contact, and provide diagnostic and treatment services. Although CPS and law enforcement may seek medical services as part of their investigation, the physician's role should always remain clear—to meet the child's medical diagnostic and treatment needs.

The presenting signs and symptoms of a child who is sexually abused may include specific complaints regarding the genitalia or anus, or the problems may be nonspecific and diffuse in nature. A child who presents with the signs and symptoms of an STI obviously needs evaluation for the possibility that he or she contracted the infection through sexually inappropriate activities. When a child presents with an STI, the clinician must presume sexual abuse until proven otherwise.[17,18]

A medical history rich in detail regarding sexually inappropriate activities without diagnostic findings to corroborate the history is the rule rather than the exception. Thus the absence of an abnormal physical or laboratory examination cannot be presumed to contradict a child's medical history reflective of experiencing sexually inappropriate activities. Behaviors that reflect age-inappropriate knowledge of adult sexual activities must be considered to have high specificity to either experiencing those activities themselves, being exposed to adult sexual activities, and/or both. In particular, when young children demonstrate behaviors or knowledge about oral-genital activities or intrusive sexual acts, the concern that this could reflect their own victimization should be paramount. The spectrum of age-appropriate behaviors considered to reflect the curiosity of children and normative behaviors, as well as those of concern, have been described by Friedrich et al and Rosenfeld et al.[19–21] Box 2.2 lists examples of the types of nonspecific physical and behavioral complaints that could suggest sexual abuse. The specificity of each of the nonspecific presenting symptoms becomes more or less specific following a detailed history.

Approach to the Evaluation of Sexual Abuse

The suspicion and/or disclosure of sexual abuse invariably precipitates a crisis for the family. Because the dynamics of sexual abuse are very different from that of classic rape, few children present immediately

BOX 2.2
Nonspecific Physical and Behavioral Complaints[a]

Physical	Behavioral
Anorexia	Compulsive or excessive masturbation[b]
Abdominal pain	Unusual sexual curiosity; repetitive sexualized play[b]
Enuresis	Excessive distractibility
Dysuria	Nightmares
Encopresis	Phobias, fears
Vaginal itching	Clinging behavior, difficulty in separation
Vaginal discharge	Aggressive behavior
Vaginal bleeding	Abrupt change in behavior
Urethral discharge	Attempted suicide
Painful defecation	

[a] Adapted from Fleisher GF, Ludwig S. *Textbook of Pediatric Emergency Medicine*. 2nd ed. p 1145.
   Copyright © 1988 the Williams and Wilkins Co., Baltimore. Used by permission.
[b] Although not specific for sexual abuse, these should be viewed as warning flags and require careful evaluation.

following the last alleged sexually inappropriate contact and are unlikely to have the acute injuries so commonly associated with rape. Thus sexual abuse usually presents primarily as a family and mental health emergency rather than a medical emergency. When the concern of possible sexual abuse arises, there is always a need for a prompt and thorough medical and psychological evaluation. Child protective services will assess whether the child is at risk for continued inappropriate contact and in need of immediate protection. The sense of urgency created by a disclosure to determine whether a child has been sexually abused can result in inappropriate triage of the suspected victim. Pressure to "know for sure" may come from a non-offending parent, CPS, and/or law enforcement. The clinician's responsibility is to ensure that the child receives the most comprehensive and skilled evaluation. When children find their way to clinical settings in which the needed evaluation cannot be provided, the responsibility of the clinician is to provide triage to the most appropriate professionals. When CPS and law enforcement are the first to receive a referral concerning alleged abuse, the child should be referred to the most appropriate institution/individual for the initial medical assessment. The child should not undergo a screening examination by his or her primary care practitioner, nor should he or she be told to go to the local ED because of expediency.

To ensure that the child receives proper support and care throughout the evaluation, the health care professional should be familiar with the criteria for evaluation and intervention.[22,23] Psychosocial support and protection take priority throughout the total examination. Because of the complex nature of allegations of sexual abuse, the medical evaluation must be considered as one component of the complete assessment. Child protective services, law enforcement, and mental health professionals will bring their discipline-specific assessment to the table and assist in developing a complete understanding of what a child may have experienced and his or her need for protection. Many communities have developed multidisciplinary teams that assist in ensuring the most comprehensive understanding of what a child has experienced and addressing the child's needs for protection and treatment. Medical professionals are an essential component of this assessment and should be active participants in their communities' multidisciplinary teams if they exist. Multidisciplinary teams may be housed in child advocacy centers or prosecutors' offices or be community based.

Determining the Urgency of an Examination

The guiding principle that underlies the timing of an examination is ensuring that children undergo only one examination by a clinician who has the requisite skills to conduct it. This principle is important for both medical and legal reasons, beyond the obvious need to see that the child does not have to experience more than one examination. The first examination of a child following a disclosure is considered by the courts to be the examination for the purpose of diagnosis and treatment. The medical history and physical assessment conducted by a physician for the purpose of diagnosis and treatment not only serves the child's medical needs, but the medical history obtained under this set of circumstances may be admissible in court under the diagnosing and treating physician's exception to hearsay. Any

subsequent examinations can be interpreted as investigative. An examination considered to have been done for the purpose of an investigation may not provide for the admissibility of out-of-court statements by the child under the diagnosing and treating physician's exception. For example, if a child is seen initially in an ED and the examining physician does not have the experience to obtain a complete history and conduct a thorough examination, it is in the child's best interest that the physician does not formulate a final diagnosis. Instead, the physician should note the concern at hand and refer to the appropriate consulting physician. The physician should note in the medical record that the purpose of the referral is for diagnosis and treatment of residua to the alleged contact, if any. This approach is consonant with the triaging of any medical subspecialty consultation and preserves the diagnosing and treating physician's exception.

Children will be well served by educating CPS workers, law enforcement professionals, and primary care and ED physicians regarding the medical diagnostic and treatment needs of child victims and when to seek immediate examinations and when they can be deferred. By providing this guidance, the potential to secure appropriately conducted examinations is more likely and minimizes the chance that a child will have to undergo a repeat examination. Some of the most important topics a physician, law enforcement official, or a CPS caseworker can question the child about to assist in determining the urgency of the examination are as follows:

1. Ask when the last time was that the child had any contact with the individual(s) alleged to have engaged the child in sexually inappropriate activities. If the contact was more than 72 hours ago, then few children will require an immediate examination. If there was a history of injury and if the injuries were superficial, they are already likely to have healed. Chronic residua to significant trauma will remain identifiable even if the examination is deferred. In those circumstances in which the history dictates the need to diagnose STIs or pregnancy, the urgency for such generally does not dictate the need for an immediate examination but, rather, an urgent examination conducted as soon as possible in the most appropriate setting.
2. If the last contact was within 72 hours, inquire whether the child experienced discomfort and whether there was contact with potentially infected genital secretions. Contact with ejaculate may require the need for prophylaxis for human immuno-deficiency virus and other STIs within this time frame even in the absence of a history of injury. If the child responds that none of the activities hurt him or her and there was no history of contact with semi-nal products, CPS and/or law enforce-ment can focus the investigation on understanding the concerns and defer the examination to a more appropriate time and setting.

3. If the last contact was within 72 hours and the child complained of being hurt, the examination should be conducted immediately in an appropriate setting whether or not there is a history of contact with seminal products.

With each of the above scenarios, there must also be an assessment of the risk of STI or pregnancy and the potential for identifying and collecting trace materials/serology (seminal products). In light of the above caveats, the generally accepted criteria that warrant an emergency evaluation are as follows:

1. History of age-inappropriate sexual contact within the past 72 hours
2. History of acute genital, anal, or extragenital trauma
3. Vaginal discharge and the possibility of an STI
4. Possibility of pregnancy when presented with a history of penile-vaginal penetration in an adolescent who has reached menarche
5. Contact with seminal products and the potential for collection of seminal products, trace materials, and/or serology

When the examination is non-emergent, CPS and/or law enforcement should focus on investigating the concerns at hand and refer for comprehensive medical evaluation in a non-emergent fashion.

When a child does not meet the criteria for an immediate examination and the caretaker insists on an immediate examination, the caretaker should explain the importance of having only one assessment. By addressing caretaker anxieties and fears, most children can avoid multiple examinations. Parents may express a desire to have their child seen at their local hospital or primary care provider if the examination can't be done immediately. It may be necessary to explain in a diplomatic manner that it is in the best interest of their child to have him or her examined by a physician who is knowledgeable and equipped to address the special needs of their child.

The clinician may find that a child is cooperative for the medical history component of the evaluation but expresses reluctance and/or outright refusal to undergo the physical examination. When the child refuses to cooperate for the physical examination, the health care professional should attempt to identify the source of the child's anxiety and address those fears prior to the examination. The child may need additional time to become comfortable with the health professional and should be given an opportunity to have any questions regarding the examination answered. Some children may not be emotionally ready for an examination and may need to receive mental health services prior to proceeding with the physical examination. If this is the case, the physician should acknowledge the child's desire not to undergo an examination and express respect for this decision; however, the physician must also explain to the child why the examination could be of benefit to him or her. It is hoped that with time and the initiation of mental health services, the child will feel more

comfortable with the idea of having an examination and will return.

The complete examination may be postponed as long as referral to the multidisciplinary team and/or a follow-up visit is scheduled and provisions are made to ensure the safety of the child. The non-offending parent's anxiety over the examination must be addressed to minimize the potential of him or her conveying anxiety to the child. Providing information about the examination that answers common child/parent concerns can go a long way toward reducing anxiety and setting the child at ease. (See the Appendix in Chapter 3.)

When it is necessary to defer a component of the complete evaluation, the health care professional should use the time in the interim to build a rapport with the child. A common fear of young children when they first appear in a physician's office is that they might be getting a shot. This fear can be readily addressed, because it is unlikely that the child will receive a shot. If the need to draw blood is apparent at the beginning of the assessment, the clinician should be up front with the child. As the examination progresses, the child may ex-press a fear of being touched by a cotton swab. Allowing the child to touch a moistened swab or having the child touch his or her genitalia with the cotton swab may reduce anxiety. If the child still cannot overcome his or her fear enough to cooperate with the examination, try sending the child home with cotton swabs and culturettes to practice on a doll or himself or herself. It is hoped that the child's mother can help the child overcome his or her fears and return for an examination at a later date.

Sometimes children have unrealistic fears that may not be verbalized and may take considerable time to identify. The physician should never use force or restrain a child to conduct an examination. Circumstances rarely require that a child be examined under anesthesia, but when this occurs, it is usually because the child has extensive acute intravaginal and/or anorectal injuries that potentially require surgical repair.

Fortunately, with the use of video colposcopy, the child can watch the examination. A skilled examiner can use the video colposcopy to demystify the examination for the child. When a child watches the examination of his own genitalia, he has a sense of participation and control throughout the examination. This approach enhances cooperativeness and increases the chances of a positive examination experience.

Contextual Details of the Medical History

The history obtained from the child is the centerpiece of the medical evaluation for suspected sexual abuse. It is, perhaps, the most important aspect of the evaluation. Children are unlikely to fabricate tales about detailed sexual activity.[24] According to Kempe,[24] the child "witnessed" his or her own victimization and is best at describing

what he or she experienced. Lay people, attorneys, and CPS workers often assume that physical evidence will confirm or deny the occurrence of sexual abuse. However, experience shows that the child's account of his or her experience is the most important information to be considered in determining what occurred. With an understanding of the full scope of a child's experience, the physician is more likely to be able to predict the potential for residua from the alleged contact and explain the reasons for the absence of such.

The medical history that the health professional obtains is vital to understanding a child's experience, and it guides the need for testing for STIs, contributes to understanding potential patterns of injury, and provides insight into the child's worries about his or her body intactness. Thus the child's account of the events is critical to understanding not only what he or she may have experienced but also his or her continued risk and need for protection. Unfortunately too few clinicians will find obtaining the medical history of alleged sexual abuse something that they are prepared for and when confronted with the need to conduct such it can be an emotionally challenging interaction. With experience, obtaining the medical history can be one of the most rewarding aspects of the medical assessment.

The Appendix of this chapter provides an outline for a structured medical history and the rationale for the questions asked.

Dynamics of Sexual Victimization Assist in Predicting Diagnostic Findings

The possibility of residua to alleged inappropriate sexual activities is gleaned through a complete medical history and an understanding of how the dynamics of sexual victimization mitigate for or against its presence. Physical findings that confirm sexual contact with medical certainty are uncommon because of the dynamics of the sexual interactions that the children experience.[25–31] As the field has garnered increasing clinical experience examining children suspected of sexual abuse and diagnostic criteria have been refined, fewer children are identified with diagnostic findings than the literature had previously suggested were diagnostic. Older studies reflect the prevalence of physical findings to be frequent, ranging from 23% to 84%.[32]

Approximately 75% of child sexual abuse is at the hands of individuals known to and trusted by the child.[33,34] Most individuals who engage a child in sexual activities do not intend to harm him or her to facilitate repeated engagement over time. Thus coercion and deceit become substitute mechanisms for engaging the child in the activities and are preferred over force and restraint. The individual engaging the child in inappropriate sexual activities avoids injuring the child to reduce the chances of disclosure. Also, a young child who experienced discomfort as a result of his or her first inappropriate sexual contact may be less likely to be deceived into the activity again.

Another critical dynamic is secrecy. By forcing the child, through direct or implicit threats, to maintain secrecy, the perpetrator may deceive himself or herself into thinking that no one will find out about the sexual activities and thus believe that the activities can be repeated as often as he or she wishes. Secrecy and the associated fear of reprisal explain in great part why few children disclose their inappropriate experiences. When they do, it is generally long after the last contact, when they feel safe. This also explains why so few children present for medical examinations immediately following their experiences.[35]

Pattern and Timing of Disclosure

Disclosures fall into the broad categories of purposeful, accidental, or prompted/elicited.[36,37] The pattern of children's disclosures can be quite variable, spanning the spectrum from full and detailed to delayed and incomplete. Children not uncommonly delay their disclosure of sexual abuse for a variety of reasons, which although not limited to can include any or all of the following: clear threats by the perpetrator; perceived/implied threats and/or consequences; embarrassment, shame, and stigmatization; fear of disbelief; close relationship of the perpetrator to the family; more intrusive events; and expected negative reactions by parents.[38–40] If the clinician understands the spectrum of factors that contribute to the difficulty of disclosing, the clinician can address those factors with the child and possibly create a supportive environment that facilitates the child's sharing of the complete details of his or her core and peripheral experience. When children are given an opportunity to provide details in a friendly context and are encouraged to share their experience using open-ended prompts, they are more likely to provide rich and detailed information about the sexual contact.[39,41] By contrast, when the historian is intimidating and asks inappropriate questions, the child's response will be less accurate and may include false-positive and false-negative information. Lamb et al[41] and Keary and Fitzpatrick[42] found that contrary to prior reports, in general older children are more reluctant to disclose because of their awareness of social norms/taboos and/or of being ashamed/embarrassed by their inability to stop their victimization.[39,41,43]

In a study by De Jong and colleagues,[44] the authors found that 49% of the children delayed reporting the incident for at least 24 hours, and another 22% reported only after multiple episodes. Another study revealed at least a 72-hour delay in reporting in approximately 55% of the cases.[45] Many children are not seen until weeks or months after the alleged abuse.[46] If delayed reporting occurs, any superficial trauma that may have been present as a result of the sexual contact is likely to have healed, leaving no signs of acute trauma.[47] Woodling and Heger[31] found that children who describe painful penetration of the vagina or anus are more likely to manifest physical findings. Findings are more common when the context of the experience involves the use of force and restraint, which is more likely when the assailant is either an adolescent family member or an extrafamilial perpetrator.[29]

The specific techniques used to conduct the physical examination are detailed in Chapter 3.

Laboratory and Evidentiary Collection in Brief

Laboratory studies may corroborate the medical history and physical examination. The Centers for Disease Control and Prevention[17] and the American Academy of Pediatrics[18,22] recommend that any child found to have an STI should be evaluated for sexual abuse. (See Chapter 5 for guidance.) Identification of seminal products on the prepubertal child is considered confirmatory evidence for sexual abuse of that child but is an infrequent finding. Palusci et al[48] reviewed 190 consecutive cases of children younger than 13 years who were urgently referred for suspected sexual abuse examinations. Semen or sperm was identified in 9% from body swabs only from non-bathed, female children older than 10 years or on clothing or objects. Christian and colleagues[26] reviewed 273 children younger than 10 years who were evaluated urgently and found that no swabs taken from their bodies were positive for blood after 13 hours or sperm/semen after 9 hours. The authors conclude that swabbing a child's body for evidence after 24 hours was unnecessary. When the history suggested the possibility of identifying forensic evidence, the investigators found that most forensic evidence (64%) was found on clothing and linens and not on the child. (See Chapter 6 for specific guidance in collecting, preserving, and interpreting forensic evidence.)

Documentation in Brief

All health care professionals who evaluate children alleged to have been sexually abused must maintain written and visual documentation of all aspects of their medical evaluation in a manner that meets acceptable medical records standards. The medical report must be formulated with objectivity and be defensible under scrutiny. The medical record can serve the interests of the suspected child abuse victim effectively if it clearly and accurately reflects all that transpires during the medical history and physical examination. As previously highlighted, it is critical to keep a record of the questions asked of the child and to document the responses, noting the exact words used by the child and accompanying affective changes. Questions should be as open-ended and non-leading as possible. (See Chapter 15.) The medical record must clearly differentiate statements made by the child from information related to the health care professional by the caseworker or parent, which is considered hearsay. Diagrams and photographs are essential tools for recording diagnostic findings. The health care professional must clearly and legibly construct a complete medical record. The preservation of such information is essential to any child protection or legal proceedings. Chapter 13 provides a more detailed set of guidelines regarding documentation and the development of a medical report in cases of suspected sexual abuse.

Summary

- Children may present with the chief complaint of suspected sexual abuse based on a child's disclosure, observed behaviors, and specific/nonspecific signs and symptoms.
- Specific criteria exist for the emergent or deferred evaluations and referral.
- The medical history obtained from the child is critical to understanding and diagnosing child sexual abuse.
- Medical evaluation involves the integration of the medical history, physical examination, laboratory studies, forensic evidence and the formulation of a balanced and objective diagnosis.
- A child with an STI must be evaluated for possible sexual abuse.
- Clear documentation of the child's statements and physical findings are an integral part of the sexual abuse evaluation.
- The medical evaluation is one part of understanding a child's experience. The medical assessment must be considered in concert with the professional insights of child protection, law enforcement, and mental health colleagues.

References

1. Finkelhor DH. *Child Sexual Abuse: New Theory and Research.* New York, NY: Free Press; 1984

2. Finkelhor DH. *Sexually Victimized Children.* New York, NY: Free Press; 1979

3. Finkelhor D, Browne A. The traumatic impact of child sexual abuse: a conceptualization. *Am J Orthopsychiatry.* 1985;55(4):530–541

4. Lentsch KA, Johnson CF. Do physicians have adequate knowledge of child sexual abuse? The results of two surveys of practicing physicians, 1986 and 1996. *Child Maltreat.* 2000;5(1):72–78

5. Ladson S, Johnson CF, Doty RE. Do physicians recognize sexual abuse? *Am J Dis Child.* 1987;141(4):411–415

6. Krugman RD. Recognition of sexual abuse in children. *Pediatr Rev.* 1986;8(1):25–30

7. Adams JA, Kaplan RA, Starling SP, et al. Guidelines for medical care of children who may have been sexually abused. *J Pediatr Adolesc Gynecol.* 2007;20(3):163–172

8. Hibbard RA, Zollinger TW. Patterns of child sexual abuse knowledge among professionals. *Child Abuse Negl.* 1990;14(3):347–355

9. Dubowitz H. Child abuse programs and pediatric residency training *Pediatrics.* 1988;82(3 Pt 2):477–480

10. Alexander RC. Education of the physician in child abuse. *Pediatr Clin North Am.* 1990;37(4):971–988

11. Herman-Giddens ME, Frothingham TE. Prepubertal female genitalia: examination for evidence of sexual abuse. *Pediatrics.* 1987;80(2):203–208

12. Paradise JE, Winter MR, Finkel MA, Berenson AB, Beiser AS. Influence of the history on physicians' interpretations of girls' genital findings. *Pediatrics.* 1999;103(5 Pt 1):980–986

13. Paradise JE, Finkel MA, Beiser AS, Berenson AB, Greenberg DB, Winter MR. Assessments of girl's genital findings and the likelihood of sexual abuse: agreement among physicians self-rated as skilled. *Arch Pediatr Adolesc Med.* 1997;151(9):883–891

14. Block RW, Palusci VJ. Child abuse pediatrics: a new pediatric subspecialty. *J Pediatr.* 2006;148(6):711–712

15. Starling SP, Sirotnak AP, Jenny C. Child abuse and forensic pediatric medicine fellowship curriculum statement. *Child Maltreat.* 2000;5(1):58–62

16. National Association of Children's Hospitals and Related Institutions (NACHRI). *Defining the Children's Hospital role in child maltreatment.* 2006

17. Centers for Disease Control and Prevention. 1998 guidelines for treatment of sexually transmitted diseases. *MMWR Recomm Rep.* 1998;47(RR-1):1–111

18. American Academy of Pediatrics Committee on Child Abuse and Neglect. Gonorrhea in prepubertal children. *Pediatrics.* 1998;101(1):134–135

19. Friedrich WN, Fisher J, Broughton D, Houston M, Shafran CR. Normative sexual behavior in children: a contemporary sample. *Pediatrics.* 1998;101(4):e9

20. Friedrich WN, Trane ST. Sexual behavior in children across multiple settings [comment]. *Child Abuse Negl.* 2002;26(3):243–245

21. Rosenfeld AA, Siegel B, Bailey R. Familial bathing patterns: implications for cases of alleged molestation and for pediatric practice. *Pediatrics.* 1987;79(2):224–229

22. American Academy of Pediatrics Committee on Child Abuse and Neglect. Guidelines for the evaluation of sexual abuse of children: subject review. *Pediatrics.* 1999;103(1):186–191

23. American Academy of Pediatrics Committee on Adolescence. Sexual assault and the adolescent. *Pediatrics.* 1994;94(5):761–765

24. Kempe CH. Sexual abuse, another hidden pediatric problem: the 1977 C. Anderson Aldrich lecture. *Pediatrics.* 1978;62(3):382–389

25. Berenson AB, Chacko MR, Wiemann CM, Mishaw CO, Friedrich WN, Grady JJ. A case-control study of anatomic changes resulting from sexual abuse. Citing article *Am J Obstetr Gynecol.* 2000;182(4):820–881; discussion 831–834

26. Christian CW, Lavelle JM, De Jong AR, Loiselle J, Brenner L, Joffe M. Forensic evidence findings in prepubertal victims of sexual assault. *Pediatrics.* 2000;106(1 Pt 1):100–104

27. De Jong AR, Rose M. Frequency and significance of physical evidence in legally proven cases of child sexual abuse. *Pediatrics.* 1989;84(6):1022–1026

28. De Jong AR, Rose M. Legal proof of child sexual abuse in the absence of physical evidence. *Pediatrics.* 1991;88(3):506–511

29. Finkel MA. The medical evaluation of child sexual abuse. In: Schety DH, Green AH, eds. *Child Sexual Abuse: A Handbook for Healthcare and Legal Professionals.* New York, NY: Brunner/Mazel; 1988:82–103

30. Muram D. Child sexual abuse: relationship between sexual acts and genital findings. *Child Abuse Negl.* 1989;13(2):211–216

31. Woodling BA, Heger A. The use of the colposcope in the diagnosis of sexual abuse in the pediatric age group. *Child Abuse Negl.* 1986;10(1):111–114

32. Heger A, Ticson L, Velasquez O, Bernier R. Children referred for possible sexual abuse: medical findings in 2384 children. *Child Abuse Negl.* 2002;26(6-7):645–659

33. Tilelli JA, Turek D, Jaffe AC. Sexual abuse of children: clinical findings and implications for management. *N Engl J Med.* 1980;302(6):319–323

34. US Department of Health and Human Services Administration on Children Youth and Families. *Child Maltreatment 2004.* Vol 2006. Washington, DC: US Government Printing Office; 2006

35. De Jong AR. The medical evaluation of sexual abuse in children. *Hosp Community Psychiatry.* 1985;36(5): 509–512

36. Alaggia R. Many ways of telling: expanding conceptualizations of child sexual abuse disclosure. *Child Abuse Negl.* 2004;28(11):1213–1227

37. Nagel DE, Putnam FW, Noll JG, Trickett PK. Disclosure patterns of sexual abuse and psychological functioning at a 1-year follow-up. *Child Abuse Negl.* 1997;21(2):137–147

38. Distel NE. Disclosure of childhood sexual abuse: links to emotion expression and adult attachment. *Diss Abstr.* 1999;60 (6-B):2938

39. Hershkowitz I, Lanes O, Lamb ME. Exploring the disclosure of child sexual abuse with alleged victims and their parents. *Child Abuse Negl.* 2007;31(2):111–123

40. Somer E, Szwarcberg S. Variables in delayed disclosure of childhood sexual abuse. *Am J Orthopsychiatry.* 2001;71(3):332–341

41. Lamb ME, Sternberg KJ, Orbach Y, Esplin PW, Stewart H, Mitchell S. Age differences in young children's responses to open-ended invitations in the course of forensic interviews. *J Consult Clin Psychol.* 2003;71(5):926–934

42. Keary K, Fitzpatrick C. Children's disclosure of sexual abuse during formal investigation. *Child Abuse Negl.* 1994;18(7):543–548

43. Saywitz KJ, Goodman GS. Interviewing children in and out of court: current research and practice implications. In: Briere J, Berliner L, Bulkley JA, Jenny C, Reid T, eds. *The APSAC Handbook on Child Maltreatment.* Thousand Oaks, CA: Sage Publications; 1996:297–318

44. De Jong AR, Hervada AR, Emmett GA. Epidemiologic variations in childhood sexual abuse. *Child Abuse Negl.* 1983;7(2):155–162

45. Rimsza ME, Niggemann EH. Medical evaluation of sexually abused children: a review of 311 cases. *Pediatrics.* 1982;69(1):8–14

46. Emans SJ, Woods ER, Flagg NT, Freeman A. Genital findings in sexually abused, symptomatic, and asymptomatic girls. *Pediatrics.* 1987;79(5):778–785

47. Finkel MA. Child sexual abuse: a physician's introduction to historical and medical validation. *J Am Osteopath Assoc.* 1989;89(9):1143–1149

48. Palusci VJ, Cox EO, Shatz EM, Schultze JM. Urgent medical assessment after child sexual abuse. *Child Abuse Negl.* 2006;30(4):367–380

Appendix

Obtaining the Medical History in Suspected Child Sexual Abuse: Suggested Rationale and Questions

Martin A. Finkel

The medical history can be one of the most challenging aspects of evaluating children and adolescents who are alleged to have experienced sexual abuse. Unlike obtaining a medical history in general pediatric practice, the emotionally charged issue of sexual abuse can be uncomfortable for both the historian and the child. When the clinician is uncomfortable, the child is most likely to sense this unease and will be reluctant to engage in a meaningful dialogue. The historian's responsibility is to engage children in a nonjudgmental, facilitating, and empathetic manner, which will increase the opportunity to understand what a child may have experienced. The key to making any diagnosis is rooted in an understanding of the clinical presentation of a given disease. The historian obtains the medical history in a logical progression that seeks elements of the chronology of the clinical presentation and accompanying signs and symptoms that lead to a diagnosis. This same tried and true process is applied to obtaining a medical history when making the diagnosis of sexual abuse. The more knowledgeable doctors are about the "disease of sexual victimization," the more likely they can convey their understanding with professionalism, enhancing their ability to develop rapport. With understanding the clinician can impart empathy. The empathetic clinician is best equipped to anticipate and then address fears and anxieties in their patient. When children sense that the clinician understands their fears and anxieties, they are more likely to entrust their worries to the clinician.

This section provides by example some how-tos for preparing both the nonoffending parent and child for the medical history and evaluation. A series of iterative questions designed to assist the historian in obtaining a medical history when sexual abuse is suspected is presented. In addition, the rationale for asking particular questions is explained. There are many ways in which questions can be successfully asked. This section is by no means intended to be the only way to obtain a medical history but rather a distillate of the author's clinical experience. Each clinician will need to develop an approach with which he or she is comfortable when engaging children in the medical history. This section is not intended to address the myriad of circumstances that children present with when sexual abuse is a concern but rather provides a framework for obtaining the medical history. Examples provided are developmentally appropriate for children 5 years and older.

Introducing the Purpose
of the Medical Examination to the Caretaker

The process of reducing a child's and caretaker's anxiety begins with the manner in which the child and caretaker are greeted beginning with the encounter in the waiting room. For example, most young children when going to the doctor have one overriding fear and that is the fear of a needle. The clinician might introduce himself or herself by first approaching the child and saying, "My name is Doctor… and I am a kids' doctor. Are you a kid? Thanks for coming to see me today. I just want you to know that there are no shots, so you don't have to worry about that. I am going to ask your mom (accompanying adult) a whole bunch of boring questions so you get a chance to play a little bit until it's your turn."

By meeting with the caretaker independent of the child there is an opportunity to explain to the caretaker the purpose of the examination and what is anticipated to be accomplished as a result of the evaluation. When caretakers understand what to expect and have their anxieties and fears addressed, they are better prepared to support their child throughout the examination. Explain that the following will be achieved:

1. A complete review will be done of their child's medical history.

2. An account will be requested of the specific details of the circumstances under which they first became aware of a concern that something inappropriate may have happened to their child and all the intervening details up until this examination in a chronological manner. The physician should show a willingness to hear everything caregivers want to say: any and all worries, concerns, observations, and questions they want to ask.

3. A medical history will be obtained from their child independent of the caretaker to learn about what the child may have experienced as well as providing an opportunity for the child to express any worries or concerns he or she may have.

4. After the child's medical history, the caretaker will return to the examination room to be with the child for a complete physical examination. Parental anxiety is often reduced by explaining to the caretaker of the prepubertal girl that the genital examination is not an adult gynecologic examination and that the child should not experience any physical discomfort. For the parent of an adolescent female, explain that the extent to which the gynecologic examination approaches a complete adult female examination will be dictated by the history and initial observed findings. State that testing for sexually transmitted infections (STIs) will be completed as clinically indicated. If based on history anoscopy is indicated, explain what this procedure entails.

5. Explain that following the examination, the results of the examination will be discussed and there will be an opportunity for the caretaker to have any

questions answered. In addition, any next steps such as follow-up examinations, recommendations for medical treatment if required, and the need for mental health services will be discussed.

By outlining the above sequence of events, parental anxiety should be reduced, which in turn allows the caretaker to focus his or her efforts on being supportive of the child. Before meeting with the child, ask the caretaker what he or she told the child the visit was for. Many parents may have not told the child anything about the examination.

Preparing for and Obtaining the Medical History

The emotionally charged nature of child sexual abuse requires that clinicians maintain an objective demeanor throughout their interactions with the child caretakers, child protective services/law enforcement, and the court, if challenged. The ability to modulate one's visceral response to this highly charged issue is not intuitive and is a learned/modeled skill that develops with time. The most challenging skill for clinicians to develop is the ability to obtain the medical history in a non-leading and non-suggestive manner that is appropriate for the child's developmental, cognitive, and linguistic capabilities.

It is important not only to be able to obtain the medical history of the child's experience but also to document the questions asked and the child's verbatim response. This can only be achieved when adequate time is allocated to allow for an unhurried assessment. The documentation should reflect contemporaneous writing of the exact questions asked and the child's verbatim response. It is the idiosyncratic statements of children and adolescents that capture both the central and peripheral details of the child experience. The details obtained during the medical history have the potential to be the most compelling information that helps in understanding the child's experience. (See Chapter 2.)

An example of a statement to the child to explain the purpose of writing down what the child has to say during the history could be

> *Everything you have to say is important to me. I am going to need to listen very carefully and will be writing down everything you tell me. I cannot write as fast as you can talk so I may ask you to stop so I can catch up. If you don't understand a question that I ask, I want you to let me know. I will ask you to explain if there is something I don't understand.*

The approach taken in engaging children in a medical history will vary depending on the child's age, development, cognitive abilities, and language skills. During the initial face-to-face interaction with the child the clinician must impart to the child a feeling that he is speaking with someone who is there to understand his experience and help put it behind him. The child should be asked if he knows why he is having an examination because the purpose of the visit may not have been clearly articulated by the parent or the referent. Taking time to anticipate and reduce a child's fears and anxieties helps set the stage for a more positive and productive interaction.

Whenever possible it is best to meet with the child independent of the caretaker. Most children will separate from the caretaker without difficulty. Caretakers sometimes express discomfort in allowing the child to speak alone with the doctor. Explain to the caretaker that, in your experience, children are generally most comfortable sharing details of their experiences with doctors and are frequently embarrassed/afraid to share specific information when caretakers are present because either they may be worried about the caretakers' response and/or don't want to upset the caretaker. When the caretaker seems comfortable and reassuring, children are more likely to be able to speak about their experiences.

If the child will not separate from the caretakers or the caretakers will not allow the child to meet independent of them for the medical history, special instructions should be provided to the caretaker independent from the child. Explain that there is the possibility that when they sit in on the history session with their child they are likely to hear new and upsetting information and may have difficulty maintaining composure. Explain to the caretaker that their role is to provide physical comfort to their child. Have the child sit in the caretaker's lap in an enface position. Ask the caretaker not to say anything unless asked and to try to remain neutral throughout the history session.

Introductory Statement to the Child

The specifics of an introductory statement will be constructed based on a preliminary understanding of the presenting concerns and the child's age and development. An example of an introductory statement when the allegations involve inappropriate sexual contact by a family member is as follows:

> My name is…and I am a kids' doctor. One of the things that I do that is a little bit different than most kids' doctors is every day I have a chance to see a lot of kids just like you, some older and younger, when there has been a worry or concern that they may have experienced something that could be very confusing or difficult to understand by someone they know and should trust. That happens to a lot of kids, and I understand something like that may have happened to you. Is that true?

This introductory statement was constructed to impart the important message that as a doctor you see many children of differing ages. The child learns from this statement that he or she is not alone in this experience and is often reassured.

When children respond "yes" to the question that something happened to them, then consider saying:

> *When kids decide to tell, this provides a chance to understand exactly what happened and get help. When kids tell, there are a lot of important things that need to be done and we are going to talk about two of them. Your visit here today is to make sure your body is OK. I want you to think about any worries or concerns that you may have about your body because of what happened. The more I hear about any questions or concerns about your body, the better the I can help to make sure your body is OK. After we are done talking, your mom (substitute appropriate person) will come back into the room, you will change into a gown, and I will take a look at you from head to toe to make sure your body is fine. Everything that will be done during the examination will be explained to you, and you can ask any questions you want.*

The child may express concerns following the above comments. Examples of expressed concerns include

1. Is it true that I can get breast cancer because he put his mouth on my breast?

2. I think people can tell by the way I walk that I had to do those disgusting things. Can they?

3. Will I get the dying disease? (AIDS)

4. I think that icky stuff is still inside of me. Will I get pregnant?

5. Can I have a baby when I am older?

A child may not articulate worries, but on completion of the examination and when reassured that his or her body is OK, he or she may breathe a sigh of relief, as will the caretaker.

> *The second thing that I want to tell you about will happen after today's examination. It will be very important for you to see what I call a "talking doctor." A talking doctor is someone who understands how kids feel when they have things happen to them that are not OK. The talking doctor can help you understand and express your feelings. Although talking about what happened can be very difficult, the more you talk about what happened and express your feelings with someone who understands, the easier it is to put those experiences behind you. Do you have any worries, concerns, or questions for me?*

If based on preliminary information it is clear that something inappropriate happened to the child, then the previous statement is appropriate. However, if based on the presenting information there is a lack of clarity as to whether anything happened, reserve this statement until there is certainty that something inappropriate occurred.

Structuring the Medical History

Sexual victimization is not a capricious activity and usually follows a rather consistent pattern that has been well conceptualized. When obtaining the medical history, using a structured approach to asking questions that follows a logical and many times predictable sequence of events allows for obtaining the most comprehensive history. The history should ask questions that address each of the following general categories:

1. Circumstances and reasons surrounding disclosure

2. Access and opportunity for the alleged perpetrator to have contact with the child

3. Details of the first inappropriate sexual interactions and the progression of the sexual contact over time

4. Statements made to the child regarding secrecy, threats, and intimidation, and/or child's perceived consequences

5. Worries or concerns about body image

6. Questions that elicit specific details surrounding sexual interactions with a focus on signs and symptoms that may have medical significance and provide insight into the potential for physical injury or contracting an STI

7. Questions that clarify the child's perception of the interaction, particularly around the issue of penetration

8. Exposure to pornography or being photographed

9. Recantation

Understanding the Disclosure Process

Children disclose for a variety of reasons, which fall into 3 general categories that can be characterized as purposeful, accidental, or elicited. In a purposeful disclosure the child's desire to tell may be primarily motivated by a simple expectation to have the sexual contact stop with no idea of the cascade of events precipitated by the disclosure. A purposeful disclosure is more likely to allow for planned intervention. An accidental disclosure can take many forms, which could include a spontaneous statement to a non-caretaker or another child, being observed in "sexual play," sexualized behaviors when asked about result in disclosure, genital or anal trauma, or an STI. Accidental disclosures or disclosures precipitated by inquiry are more likely to create a crisis response, which is more challenging to manage. An elicited disclosure is generally precipitated by an observed behavior, a spontaneous or overheard statement of concern, a constellation of observations, or information from a third party that results in an individual asking a child directly whether she experienced anything inappropriate.

Example questions are

1. Most kids never tell about those kinds of experiences. Why did you decide to tell?

2. What do you want to happen now that you told?

3. Most kids find it difficult to tell about those kinds of experiences. What made it so difficult for you to tell?

4. How do you feel now that you told?

5. If you could say something to the person who did that, what would want to tell him/her?

Each of the above questions in many ways begins the process of giving control back to the child by eliciting his or her decisions and desires. Children who experience sexual abuse are not given choices, so wherever the clinician can demonstrate through example that the child can have choices it is best to do so.

Access and Opportunity

Under most circumstances, child and adolescent victims experience their victimization by someone they know; someone who is in a position of power/authority and control over them and has relatively easy access to the child or is capable of creating opportunities to have independent contact with the child. It is important to try to understand the contextual details surrounding how the alleged perpetrator had access or what he or she did to secure access. When the individual is known to the child and most likely trusted by the child, creating opportunities for independent time is relatively easy.

Example questions are

1. Who was the person(s) who did something that just didn't seem OK?

2. How do you know this person(s)?

   — Question modified depending on relationship.

3. Where did this happen the first/subsequent time(s)?

   — Additional questions regarding place and within specific place which
     room(s). Was anyone else present?

4. When was the first/last time something happened?

   — With young children who cannot provide specific dates, questions that try
     to relate an experience to an important life event such as a birthday, starting
     or ending school, a family trip, or before or after a holiday help narrow the
     time.

5. How often did it happen? Why did it stop?

Sexual Interaction and Progression

The most difficult questions will be those that attempt to elicit idiosyncratic
details of the sexual interactions. These questions need to be formulated to reflect
sensitivity and care and are skillfully asked in a nonjudgmental and supportive
manner. As a historian, one's ability to facilitate and reassure throughout the
questioning enhances the likelihood of the child sharing information. Most perpetrators who engage children and adolescents in sexual activities intend to do so
in a manner that is engaging, progressively more intrusive, and repeated over time.
Unlike sexual assault, physical force and restraint are less likely to be used to
initiate or continue the activities over time. Substituting for physical force will be
coercion, deceit, intimidation, bribery, or representing the activities as loving and/
or playful interactions. The historian should attempt to elicit details regarding how
the activities were represented to the child at the initiation of sexual interaction
and how the activities progressed and were maintained over time.

The following introductory statement can be helpful in setting the stage for why
questions are being asked about the specific sexual experiences. This approach is
generally helpful for children 5 years and older.

Question (Q) or Statement (S)

*When you have gone to the doctor and you haven't felt well, the doctor
asks all kinds of questions about whether you have a fever, your head
hurts, or your belly hurts. The reason the doctor asks those questions
is that the doctor is trying to understand what's bothering you so the
doctor knows what to look at and see if you need any tests or medicine to
get you better. I am going to ask some questions about what happened,
not to make it difficult for you but to help me understand before I
examine you.*

Q: Is it important to tell the doctor the truth?

A: Most kids answer "yes."

Q: Why is it important to tell the truth?

A: The common response is: "That way the doctor can help me get better."

S: It is always important to tell the truth, but it is particularly important to tell the doctor the truth. If you told me that your toe hurt and it was really your thumb that hurt, would that make it easier or harder for me to help?

A: Most respond "harder."

S: One of the things that is special about doctors is that you can tell doctors anything, anything that worries you, upsets you, or confuses you. The more you share with the doctor, the better the doctor understands and the better he or she can help. Doctors and kids work together to solve problems.

This above introduction sets the stage for a series of questions that is focused on the what, when, and where details as well as specific questions that elicit signs and symptoms associated with the contact. It is best to try to sequence the questions in a chronological manner.

Example questions are

1. Who was the person who did the things that weren't OK?

2. How did you know this person?

   — Access and opportunity questions? Caretaking role of individual?

3. Where did this happen?

   — Additional questions are asked pending circumstances, as may have occurred in multiple environments.

4. Did the person who did this have a name for what he/she was doing?

   – If so, have the child explain and describe the activity. Rewards and bribery are commonly a component of engaging and ensuring continuance of the sexual contact. Ask questions to elicit details of rewards/bribes.

5. What was the first thing the person did that just didn't seem OK?

   — Subsequent questions can be as simple as "And then what?" or "Tell me the next thing that happened that wasn't OK." and "What did you do or say?"

6. When that (insert specific) happened, how did that feel?

— Ask the same question for all of the inappropriate sexual interactions. For any contact form of sexual interaction consider the following questions:

a. If, for example, the child responds that what happened was uncomfortable, a follow-up question might be: "Was it your body that was feeling uncomfortable or your feelings or both?" Then have the child explain.

b. If the child responds by saying that what happened "hurt," ask the child to clarify what is meant by "hurt" as above before asking more specific questions. If the "hurt" was physical, ask if it hurt just while she was being touched or after or both and to explain.

c. Ask, "Did you see anything that made you know that you were hurt?" The child might respond "blood." Then follow up with where there was bleeding and more specific questions regarding what she did and how long the bleeding lasted.

d. If the child states that it hurt after the touching stopped ask: "Did it hurt to do anything? What did it hurt to do?" The child might respond that it hurt to go to the bathroom. If so then ask: "To do what in the bathroom?" The child might respond "to pee." Ask: "What did that feel like?" The child might respond that there was a burning or stinging sensation. If so ask: "Did you ever have that feeling before?" The child might respond "no." Ask: "Did you ever feel that again?" The child might respond: "The next time he put his finger in my pee pee and rubbed it or put his pee pee in my pee pee."

e. After the child responds to the above set of questions consider asking: "What happened next?" The child might respond that she had to clean herself. If so ask her to describe what she cleaned and what part of her body she cleaned. Through these questions the focus is on trying to elicit idiosyncratic details that provide insight into whether there was contact with ejaculate, increasing the risk for an STI and the potential identification of DNA.

For eliciting a history that involves oral contact it's important to recognize the following:

— Younger children often spontaneously make statements about someone sucking their "wee wee" or licking their "coochie." Sometimes the activity is viewed by the child with excitement, and the child may share the excitement by stating that, "John let me suck his pee pee," as if it was something special.

Oral activities may be particularly difficult and embarrassing for older children to talk about. Older children may not spontaneously offer details about oral-genital contact.

a. Obtaining details regarding possible oral contact if not spontaneously provided can be introduced by asking such questions as follows: "Did the person kiss you?" If the child says "yes," ask:"Can you tell me where he/she kissed you or placed his/her mouth on you?" The child may point to her lips, genital/anal area, or breast; may not respond; or may seem hesitant and embarrassed. If she points to her face/lips, you may follow up with: "Did he/she put his/her mouth anywhere else?" She may say "no." A follow-up question to consider is: "If the person (substitute name) who did this put his/her mouth someplace else would you tell me or be too embarrassed or afraid to tell me?" She might respond: "Too embarrassed or afraid." Follow up with: "Did the person put his/her mouth somewhere else and you are just too embarrassed to tell me?" The child might respond "yes." Reassure and ask the child to then either tell you where the person placed his or her mouth or point to the area.

b. The same line of questioning can be used when asking about a child being made to place his or her mouth on someone's body by beginning with: "Did you have to kiss him/her? Were you made to place your mouth on any part of him/her?" If the child spontaneously states that she had to put her mouth on someone's genitalia then ask: "When you were made to do that, what did you do?" Try to have the child express what that felt like and anything that was observed as a result of those interactions.

If the child acknowledges that she was made to place her mouth on an individual's genitalia, then ask her to describe what she was made to do, whether anything happened, and what she did afterward. Children may respond with statements such as: "He peed in my mouth. He made drink that icky spit." Follow-up questions might be: "And what did you do after that?" The child might respond that she spit it out, went to the bathroom and brushed her teeth, wiped the stuff from a particular area of the body, or felt dirty and took a shower.

Depending on the time between the sexual contact and the disclosure, it may be possible to obtain the cloth or piece of clothing used to wipe away the seminal products. It may be appropriate to ask the child to describe what was used to wipe them and what was done with that item. A child's idiosyncratic description of semen through either what was observed or the character of semen based on contact provides details that a child would not be expected to know about unless he or she had such an experience.

7. Try to clarify the child's perception of the interaction around the issue of vaginal penetration.

When a child or adolescent discloses that someone put an object inside of a part of his or her body, there should be an attempt to clarify what is meant by "inside." Depending on the child's age and developmental level, there could be very different understandings of "inside." Parents and/or the child may have worries or concerns about body intactness. Those worries may be either expressed or not expressed regarding the issue of virginity. Clearly any genital/anal touching other than in the context of care is inappropriate regardless of the degree of penetration. Law enforcement might seek to know the depth of penetration because there may be differences in the "degree of the crime." The legal definition of penetration varies from state to state. Some states define penetration of the female genitalia as "between the labia no matter how slight," whereas others might define penetration as being in the vagina.

A purpose of the medical examination is to attempt to determine whether an object penetrated into the vagina or any orifice stated to have been touched and then to explain any discrepancy between the child's perception of the degree of penetration and what was actually experienced should that be necessary. Making this determination is clinically less complicated in prepubertal children than in pubertal children, where the estrogenized hymen demonstrates elasticity and distensibility. Because the prepubertal hymen is thin, relatively nonelastic, and sensitive to the touch if a large-diameter object such as a penis or a finger penetrated through the hymenal orifice, residual would be anticipated. The potential for signs and symptoms as well as residual findings, such as transections to the edge of the hymen, are more likely to be found in a prepubertal child than in a pubertal child with the same experience. However, because most children do not disclose immediately following the sexual contact and because most perpetrators have no intent to physically harm the child, most examinations will not demonstrate any acute or healed residua to the contact.

One way of clarifying the child's perception of whether an object was placed between the labia or into the vagina is by showing the child a model of the female genitalia (Ortho-McNeil Pharmaceutical, Raritan, NJ). Using an anatomical model, demonstrate to the female child where she pees from, where she has a bowel movement, and if she is menstruating where she would place a pad or how a tampon would go inside. Explain that when she goes to the bathroom and pees, she wipes herself (demonstrating) between the labia. Demonstrate the same regarding bowel movements. Then state that there are different kinds of "inside" and you would like her to show you what kind of inside she thought she experienced. This can be accomplished by then taking the index finger and placing it between the labia and then say: "Inside can be like this when you wipe yourself or inside can be like this" (demonstrating inside in the adult sense of penetration). Continue with: "Some kids aren't really sure what kind of inside they experienced" and ask the child to demonstrate what she perceived the "inside" to be. The child may demonstrate with bravado in the adult sense of penetration when in fact, based on the physical examination, it is evident that no object penetrated into the vagina, or she may say she is not sure. With an understanding of the child's perception of the degree of contact the clinician is better equipped to explain why there can be a discrepancy between the child's perception and what she actually experienced.

8. Questions that clarify the child's perception of the interaction around the issue of anal penetration

   a. When anal contact occurs, history questions as previously outlined should be asked regarding how the contact felt both during and afterward. When children disclose insertion of an object into the anorectal canal, the mucosal area between the intersphincteric line and the pectinate line may be abraded and the child may then complain of a burning sensation with passage of a bowel movement, which is a symptom that the child is unlikely to know of without having experienced trauma to this mucosal surface. If lubrication is used, this symptom will likely be absent.

      Where allegations of anal penetration arise there also are challenges in identifying residual physical findings on examination, even when there is a detailed history of symptom-specific complaints. The anal sphincter is designed to pass large-diameter objects every day. In cases of encopresis children pass what are frequently described as huge bowel movements without any residual findings. The variables that determine the potential for anal findings following penetration into the anorectal canal may be dependent on the size and type of object introduced, use of lubricants, and "cooperativeness" of the child. When questioning children regarding anal penetration, attention to these variables may help predict and/or explain the presence or absence of findings.

      The Ortho-McNeil Pharmaceutical anatomical model can be used with the same approach as illustrated with genital contact when attempting to understand the degree of anal penetration. Under most circumstances anal penetration with an object such as a penis is limited to penetration between the gluteal cleft and rubbed over the anal verge tissues, providing a sensation of "inside." Children may also experience anal penetration or anal contact with a finger, a foreign body, or a mouth.

9. Additional sexual interactions to be considered

   a. Just as children can experience anal penetration, they may be forced/coerced into performing the same on the other person. If so, ask questions to elicit details.

b. The child victim may be made to touch the genitalia of the other person.

c. The child may be made to watch the other person engage in masturbation.

d. The child may be made to engage other children in sexual activities orchestrated and observed by the adolescent/adult.

Exposure to Pornography or Being Photographed

Adult or child pornography may be used by the alleged perpetrator to normalize the sexual activity. Children may be exposed to pornography either because of direct actions on the part of the perpetrator or because of failure to protect children from exposure to this material. Adolescent males may access pornography either accidentally or volitionally on the computer or through cable television, or they seek or are provided sexually explicit print materials by age mates or grown-ups. When adolescents are exposed to sexually explicit materials they then may act out what they have seen with younger children that they have easy access to and control over, usually siblings and/or cousins.

Perpetrators may also take still photographs in digital or 35-mm format and/or videotape the sexual activities. If the child is aware that such images have been obtained, he or she can have anxiety regarding where and when this material may appear. The production of child pornography can occur with or without physical contact. When images are captured, to the child victim they represent a permanent reminder of an abusive event. Children have a desire to know that any and all recorded images have been destroyed.

Example questions to explore exposure to and/or participation in pornography production

1. "Have you ever seen any pictures or movies of people doing things that are confusing?" If there isn't a response to this question follow up with a more specific question: "Have you ever seen any pictures of people without their clothing on?"

2. If there is a positive response, ask the child: "Can you tell me where you saw that?" Ask questions regarding circumstances of exposure (who showed, when, did anyone else see) and ask the child to provide specific details of what he or she was exposed to.

3. "Has anyone ever taken any pictures or videos of you that made you uncomfortable?" If yes, ask specific questions such as, "Did you see the pictures? Did anyone else see the pictures? Was anyone else in the pictures? What was the explanation provided for taking the photographs/video? Were there any rewards/threats?" Ask the child to describe the setting in which photographs were obtained.

4. If images exist, ask the child if he or she knows where they are.

Secrecy

Once a child has experienced something of a sexually inappropriate nature, the primary task of the offender is to either directly or indirectly deliver a message to the child that he is not to tell, to maintain secrecy regarding the interaction. From the offender's perspective the use of secrecy plays a role in ensuring the progression of the activities over time and removes a sense of accountability. Children maintain secrets for numerous reasons that might include (a) the sexual interaction is represented as special and loving and the child wants to continue the "special time" with the offender, (b) the child simply recognizes that there is something wrong about the interaction and decides to maintain secrecy, (c) the offender uses nonverbal signs that implicitly provide a message not to tell, (d) the offender makes clear threats to the child regarding the consequences of telling, (e) the child feels embarrassed or ashamed, (f) the child might think it is his fault, (g) the child believes he is going to get into trouble.

Clearly, offenders are individuals not interested in the welfare of the children they engage in sexual activities and thus frequently use threats to maintain secrecy. The mechanism to maintain secrecy may change over time. Initial special attention or rewards may predominate with statements to the effect that what is happening is "special" and the child might be excited about this "special" interaction. As the activities progress over time the use of increasingly intimidating threats will be used to maintain the activities. Examples of threats might include (a) don't tell anybody, and if you do I will beat you; (b) if you tell, no one is going to believe you and you will be in a lot of trouble; (c) if you tell, I will do even more; (d) if you tell, you will be taken away from your mother; (e) if you tell, I will do the same to your sister; (f) if you tell, I will kill your mother; (g) if you tell, no one will love you.

These threats and any possible permutation or combination of them are routinely used to maintain secrecy. It is important to understand how threats and/or intimidation were used to maintain secrecy. If the child doesn't spontaneously state that he was told not to tell, consider asking the following: "Did the person who did this want you to tell?" The typical response to this question is "no." Then ask: "How did you know that he/she didn't want you to tell? Did he/she say what would happen if you told?" If there were no specific threats then ask: "What did you think/worry would happen?"

Additional insights can be obtained by asking the following questions: (a) Why did you find it so difficult to tell? (b) What do you want to happen now that you told? (c) How do you feel now that you told? (d) If you could say something to the person who did this what would you want to say to him/her? These questions also serve to empower the child and may provide idiosyncratic details that express the reality of the child's experience.

Recantation

When children and adolescents disclose sexually inappropriate experiences, they generally have not considered the possibility that they might not be believed nor anticipated the cascade of events that follows their disclosure. If asked why they disclose, most commonly it is simply because they want the inappropriate contact to stop. When children recant it is most likely based on fears and anxieties that are either real or imagined, but the end result is that the child states that what they initially said wasn't true. Some children may be fearful that the perpetrator will go to jail, they will be responsible for breaking up the family, their mom will not have any way of supporting the family, and the family will become homeless.

Although it may be difficult to fully understand all of the contributing factors to a recantation, the physician can potentially reduce the chances of recantation by asking questions that assist in understanding who the child perceives as responsible for what happened and what she wants to happen now that she has disclosed. Wherever possible ask a question in a manner that affords the child the opportunity to make choices. Choices are empowering and respectful; children who experience victimization were not given a choice regarding the sexual interactions.

Summary

The most difficult aspect of the medical evaluation of child sexual abuse is obtaining the medical history from the child in an objective, nonjudgmental, and empathetic manner; all critical to understanding the child's experience. A successfully obtained history stems from an understanding of the "disease" of sexual victimization. There is little that is intuitive about sexual victimization, and the clinician can only become competent in assessing children suspected of abuse when they have a grasp of the manner in which sexual victimization presents itself clinically and can then obtain a defensible medical history with objectivity. As challenging and emotionally charged as this issue is, the clinician can still find this work professionally rewarding because a correct diagnosis is the first step to protecting children, effectively intervening, and providing treatment.

Chapter 3

Physical Examination

Martin A. Finkel

A medical diagnosis is the result of a successful marriage of the medical history, physical examination, and laboratory results. A medical evaluation of the child suspected of being sexually abused includes the child's account of his or her experience; a medical history; a review of systems, with particular attention paid to the genitourinary (GU) and gastrointestinal systems; a thorough physical examination; and appropriate laboratory testing. In the evaluation of alleged sexual abuse, the genitalia and anus deserve special attention, but they are examined only within the context of a complete physical assessment. This chapter reviews genital and anal anatomy; appropriate terminology; preparation of the child for an examination; examination techniques; and the interpretation of genital, anal, and extragenital residua to sexual contact.

Genital Anatomy

Basic Anatomy and Development

Familiarity with genital and anal anatomy is a prerequisite to conducting an examination, identifying normal anatomical variants, identifying clinical residua, and describing findings with accurate and preciselanguage. This section presents basic information about anogenital anatomy in preparation for a detailed discussion of the genital examination.

An examination of the external genital structures of the female includes each of the following structures: (a) mons pubis, (b) labia majora, (c) labia minora, (d) clitoris, (e) urethra, (f) vaginal vestibule, (g) hymen, (h) Skene glands/ducts and Bartholin glands/ducts (i) fossa navicularis, and (j) posterior fourchette.[1] All of the external genital structures of the female are referred to collectively as the *vulva*. Because of the lack of specificity of the term *vulva,* it is preferable to describe each of the component parts. It is important to keep in mind that the dividing line between the internal and external genital structures is the hymenal membrane. Even though the structures of the vaginal vestibule are considered a part of the vulva and thus external, the vestibule is covered by mucosa and thus reflects an internal environment. Examination of the "internal" struc-tures found within the vaginal vesti-bule usually can be completed without instrumentation or anesthesia. The examination of the innermost aspects of the vagina is generally reserved for pubertal children and requires the use of instrumentation. In circumstances where it is necessary to assess the prepubertal child for intravaginal trauma or a foreign body, it is best to use anesthesia or conscious sedation. A bimanual or speculum examination is indicated in most pubertal children with a history involving penetration into the vagina. The examination of the pubertal child is described in detail in Chapter 7.

In the male, the genital examination includes (a) the glans and frenulum (prepuce, or foreskin, if uncircumcised); (b) shaft; (c) scrotum; (d) testicles and epididymis; (e) inguinal region, for adenopathy and hernias; and (f) perineum.

The anal examination is completed in both male and female children, with attention to (a) anal verge tissues, (b) the anorectal canal, and (c) the perianal region and gluteal cleft.

Assessment of Pubertal Development

The following discussion includes 2 developmental staging systems. The first system, developed by Huffman,[2] consists of 4 stages. The stages differ according to the relative estrogen effect on the female. The second staging system, described by Tanner,[3] delineates obvious sexual characteristics, such as pubic hair and breast development in the female and pubic hair and external genital appearance and size in the male.

Estrogen Effect on Female Genitalia: Huffman Stages

The 4 Huffman[2] stages are as follows:

Stage 1: Postneonatal regression
(0–2 months)

Stage 2: Early childhood
(2 months–7 years)

Stage 3: Late childhood
(7–11 years)

Stage 4: Premenarche
(11–12 years)

Because female children grow and mature at differing rates, sexual maturity ratings (SMRs) more accurately reflect developmental stages than does chronological age. Huffman staging is helpful in delineating the changes that occur in the external structures of the female child on her path to sexual maturity. In Stage 1, the child's external genitalia show evidence of a profound estrogenic effect due to maternal hormones. These changes include a thick, pink, lubricated hymenal membrane. These effects recede over the first several weeks to months. At Stage 2, the female genitalia take on the immature appearance that they manifest throughout the entire stage of early childhood. At this point, there is little endogenous estrogen evident. At the end of this somewhat quiescent period, the child enters Stage 3, the late childhood stage, during which the body begins to slowly increase its production of estrogen. This sets the stage for the rapid changes that are evident during Stage 4, the premenarche.

Outward Sexual Development: Tanner Stages

The Tanner stages make up an SMR system that tracks the normal appearance and pattern of pubic hair in the female and male (Figures 3.1 and 3.2); breast development in the female (Figure 3.3); and testicle size and scrotum and phallus development in the male. These stages provide a useful common language for communication among health practitioners.

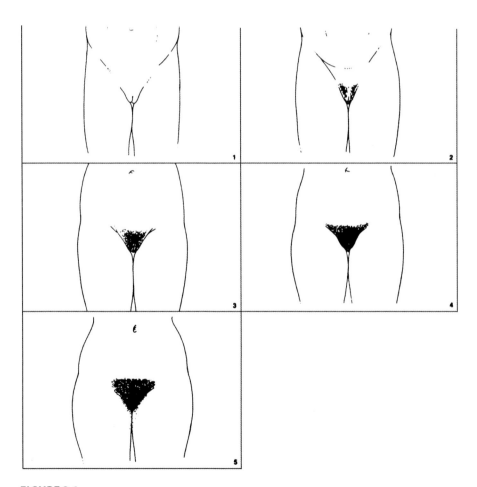

FIGURE 3.1
Tanner stages: female pubic hair.

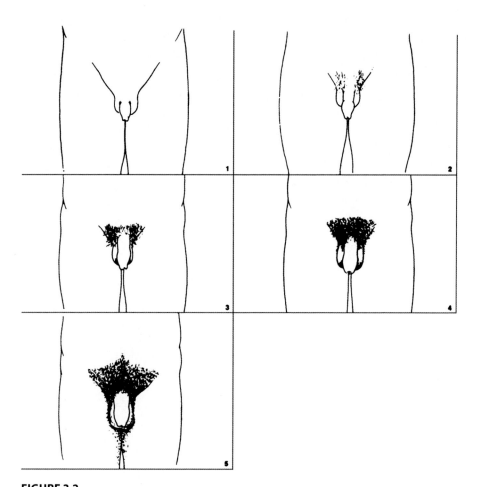

FIGURE 3.2
Tanner stages: male pubic hair.

The Tanner[3] stages are as follows.

Pubic Hair: Male and Female
- *Stage 1:* Preadolescent. No pubic hair. Fine vellus type hair similar to that over the abdomen.
- *Stage 2:* There is the appearance of sparse, long, and slightly pigmented hair. Straight or slightly curled hair develops at the base of the penis or along the labia.
- *Stage 3:* Hair darkens and becomes more coarse and curled. It increases in density.
- *Stage 4:* Hair is of the adult type, but the area covered by it is considerably less than in the adult. No hair spread to the medial surfaces of the thighs.
- *Stage 5:* Adult hair characteristics in quantity and type. There is distribution of the horizontal pattern and hair spread to the medial surface of the thighs.

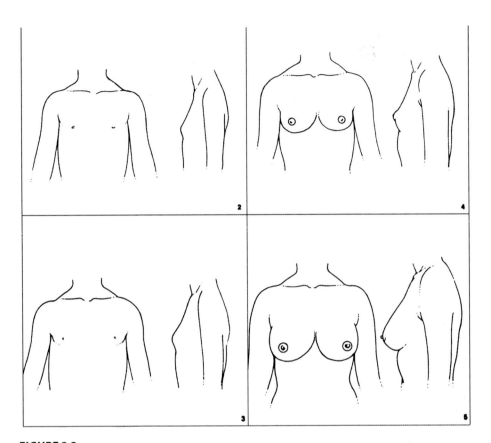

FIGURE 3.3

Tanner stages: breast development.

Reproduced with permission from *Patient Care*, May 30, 1979, copyright © Medical Economics Co., Inc., Montvale, NJ. All rights reserved.

Originally, Tanner also described a Stage 6, which occurred when the pubic hair extended up the linea alba, but this has since been dropped because of its ethnic variability.

Breast Development

- *Stage 1:* Preadolescent. Elevation of papilla.
- *Stage 2:* Breast bud stage. Elevation of breast bud and papilla as a small mound with enlargement of the areolar diameter.
- *Stage 3:* Further enlargement and elevation of breast and areola, with no separation of their contours.
- *Stage 4:* Projection of areola and papilla to form a secondary mound above the level of the breast.
- *Stage 5:* Mature stage projection of the papilla only, due to recession of the areola to the general contour of the breast.

Male Genitalia

- *Stage 1:* Preadolescent. Testes, scrotum, and penis are small. Size and proportion as that in early childhood.

- *Stage 2:* Enlargement of scrotum and testes. Skin of scrotum reddens and changes in texture. Little or no change in size of penis.
- *Stage 3:* Further growth of testes and scrotum, with lengthening of penis.
- *Stage 4:* Growth in breadth and development of the glans, with increased size of the penis.
- *Stage 5:* Adult size and shape of penis.

Terminology

When describing anogenital structures, it is critically important to use only those terms that are appropriate and descriptive.[4,5] When the issue of child sexual abuse began to be addressed by medicine, physicians began to look at the genitalia with greater scrutiny. They coined terms to describe anatomical features thought to potentially represent residua to inappropriate contact. Many of these early descriptions of anatomical findings interpreted as residua to abuse have since proved to be normal anatomical variants.[6-8] Illustrative of this point was the recognition that synechiae in the superior quadrants were more likely not to be residual to sexual abuse but rather pubo-urethral supporting ligaments, and midline avascular areas in the fossa navicularis were more likely to be linea vestibularis than scar tissue. The early literature also reflects the use of a myriad of terms describing examination findings, which has resulted in some confusion and difficulty in comparing studies.[9-11] Some terms create the impression that a specific finding also suggests a contributing mechanism that could explain the presence of that finding. For example, the reference to the term *rounding* of the edge of the hymen was often interpreted as residual to the introduction of a foreign body. Rounding of the hymenal orifice edge was presumed to be the result of the repeated introduction of an object that would wear down the edge, resulting in a rounded appearance. With improvements in examination techniques, it became apparent that the appearance of the edge could change in the knee-chest position or with the use of saline to float the hymen.[12] Following the use of additional examination techniques, many rounded edges demonstrated an unfolding of the edge and a normal-appearing hymen. The term *attenuated* also has created confusion. By definition, attenuated implies that the hymen has been narrowed from a preexisting condition. This term should not be used to describe a narrow posterior rim, implying a change in the hymen, without knowledge of the premorbid state. The American Professional Society on the Abuse of Children has developed a consensus statement on descriptive anogenital terminology.[13] This consensus statement is an excellent reference that has contributed to the standardizing of descriptive terminology for the field.

Normal Female Genitalia

This section describes the characteristics of the normal external genital structures (vulva). The external geni-talia consist of the mons pubis, labia majora, labia minora, clitoris, hymenal membrane/orifice, urethral meatus, vaginal vestibule, Skene glands/ducts, Bartholin glands/ducts, fossa navicularis, and posterior fourchette (commissure in prepubertal children) (Figure 3.4).

Mons Pubis
The mons pubis is the skin-covered mound of fatty tissue above the pubic symphysis at the anterior commissure of the labia majora. In the neonate, the maternal estrogen effect causes the area to appear plump at birth. With the loss of maternal estrogen, the mons pubis loses its roundness. During the late childhood stage, the mons pubis begins to thicken and assume a more adult form based on endogenous estrogen

production. During puberty, the mons pubis will be a site for pubic hair.

Labia Majora
The labia majora are longitudinal folds of both fatty and connective tissue that are covered by skin. This structure is analogous to the male scrotum. The labia are relatively larger and thicker at birth and remain so for several weeks to months afterward. Anteriorly, the folds are united by a commissure. Posteriorly, the folds may appear united but in actuality they are not. If actual posterior fusion occurs, signs of actual virilization may also be evident.

In the prepubertal child, the labia majora do not completely cover the

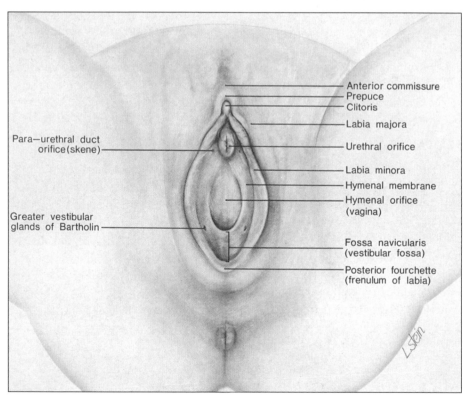

FIGURE 3.4
A. External structures of the female.

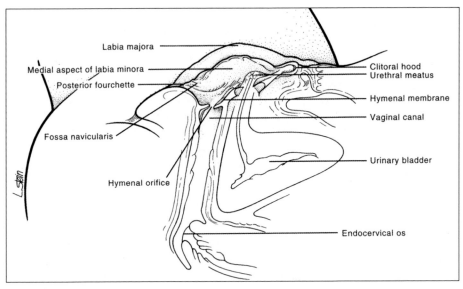

FIGURE 3.4
B. Midsagittal view of external female genitalia.

external genital structures. The labia majora change with growth. Eventually, the labia of the child are completely opposed and offer protection to the other vulvar structures. During puberty, the labia majora and mons pubis become covered with pubic hair as well.

Labia Minora

The labia minora are thin folds of tissue, with the innermost aspect lined and with the urogenital sinus epithelium forming the mucosal aspects of the labia minora. The labia minora are protected by the labia majora. In the neonate, the labia minora are relatively large and may protrude beyond the labia majora. Anteriorly, each labium divides into lateral and medial wings. The lateral labia fuse anteriorly and form the prepuce of the clitoris. The medial labia then fuse to form the clitoral frenulum. Posteriorly, the labia fuse to form the posterior fourchette. There are no hair follicles on the labia minora.

Clitoris

The clitoris is a cylindrical erectile structure that consists of a glans, prepuce, frenulum, and body. It is analogous to the penis of the male. In the neonate, the glans is disproportionately large. During growth and development, the clitoris grows at a slower pace than surrounding structures, and its relative size decreases. The glans is visible, whereas the body extends upward toward the pubis under the skin. Clitoromegaly is a clinical diagnosis made in the prepubertal child if the length of the glans is greater than or equal to 5 mm in length or 6 mm in width.

Urethral Meatus

The urethra forms the outlet of the urinary system, and its opening forms the urethral meatus. The urethral meatus is surrounded by several mucoid secreting glands and ducts that are rarely visible. The Skene glands form an extensive network that ends in Skene ducts. Skene ducts are found at either side of the urethral floor. These glands and ducts do not begin to secrete until menarche, when they produce a mucoid secretion that offers protection to the urethral meatus during coitus.

Vaginal Vestibule

The word *vestibule* means "entranceway" and is the space in front of the hymenal membrane enclosed by the labia minora. The vestibule is a space that must be passed through for an object to enter into the vagina. The vestibule is considered to be a part of the external genital structures and the hymen is the dividing structure between the internal and external anatomy. The vestibule is formed by the following structures: (a) the clitoral hood superiorly, (b) the inner aspects of the labia minora laterally, (c) the commissure/fourchette posteriorly, and (d) the external surface of the hymenal membrane internally. The vaginal vestibule is lined by urogenital sinus epithelium.

Hymen

The hymen (urogenital septum) is a mucous membrane with the external surface covered by urogenital sinus epithelium and the internal surface covered by vaginal epithelium. It is a recessed structure that sits at the entrance to the vagina. Embryologically, the urogenital septum is cannulized to form the hymenal orifice.[14,15] Although there have been colloquialisms that reference the absence of the hymen, the breaking of the hymen, or the hymen being lost or missing, the hymen is present in all children except for rare circumstances.[16-18] Some unusual circumstances in which the hymen is not developed include ambiguous genitalia, transverse vaginal septum, and distal vaginal agenesis.[5] The hymen should have an opening to allow genital secretion and/or menstrual blood to escape. In the unusual circumstance in which there is an imperforate hymen, the conditions of either mucocolpos in the prepubertal child or hematocolpos in the adolescent will present.[19-21] When referring to the opening in the hymen, it is best to describe the opening as the *hymenal orifice* rather than using the term *introitus*. Although introitus is a synonym for the hymenal orifice, some clinicians have inadvertently called the vaginal vestibule the introitus. The appearance of the hymenal membrane and the orifice will change with age and the influence of estrogen.[22-24]

An assessment of the hymen includes the shape and size of the orifice, degree of estrogen effects, and any signs of trauma or scar tissue. The hymenal orifice edge is usually smooth and uninterrupted in the inferior quadrants except when the orifice has a fimbriated appearance. The membrane edge in the prepubertal child may have some translucency and can appear similar to the edge of a feather when held to the light. This appearance has been referred to as *velamentous.* The hymen is estrogen sensitive, and its appearance changes over time. The first evidence of estrogen sensitivity is in the newborn, when the hymen may appear "succulent," prolapsed from the labia, and accompanied by a milky mucoid discharge. Shortly thereafter, with the natural withdrawal of maternal estrogen, the hymen involutes and takes on the appearance of the unestrogenized thin and vascular hymen until endogenous production begins with the onset of puberty. In the newborn, the loss of maternal estrogen can result in withdrawal vaginal bleeding.

In the prepubertal child, the external surface of the hymen and the mucosal surfaces of the structures that form the boundaries of the vaginal vestibule are very vascular, resulting in a reddened appearance. The degree of redness varies from child to child. Redness is nonspecific, and caution must be exercised not to overinterpret this observation. In puberty, the hymenal membrane undergoes significant changes that are secondary to estrogen. Estrogen results in thickening of the hymenal membrane, increased elasticity, and decreased pain sensitivity. Also, puberty results in a change in the appearance of the mucosal surfaces, the now estrogenized tissues lose their prominent vascular appearance and

become increasingly pinkish-white in coloration. Crescentic-appearing orifices in the prepubertal child may appear to take on an annular configuration with the onset of puberty as tissue in the superior quadrants responds to estrogen.

The medical literature reflects a variety of terms to describe the appearance of the hymenal membrane orifice. Although there is a spectrum of variability regarding the appearance of the hymenal membrane and its orifice shape, several clearly defined orifice configurations exist that may be further characterized by small variations.[25-27] The most common descriptions of the fundamental hymenal orifice shapes are crescentic, annular, fimbriated, septate, cribriform, and microperforate. Other classification systems existthat are equally valid. Each of the aforementioned shapes can be modified further by the presence of clefts, bumps, notches, tags, thickening, thinning, estrogen effect, elastic character, and variability in the orifice size.[27-32]

The "normal" size of the hymenal orifice varies with age, body habitus, and pubertal development.[33-36] The size of the orifice may vary during the examination depending on positioning (supine frog-leg vs knee-chest), the state of relaxation of the patient, and examination technique. Clearly, there is a range of normal variability.[6] The transverse diameter of the hymenal orifice alone cannot be relied on as a sole diagnostic finding of vaginal penetration. The terms *intact hymen, virginal hymen,* and *marital hymen* are inexact and lead to confusion.[37]

As such, these terms should not be used, either in conversation or in documentation of the findings.

Fossa Navicularis

The fossa navicularis is a concave area between the posterior attachment of the hymen to the vaginal wall and the posterior fourchette.

Posterior Fourchette

The posterior fourchette is the point at which the labia minora meet posteriorly. The structure is sometimes referred to as the *frenulum of the labia*. In the prepubertal child, the labia minora do not fuse, and the corresponding location is referred to as the *posterior commissure*.

Colpophotographic Images

A section of colpophotographic case slides can be found at the end of this chapter.

Male Anatomy

The following background anatomy is offered with regard to the examination of the male external genitalia (Figures 3.5, 3.6, and 3.7).

Penis

The penis is a cylindrical, erectile structure composed of a glans, body and prepuce, and frenulum. The body is composed of 3 erectile structures, 2 corpora cavernosa, and one corpus spongiosum. The erectile bodies are covered by thin, loosely attached skin without fatty tissue or hair, except at the base. The prepuce is a fold of similar tissue with no subcutaneous fat whose interior surface appears more like a mucous membrane. The prepuce encircles the glans and has an apical orifice that allows for retraction over the glans.

In the uncircumcised male child, the foreskin can be retracted over the glans by approximately 5 years of age. Post-inflammatory adhesions may lead to phimosis of acquired etiology, making it impossible to retract the foreskin. A constricting paraphimosis may develop if the foreskin is retracted and not repositioned over the glans.

The prepuce is attached to the underside of the penis by a frenulum that contains its own artery. Circumcision involves the removal of both the prepuce and frenulum and cautery of the artery. The urethral meatus is present at the apex of the glans. The opening of the meatus may be displaced either superiorly or interiorly, in which case epispadias or hypospadias results.

Scrotum

The scrotum is a saclike structure composed of skin, muscle, and connective tissue. It serves to protect the testicles and associated structures. The scrotal skin is thin and elastic and has obvious rugae. During puberty, the scrotum develops a thin covering of pubic hair and increased pigmentation.

Testes

The testes are oval structures composed of a compact array of tubules, connective tissue components, hormone-secreting cells, and sperm-producing cells. Testicles are readily palpated through the thin skin of the scrotum. In the normal male, both testes are descended and palpable. The right testis generally hangs lower than the left because the arterial supply to the left testis comes from the renal artery, as opposed to the aorta.

In young children, an unusually brisk cremasteric reflex causes a retractile testis. A retractile testis is descended but difficult to palpate. Undescended testes imply abnormal gonadal development. In such cases, the testes must be surgically approached to avoid infertility and possible undetected testicular cancer in the future.

Epididymis

The epididymis is a long, narrow, tubelike structure that carries sperm from the testicle to the seminal vesicle. It is composed of a head, body, and appendix. The epididymis may be palpated through the thin skin of the scrotum until it enters the inguinal

canal. Inflammation of the epididymis is called *epididymitis.*

Anal Anatomy

The anus is the opening of the rectum through which feces are extruded. The opening is surrounded by both internal and external sphincter mechanisms that collectively make up the anal sphincter (Figure 3.8). The tissue that overlies the external anal sphincter is referred to as the *anal verge.* This loose cutaneous tissue extends internally to the pectinate line, where the anal papilla and columns interdigitate with the anal verge tissues. The typical perianal appearance on examination is that of a circumferentially symmetrical, pigmented, puckered tissue (rugae) that has a natural tone and reflexively tightens when the buttocks are separated. When the anus is examined in

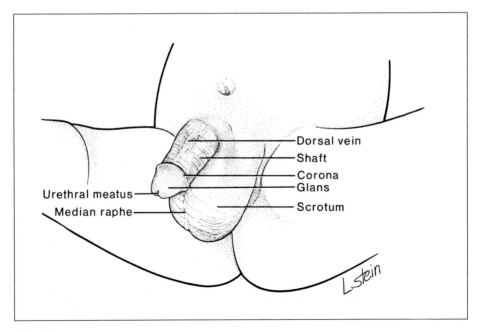

FIGURE 3.5
External structure of the male, circumcised.

the dependent position for any length of time, it is possible for hemorrhoidal veins to engorge, creating a purplish appearance that can take on a color similar to acute bruising. Differentiating bruising from venous engorgement can be done easily by changing the child's position and/or constricting the anus during external palpation. During puberty, coarse, pubic-like hair surrounds the pigmented tissue in both males and females.

The Physical Examination

Preparing for the Physical Examination of the Child

The minimal prerequisites for a thorough examination of a child suspected of being sexually abused are time and patience. The examiner must anticipate that the child and/or

caretaker will most likely have an inaccurate preconception of what the physical examination entails. These preconceptions can be barriers to conducting the examination and must be anticipated and addressed before proceeding. This chapter's Appendix provides a number of frequently asked questions and answers regarding the examination of the child suspected of being sexually abused. These questions and answers, provided in a handout form to the caretaker prior to the examination, will address many fears and anxieties, enabling the caretaker to be supportive of the child and increasing the chances that the child will be cooperative.[38,39] Also, this same information, when provided to caseworkers and law enforcement officials, serves as a way of disseminating accurate information regarding the

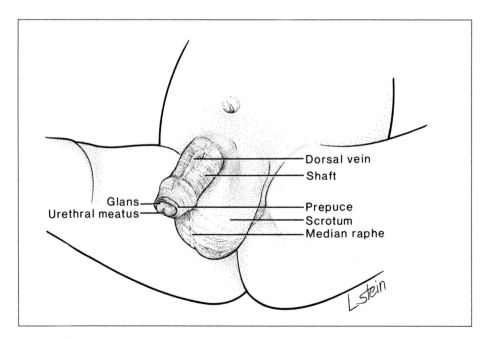

FIGURE 3.6
External structure of the male, uncircumcised.

examination to nonmedical professionals who need to understand what the examination entails and are in a position to explain it to others.

Taking the time to explain the importance of the examination helps to earn the child's confidence and trust and sets the stage for the physical examination and the collection of laboratory specimens. The rapport developed with the child during the medical history will serve the examiner well as the examination proceeds. No coercion, deceit, or force should be used, either directly or indirectly, to convince a child to submit to an examination of his or her body. The child must be fully informed and cooperative. Under no circumstances should an uncooperative child be physically restrained for an examination. Abused children are already victims of the abuse of authority and control and should not be subjected to force during a medical examination. In the unlikely event that an emergent evaluation is essential for the child's well-being and the child is unable to cooperate with the examination, use of anesthesia or conscious sedation may be necessary.[40,41] A coerced examination represents yet another assault to the child and demonstrates an abuse of the adult clinician's position of authority.

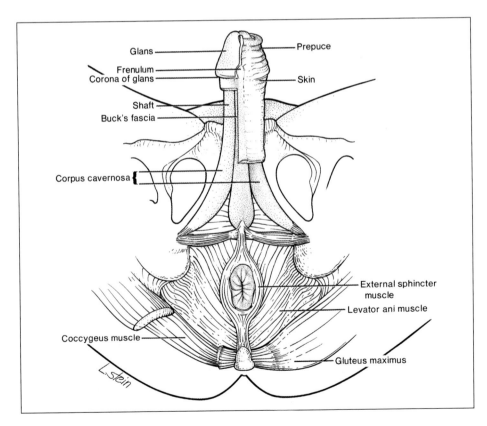

FIGURE 3.7
Basic anatomy of male genitalia, with anus.

Children who have been engaged in sexually inappropriate activities have had little or no control over what they have experienced. Once disclosure occurs, it is important for children to begin to feel as if they will now have a say in and control over what happens next to their bodies. Allowing the child to have choices, such as where to sit during the examination (eg, in an ally's lap, in a chair, or on a table on which the adult ally is present during the examination) helps give the child some control and demonstrates respect for his or her desires. Such gestures build confidence, provide the child with options, and may have considerable therapeutic value. In addition, the examiner may give the child a choice as to which gown he or she would like to wear. Older children may leave on their socks and underwear until the examination requires their removal. The examiner should answer any questions that the child or caretaker has as they arise during the evaluation.

Tools of the Physical Examination

The examination should proceed in a head-to-toe manner, leaving the ano-genital examination until the end except for the cutaneous assessment for extragenital trauma and structural evaluation. The reason for incorporating the genital and anal examination in the context of a complete evaluation is to make a statement to the child that all parts of his or her body are important.

Children are most familiar with an annual checkup. Conducting those components of the routine examination with which they are most familiar first serves to help the child transition to the

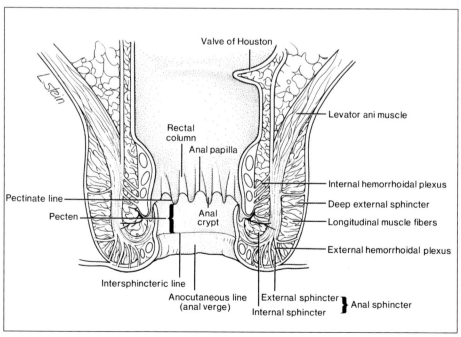

FIGURE 3.8
Anal anatomy.

anogenital examination. The genital and anal examination may be perceived as uncomfortable or embarrassing for the child. Thus the rapport developed during the initial components of the examination should help the transition to the anogenital examination. Many of the basic principles that follow also apply to the pubertal child; examination of the pubertal child is described in Chapter 7.

If possible, the examination room should be one that is dedicated for the purpose of examining children suspected of being abused. The examination area must have good lighting and, preferably, video colposcopy or similar equipment to facilitate the examination and the recording of findings.[42] Alternative tools to enhance visualization, such as lighted magnifying glasses, are acceptable but suboptimal and do not allow for appropriate documentation.[43,44] (See Chapter 4.)

In the prepubertal child, an examination of the external and internal vestibular structures and anus usually can be accomplished with the use of the palpatory techniques of labial and buttocks separation, labial traction, and positioning rarely requiring the use of instrumentation. Use of a vaginal speculum in the prepubertal child is rarely indicated unless trauma to the hymenal membrane suggests that an object was placed through the orifice and intravaginal trauma is suspected. A speculum examination, when warranted in a prepubertal child, is best accomplished with either conscious sedation or anesthesia. If a foreign body is suspected, irrigation of the vagina with sterile distilled water using a soft feeding tube is generally successful in dislodging most foreign bodies, and the use of instrumentation/anesthesia generally can be avoided. In the prepubertal child, toilet tissue is the most common foreign body. Anoscopy is most commonly of value when assessing acute injuries to the anorectal canal. Without external signs of either acute or healed trauma, anoscopy is unlikely to be of value.

The colposcope is an instrument originally designed for gynecologists to examine the cervix. Clinicians have since adapted the colposcope to assist in the visualization of external anogenital structures. The colposcope provides an excellent light source, magnification and, when attached to a still and/or video camera, the ability to document the examination through digital or 35-mm photography or recorded to a DVD or videotape. The colposcope is a noninvasive tool that, when attached to a video monitor, can assist in demystifying the examination by allowing the child to observe what the examiner is doing throughout the experience. As a result, the child may achieve a sense of participation and control that enhances his or her cooperativeness.[28,42,45-58]

Method of Evaluation

Children who experience sexual abuse may experience other forms of maltreatment as well. Therefore, the health care professional should use the opportunity to examine the child to identify any signs of physical abuse or neglect. Physical evidence of injury should be documented with diagrams, photographs, and descriptions in the medical record. Extragenital trauma such as grasp marks, ligatures, and bite marks reflect the use of force or restraint. DeJong and colleagues[49] report that approximately 10% of the children in their study, and Rimsza and Niggemann[10] report that 16% of the children in their review, have concomitant signs of extragenital trauma. Children abused by strangers have a higher incidence of physical trauma compared with those abused by individuals who are known to them.[50,51]

When there is a history of recent contact with seminal products, there should be an effort made to identify and collect such products on internal structures (vaginal, anal, pharyngeal), the skin, or on items such as clothing or bedding. Recent literature has demonstrated that the time-honored screening of body surfaces with a Wood light to identify "fluorescing" semen is not reliable.[52-54] If there is a history of oral contact, then the clinician may be able to swab such areas for saliva to possibly identify blood type–specific secretors.

Children are frequently engaged in oral-genital activities that may be difficult for them to talk about. The idiosyncratic details that children present when recounting this form of sexual interaction can be particularly graphic. Statements such as, "He made me drink icky spit" and "He peed in my mouth" are typical and suggest risk for contracting a sexually transmitted infection (STI). Under most circumstances, force and restraint

are not a part of the dynamics of oral-genital contact. Exceptions do exist, however, and trauma to the oropharynx can occur when force is used to complete the act. Thus it is important to thoroughly examine the oropharynx. The examiner should look for evidence of soft tissue and dental trauma, including palatal petechiae and tearing of the delicate labial frenulum.[55-57]

Genital and Anal Examination

Once the general examination is complete, the examiner should make a smooth transition to the genital examination. Continued explanation to the child as to what is occurring helps to ensure the child's cooperation as the examination proceeds.

Lighting and Privacy

An optimal examination of the genitalia and anus requires proper lighting, privacy, adequate positioning, and cooperation. It is appropriate to drape the older child. The younger child may be more frightened by drapes and may not want his or her view of what is happening to be obscured during the examination. A video colposcope allows for a magnified view and the ability for the child to observe the genital and anal examination on a video monitor as the examination proceeds, which helps demystify what the child is experiencing. When using video colposcopy, the clinician no longer is required to place his or her eyes in the ocular, freeing them up to observe the child's emotional state while at the same time allowing the child to observe the examination on the monitor. While monitoring the child's emotional

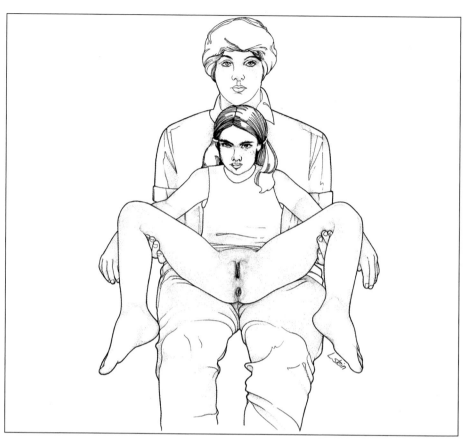

FIGURE 3.9
Supine frog-leg position while in the mother's lap.

state throughout the examination the examiner can respond immediately to any change in the child's demeanor.

Positioning

A number of positions have been described for conducting the anogenital examination of the prepubertal child. This section describes the supine frog-leg, the prone knee-chest, and the lateral decubitus positions. There are benefits to each of the examination positions, and the examiner will need to decide whether one or a combination of positions is necessary. The supine frog-leg position offers the child relative comfort and provides the examiner with a clear view of the genitalia and anus. This position may be assumed in the lap of a parent or supporting adult or on the examination table (Figure 3.9). Stirrups (the lithotomy position) may enhance the examiner's ability to obtain adequate abduction of the legs to visualize the child's genitalia (Figure 3.10).

The prone knee-chest position offers an excellent view of the anus and allows for a different perspective of the hymenal

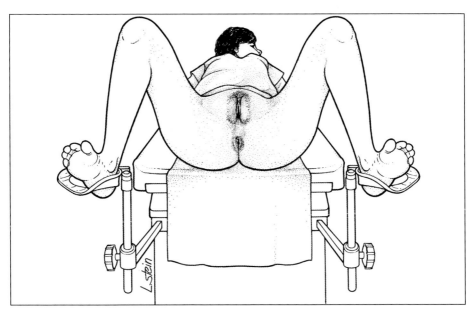

Figure 3.10
Lithotomy positioning of older female patient for genital examination.

membrane and vestibular structures (Figure 3.11). In this position, the anterior wall of the vagina falls forward and allows the hymen to splay out for easy viewing. Although the prone knee-chest position is both awkward and uncomfortable for most children, it can help clarify findings that in the frog-leg position alone are concerning. The knee-chest position can be particularly uncomfortable for the child who was sodomized in this position. As a general rule in prepubertal children, both the frog-leg and knee-chest positions may be needed to examine the genital structures fully. When children are positioned with their legs either in stirrups or in adduction with the soles of their feet touching, explain that you would like them to relax and, for a moment, hold their legs out like a frog or like a butterfly with its wings apart.

Using an age-appropriate humorous analogy, such as asking the child to lay on the examination table like Kermit the Frog when he visits the office to have his private parts examined, is helpful for young children.

The examination is an exercise in look- ing, touching, and sampling. The examiner relies on inspection and gentle palpation to view all of the necessary structures. Most examina-tions do not require instrumentation. Occasionally, the use of saline to "float" the hymen when there is redundancy or cohesiveness of the tissue is indicated. If the examiner needs to run a cotton swab along the internal edge of the hymen, a small-diameter, saline-moistened swab should be used. The unestrogenized hymen is exquisitely sensitive to touch, so any manipulation of the tissues should be done only when positioning and saline techniques fail to allow full visualization of the membrane edge. If available, a colposcope can be of enormous value in enhancing visualization of the anogenital tissues and, if connected to a video monitor, serves to record examination findings.

Examining the External and Internal Structures

Rectovaginal bimanual, speculum, or anoscopic assessment of internal structures in prepubertal children is not routinely indicated because it is unlikely to provide valuable diagnostic information. In the pubertal child, an internal examination is more appropriate if visual examination and/or history suggests that penetration with a penis or foreign body has occurred. (See Chapter 7.) A digital rectal examination is not routinely necessary; its primary value is to assess sphincter tone and the presence of stool in the ampulla. External palpation and traction on the buttocks is generally sufficient to assess tone. If a fissure or laceration of the external sphincter or anorectal canal is suspected, then the use of test tube proctoscopy or anoscopy is warranted.

When examining the female genitalia with the child in the frog-leg position, 2 techniques assist in observing the internal aspects of the genitalia. The first of these techniques is labial separation (Figure 3.12). Labial separation is accomplished by gently placing the examiner's thumb and index finger at the 10 o'clock and 2 o'clock positions on the labia majora. With lateral movement of the fingers, the labia majora will separate to improve visualization of the labia minora and the superior portions of the vestibule. The second technique is labial traction (Figure 3.13). When using labial traction, the examiner gently

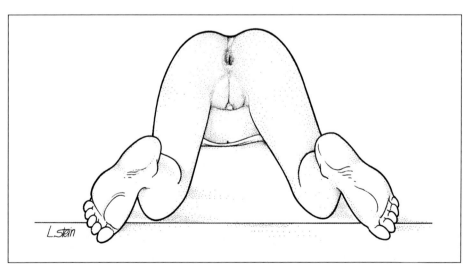

FIGURE 3.11
The prone knee-chest position for genital examination.

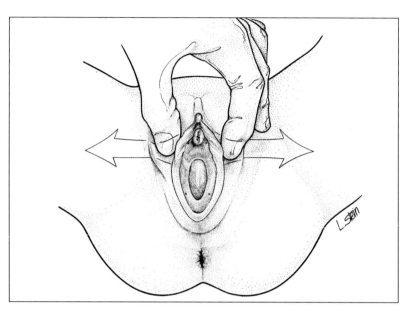

FIGURE 3.12
Labial separation technique for examination of female genitalia in the supine
frog-leg position.

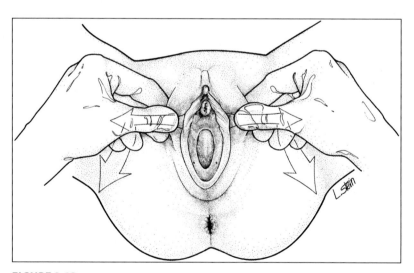

FIGURE 3.13
Labial traction technique for examination of female genitalia in the supine
frog-leg position.

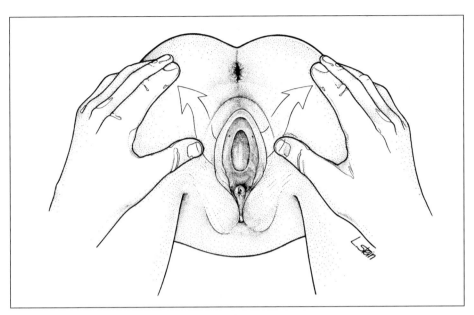

FIGURE 3.14
Technique for examination of female genitalia in prone knee-chest position.

grasps the left and right labia with the thumb and index finger of each hand and applies downward and lateral traction on the labia majora. Traction will open the vestibule for visual inspection of all of its component parts. Sustained traction may be necessary to break the cohesive forces of the moist hymenal membrane and allow full visualization of the edge of the hymenal membrane orifice. When the child is in the prone knee-chest position, upward and lateral pressure applied with the thumbs at the 3 o'clock and 9 o'clock positions will accomplish the same (Figure 3.14).

Vaginal Vestibule

The structures surrounding the vaginal vestibule are inspected visually first prior to applying separation or traction. After observing the labia majora, labia minora, and clitoral hood in apposition, the examiner separates the labia and

applies traction to observe all aspects of the tissues that form the component parts of the vestibule.

Acute injuries—as evidenced by tissue edema, abrasions, lacerations, puncture wounds, hematomas, bruising, and bleeding of the structures that form the boundaries of the vestibule—should be noted, described appropriately, and documented. In blunt force trauma with or without penetration through the hymenal orifice it is possible to incur injuries to the inner aspects of the labia minor, urethra, fossa navicularis, and posterior fourchette. The examiner should also record information on the shape and contour of the hymenal orifice; the appearance of the external surface of the hymen; the variability of the hymenal orifice diameter; any transections, distortions, redundancy, or signs of healed injury;

the appearance of the periurethral area, fossa, and fourchette; and any vaginal discharges, abnormal erythema, or malodor. When describing physical findings, it is best to reference their location with the use of a clock face, as illustrated in Figure 3.15.

Hymenal Orifice Size

The significance of the size of the hymenal orifice has generated considerable controversy in the literature.[36,58,59] The orifice diameter may vary considerably, depending on the age of the child, the position in which the child is examined, the degree of relaxation, and the amount of traction used on the labia during the examination. The transverse diameter alone is rarely sufficient to determine whether a child has or has not been sexually abused and should not be used as the sole criterion for such a determination.

From a practical perspective, the only purpose for assessing the maximal

transverse hymenal orifice diameter is to make a judgment whether the opening is sufficient to have allowed intromission of the object stated to have been introduced. Clinically, children will commonly state that someone has put something inside them, and "inside" is interpreted as entering the vagina. Making the determination as to whether an object penetrated into the vagina per se can be assessed most confidently in prepubertal girls because of the limited elasticity of the membrane and the likelihood that diagnostic findings of blunt force trauma will be found. In the adolescent, however, making this determination is more challenging in the absence of diagnostic findings such as a transection and/or acute injury. Thus an estrogenized hymenal membrane whose edge is uninterrupted does not mean that the orifice could not dilate sufficiently to allow introduction of an object such as a digit or penis. By the same token, just because the opening is sufficient to have allowed introduction of a given object does not mean that penetration can be stated definitively to have occurred. In the absence of definitive physical findings, the child's history regarding signs and symptoms associated with the contact as well as any excited utterance may assist in concluding whether vaginal penetration occurred.

The following example describes a circumstance in which an adolescent made a statement in association with a specific event (speculum examination) that resulted in a change in emotional state and the rekindling of memories

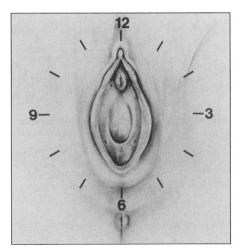

FIGURE 3.15
Face of clock orientation with patient in frog-leg supine position.

of a prior event. While introducing a vaginal speculum or conducting a digital vaginal examination, the child becomes visibly upset, begins to emote, and says, "Stop! That feels just like when John put his penis inside me." This type of statement—because of its spontaneous nature and the fact that a specific sensation/experience triggered a memory of a prior event—might be considered an excited utterance and is generally presumed to speak to the truth of an experience. The courts usually consider an excited utterance to be an exception to hearsay. Specific legal criteria apply to this determination. When a child makes such a statement, both the statement and the context in which the statement was made must be documented verbatim.

Anus and Perianal Area

The anus and perianal area are examined with the child placed in any of the following positions: (a) supine with the legs flexed onto the abdomen, (b) lithotomy with buttocks separation, (c) lateral decubitus with buttocks separation (Figure 3.16), or (d) knee-chest position. When examining the external anal verge tissues, the rugae usually appear to have a symmetrical puckered appearance radiating from the anal orifice. Gentle traction or stroking of the perianal area should elicit reflex contraction of the sphincter muscle. Asymmetry of the rugal folds, changes in pigmentation, rectal discharge, stigmata of STIs, signs of trauma, dilation, and tags should all be noted.[60] Before interpreting rectal dilation as a response to buttocks traction as a pathologic condition, the examiner should be sure that the ampulla is free of stool, because the anus may naturally relax to evacuate stool under such circumstances.[61–64] Controversy exists concerning the significance of anal dilation in response to traction.[65] Rectal dilation should be interpreted cautiously when observed in isolation.

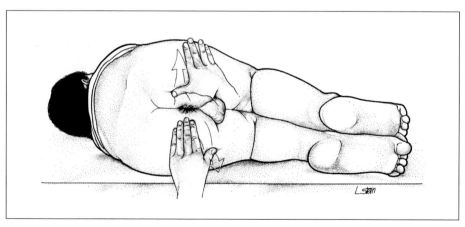

FIGURE 3.16
Position and technique for examination of male child in left lateral decubitus (cannonball) position.

Presence or Absence of Diagnostic Findings

Physical findings that reflect acute or chronic residua to sexual contact are infrequent.[66-71] For the most part, this is the result of 2 dynamics: (a) The individual engaging the child does not intend to hurt the child physically, and (b) most children do not disclose immediately following their last contact for fear of harm. The lack of physical evidence alone should not lead to the conclusion that inappropriate sexual contact did not occur. Clinicians must be as adept at preserving the child's spoken word as they are at recognizing residua to sexual contact and collecting physical evidence and laboratory specimens.

In many cases of child sexual abuse, there are no confirmatory physical or laboratory findings to corroborate the child's history.[72,73] The original research on the healing chronology of acute anogenital trauma published in *Pediatrics* by Finkel[74] in 1989 provides insight into why even with a history of genital or anal trauma physical findings are not likely to be observed on examination unless acute. These observations have been confirmed in larger case series by Heppenstall-Heger[75] in 2003 and in a longitudinal study of 239 girls by McCann in 2007.[76] The most reasonable predictor that diagnostic physical findings will be found is the child's verbal description of the sexual interaction. Children who complain of being hurt during the sexual contact are more likely to present with physical findings depending on the temporal relationship between the contact and the examination. If the child incurred an injury that was superficial, and the time interval since the last contact is more than 72 hours, it is unlikely that any residua will be identified.[73] If the child complained of significant pain and observed bleeding associated with the event(s), more significant residua might be present. Healed diagnostic genital and anal findings that can stand alone to confirm sexual contact are present in approximately 5% of cases. With some caveats, STIs can be diagnostic of sexual contact and are present in approximately 2% to 7% of sexually abused children.

When children disclose immediately following the last inappropriate contact, the potential to diagnose acute and/or chronic residua or to collect forensic evidence is increased. Christian et al[73] found that 24.9% of 293 prepubertal children presenting to the emergency department within 44 hours of their last contact had some form of forensic evidence identified. Ninety percent of the evidentiary collection of seminal products occurred in children seen within 24 hours of the last contact. Most of the evidence identified (64%) was found on either the child's clothing or his or her linens, although only 35% of the children had clothing/linens collected. Twenty-three percent of the children had findings of acute genital injury.

When physical findings are present, the clinician must attempt to corroborate the observed findings with the history from the child. The absence of findings, however, does not deny the occurrence of sexual interaction, because many activities typically do not have residua. Also, it is common for the child to initially disclose only a portion of the details of his or her experience(s). A complete examination of the child is always indicated to avoid the need for reexamination should additional details surface.

A number of variables may affect the likelihood of finding physical evidence of sexual abuse, such as the following[74]:

1. Use (or absence) of force
2. Age difference between child and perpetrator
3. Size of object introduced into body orifice
4. Level of resistance by the child
5. Use of lubricants
6. The specific abuse activity
7. Position of the child during the victimization
8. Chronicity and acuity of the abuse

Spectrum of Diagnostic Findings in Sexual Abuse

This section focuses on the findings that may be noted in cases of acute or chronic sexual abuse. Although many children will neither complain of injury nor present with signs or symptoms suggestive of STIs, certain characteristics must be considered in differentiating inflicted trauma from the infrequently seen accidental injuries to the genitalia.[77-83]

The manner in which children are engaged in sexual contact helps to explain why residual findings as a result of physical force and restraint are unusual in child sexual abuse.

Sexual abuse often involves a pattern of ever-increasing contact between perpetrator and victim.[84] By minimizing the physical harm to the child—which could lead to disclosure and discovery if the injuries required medical attention—the perpetrator hopes to ensure the child's continued cooperation. However, the perpetrator may also use both implicit and explicit threats and rewards to maintain secrecy around the contact.

Most injuries that do occur are superficial and heal without residual findings because most children disclose long after the last contact and are well beyond the 72 to 96 hours necessary for superficial trauma to resolve.[85-87] In addition, more serious injuries can heal with unanticipated residual findings based on the initial appearance of the acute injuries. The retrospective interpretation of such residual findings can be difficult without knowledge of the premorbid state. Physical force is more common in cases that involve adolescents or perpetrators unknown to the victim.[74]

Through a consensus-building process, experienced child abuse pediatricians developed the following categorization of physical findings and laboratory tests when sexual abuse is suspected. In general findings can be described as falling into one of the following categories[88]:

1. Findings documented in newborns or commonly seen in non-abused children
2. Findings commonly caused by other medical conditions

3 Indeterminate findings: insufficient or conflicting data from research studies to support significance with certainty

4. Findings diagnostic of trauma and/ or sexual contact

See Table 3.1.

TABLE 3.1
Approach to Interpreting Physical and Laboratory Findings in Suspected Child Sexual Abuse: December 2006[a]

A Product of an ongoing collaborative process by child maltreatment physician specialists, under the leadership of Joyce A. Adams, MD

(Numbering of findings is for ease of reference only and does not imply increasing significance)

Findings documented in newborns or commonly seen in non-abused children:
(The presence of these findings generally neither confirms nor discounts a child's clear disclosure of sexual abuse)

Normal variants
1. Periurethral or vestibular bands
2. Intravaginal ridges or columns
3. Hymenal bumps or mounds
4. Hymenal tags or septal remnants
5. Linea vestibularis (midline avascular area)
6. Hymenal notch/cleft in the anterior (superior) half of the hymenal rim (prepubertal girls), on or above the 3 o'clock – 9 o'clock line, patient supine
7. Shallow/superficial notch or cleft in inferior rim of hymen (below 3 o'clock – 9 o'clock line)
8. External hymenal ridge
9. Congenital variants in appearance of hymen, including: crescentic, annular, redundant, septate, cribiform, microperforate, imperforate
10. Diastasis ani (smooth area)
11. Perianal skin tag
12. Hyperpigmentation of the skin of labia minora or perianal tissues in children of color, such as Mexican-American and African-American children
13. Dilation of the urethral opening with application of labial traction
14. "Thickened" hymen (May be due to estrogen effect, folded edge of hymen, swelling from infection, or swelling from trauma. The latter is difficult to assess unless follow-up examination is done)

Findings commonly caused by other medical conditions:
15. Erythema (redness) of the vestibule, penis, scrotum or perianal tissues. (May be due to irritants, infection or traumab)
16. Increased vascularity ("Dilatation of existing blood vessels") of vestibule and hymen. (May be due to local irritants, or normal pattern in the non estrogenized state)
17. Labial adhesions. (May be due to irritation or rubbing)
18. Vaginal discharge. (Many infectious and non-infectious causes, cultures must be taken to confirm if it is caused by sexually transmitted organisms or other infections.)
19. Friability of the posterior fourchette or commissure (May be due to irritation, infection, or may be caused by examiner's traction on the labia majora)
20. Excoriations/bleeding/vascular lesions. These findings can be due to conditions such as lichen sclerosus, eczema or seborrhea, vaginal/perianal Group A Streptococcus, urethral prolapse, hemangiomas)

TABLE 3.1
Approach to Interpreting Physical and Laboratory Findings in Suspected Child Sexual Abuse: December 2006,[a] continued

21. Perineal groove (failure of midline fusion), partial or complete
22. Anal fissures (Usually due to constipation, perianal irritation)
23. Venous congestion, or venous pooling in the perianal area. (Usually due to positioning of child, also seen with constipation)
24. Flattened anal folds (May be due to relaxation of the external sphincter or to swelling of the perianal tissues due to infection or trauma[b])
25. Partial or complete anal dilatation to less than 2 cm (anterior-posterior dimension), with or without stool visible. (May be a normal reflex, or may have other causes, such as severe constipation or encopresis, sedation, anesthesia, neuromuscular conditions,)

INDETERMINATE Findings: Insufficient or conflicting data from research studies: (May require additional studies/evaluation to determine significance. These physical/ laboratory findings may support a child's clear disclosure of sexual abuse, if one is given, but should be interpreted with caution if the child gives no disclosure. In some cases, a report to child protective services may be indicated to further evaluate possible sexual abuse.)

Physical Examination Findings
26. Deep notches or clefts in the posterior/inferior rim of hymen in pre-pubertal girls, located between 4 and 8 o'clock, in contrast to transections (see 41)
27. Deep notches or complete clefts in the hymen at 3 or 9 o'clock in adolescent girls.
28. Smooth, non-interrupted rim of hymen between 4 and 8 o'clock, which appears to be less than 1 millimeter wide, when examined in the prone knee-chest position, or using water to "float" the edge of the hymen when the child is in the supine position.
29. Wart-like lesions in the genital or anal area. (Biopsy and viral typing may be indicated in some cases if appearance is not typical of Condyloma accuminata)
30. Vesicular lesions or ulcers in the genital or anal area (viral and/or bacterial cultures, or nucleic acid amplification tests may be needed for diagnosis)
31. Marked, immediate anal dilation to an anterior-posterior diameter of 2 cm or more, in the absence of other predisposing factors

Lesions with etiology confirmed: Indeterminate specificity for sexual transmission
(Report to protective services recommended by AAP Guidelines unless perinatal or horizontal transmission is considered likely)
31. Genital or anal Condyloma accuminata in child, in the absence of other indicators of abuse.
32. Herpes Type 1 or 2 in the genital or anal area in a child with no other indicators of sexual abuse.

Findings Diagnostic of Trauma and/or Sexual contact (The following findings support a disclosure of sexual abuse, if one is given, and are highly suggestive of abuse even in the absence of a disclosure, unless the child and/or caretaker provide a clear, timely, plausible description of accidental injury. (It is recommended that diagnostic quality photo-documentation of the examination findings be obtained and reviewed by an experienced medical provider, before concluding that they represent acute or healed trauma. Follow-up examinations are also recommended.)

TABLE 3.1

Approach to Interpreting Physical and Laboratory Findings in Suspected Child Sexual Abuse: December 2006,[a] continued

---

Acute trauma to external genital/anal tissues

33. Acute lacerations or extensive bruising of labia, penis, scrotum, perianal tissues, or perineum (May be from unwitnessed accidental trauma, or from physical or sexual abuse)
34. Fresh laceration of the posterior fourchette, not involving the hymen. (Must be differentiated from dehisced labial adhesion or failure of midline fusion. May also be caused by accidental injury or consensual sexual intercourse in adolescents)

Residual (healing) injuries

(These findings are difficult to assess unless an acute injury was previously documented at the same location)

36. Perianal scar (Rare, may be due to other medical conditions such as Crohn's Disease, accidental injuries, or previous medical procedures)
37. Scar of posterior fourchette or fossa. (Pale areas in the midline may also be due to linea vestibularis or labial adhesions)

Injuries indicative of blunt force penetrating trauma (or from abdominal/pelvic compression injury if such history is given)

38. Laceration (tear, partial or complete) of the hymen, acute.
39. Ecchymosis (bruising) on the hymen (in the absence of a known infectious process or coagulopathy).
40. Perianal lacerations extending deep to the external anal sphincter (not to be confused with partial failure of midline fusion)
41. Hymenal transection (healed). An area between 4 and 8 o'clock on the rim of the hymen where it appears to have been torn through, to or nearly to the base, so there appears to be virtually no hymenal tissue remaining at that location. This must be confirmed using additional examination techniques such as a swab, prone knee-chest position or Foley catheter balloon (in adolescents), or prone-knee chest position or water to float the edge of the hymen (in prepubertal girls). This finding has also been referred to as a "complete cleft" in sexually active adolescents and young adult women.
42. Missing segment of hymenal tissue. Area in the posterior (inferior) half of the hymen, wider than a transection, with an absence of hymenal tissue extending to the base of the hymen, which is confirmed using additional positions/methods as described above.

Presence of infection confirms mucosal contact with infected and infective bodily secretions, contact most likely to have been sexual in nature:

43. Positive confirmed culture for gonorrhea, from genital area, anus, throat, in a child outside the neonatal period.
44. Confirmed diagnosis of syphilis, if perinatal transmission is ruled out.
45. Trichomonas vaginalis infection in a child older than 1 year of age, with organisms identified by culture or in vaginal secretions by wet mounts examination by an experienced technician or clinician)
46. Positive culture from genital or anal tissues for Chlamydia, if child is older than 3 years at time of diagnosis, and specimen was tested using cell culture or comparable method approved by the Centers for Disease Control.
47. Positive serology for HIV, if perinatal transmission, transmission from blood products, and needle contamination has been ruled out.

Diagnostic of sexual contact

48. Pregnancy
49. Sperm identified in specimens taken directly from a child's body.

---

[a]Reprinted with permission from Adams JA, Kaplan RA, Starling SP, et al. Guidelines for medical care of children who may have been sexually abused. *J Pediatr Adolesc Gynecol.* 2007;20:163–172.
[b]Follow-up examination is necessary before attributing these findings to trauma

Degree of Physical Contact

The legal definition of rape includes the act of sexual intercourse, although the specifics may vary from state to state.[89] Some states use a strict legal definition of rape, which is any genital-to-genital contact that penetrates between the labia, no matter how slight. In other states, the legal definition of penetration requires entry into the vagina. Thus, in some jurisdictions, when a child experiences genital-to-genital contact limited to rubbing between the labia minora within the vaginal vestibule, rape has not occurred.

Children may be exposed to sexually inappropriate circumstances that do not involve actual physical contact but are psychologically intrusive and fall under the legal definition of "debauching the morals of minors." Examples may include a child being exposed to an adult's genitals or observation of an adult stimulating himself or herself. Children may be forced into observing adults engaged in sexual activities or made to look at adult or child pornography. Exposure to pornography is sometimes used to normalize the activities for the child. Children may be exploited for pornographic purposes themselves without any physical contact. Children who have their sense of personal space and privacy invaded by an adult observing them bathing, toileting, or dressing can be affected profoundly by these noncontact activities.

Fondling and Digital Penetration

In situations where the primary activity of the perpetrator involves fondling the child's genitals, the degree of force employed will be a prime determinant of the findings. Under most circumstances, force is not used, and thus residua to genital fondling is unusual and, when present, is usually nonspecific. When increasing force is used, findings may include erythema of the fondled area, edema, superficial abrasions, and contusions. Figure 3.17 illustrates how, in cases of genital fondling, the finger(s) can penetrate into the space of the vaginal vestibule without entering into the vagina per se and yet be perceived by the child as being inside. Within the context of rubbing during fondling, the child may experience superficial trauma to the urethra and the mucosa of the vestibule. As the level of inappropriate contact progresses, the child may experience increasingly forceful introduction of fingers or objects into the vagina or anus. In such cases, significant findings may include lacerations to the hymen and vaginal wall. Clinically, injuries due to fondling and digital penetration are most likely to be observed between the 9 o'clock and 3 o'clock positions (with the child in the supine frog-leg position) as the finger enters over the mons pubis between the labia minora and is rubbed over the urethral meatus. In the context of fondling/digital penetration of the vagina or anus, superficial laceration may result from the perpetrator's fingernails. However, under most circumstances, there is little

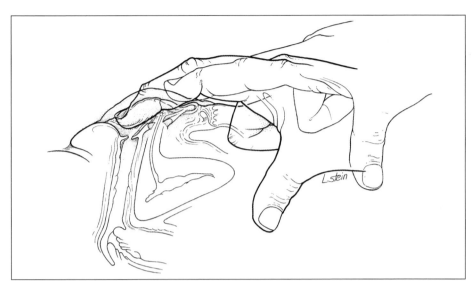

FIGURE 3.17
Index finger placed between the labia minora penetrating into the vaginal vestibule,
demonstrating the anatomical relationship of finger to genital structures during fondling.

residual to fondling, and the residual is nonspecific when present.

A history of dysuria following fondling may help corroborate the child's story. This history indicates periurethral/vestibular trauma and can be readily differentiated from a urinary tract infection (UTI). If the historical details concerning dysuria are obtained in a manner that lacks suggestibility and is non-leading, the physician can conclude with medical certainty that the history reflects knowledge of symptoms temporally related to a specific event of which the child could have no knowledge unless he or she had experienced it. Urogenital signs and symptoms in girls who experience genital contact reflect the most common residual to inappropriate touching. DeLago and colleagues[90] in a retrospective studied the medical

histories of girls 3 to 18 years old who experienced inappropriate genital contact. Sixty percent of the girls who experienced genital contact reported one or more symptoms/signs as a direct result of the genital contact, 53% had genital pain, 37% dysuria, and 11% genital bleeding. Symptoms/signs were highly associated with genital-genital contact, with 48% of the girls reporting genital-genital contact having dysuria compared with 25% of the girls not reporting genital-genital contact, 72 % had genital pain/soreness compared with 32% not reporting genital-genital contact, and 16 % had bleeding compared with 4% of those not reporting genital-genital contact.[90]

As in all aspects of medicine, this study reinforces the importance of the physician obtaining a detailed medical history. The history of signs and symptoms associated with genital contact is unlikely to be obtained in the process of a "forensic interview" by nonmedical professionals.[91]

A complete GU review of systems should eliminate differential considerations; in general, dysuria in cases of sexual abuse is infrequently associated with a documented UTI.[92,93]

Oral-Genital Contact

In cases where a history of oral-genital contact has been provided, some specific findings may be present.[57,94] A child who is forced to perform fellatio may have dental trauma and petechiae to the palate and/or posterior pharynx. Tears to the labial frenulum may result from forceful traction on the upper lip. When the child's scalp hair is grasped forcibly during the act of fellatio, traction alopecia may be evident. The examiner should look for evidence of seminal products in the oral and nasal pharynges. Such evidence will be dependent on the time since the contact and a history of ejaculation.

If the child has had fellatio or cunnilingus performed on him or her, possible acute signs would include petechiae, abrasions, or bite marks to the genitalia. The presence of these findings will depend on the time interval between the alleged contact and the examination.

Penile Contact With Genitalia Without Vaginal Penetration

Characteristic findings may result when the sexual interaction involves penile contact without introduction of the penis through the hymenal orifice (Figure 3.18). This form of contact is referred to as *vulvar coitus.* Vulvar coitus is the placement of the penis between the labia minora and generally involves rubbing the penis between the labia minora. The lateral aspects of the penile shaft may cause injury to the medial aspects of the labia minora, and the proximal and distal aspects of the shaft may cause trauma to the periurethral area and fourchette, respectively. In such contact, trauma may also be evident to the anterior commissure, fossa, and external surface of the hymenal membrane without injury to the orifice edge. Acutely, lacerations, abrasions, erythema, and edema are most evident. Children may provide a history of dysuria following vulvar coitus. In adult women, this symptom, in association with coitus, is commonly referred to as *honeymoon cystitis.*[95–97]

In vulvar coitus, the perpetrator may ejaculate on the child's abdomen or within the intracural region. If a history of ejaculation is provided and the examination is conducted within 72 hours following disclosure, there may be the potential to identify and collect seminal products. If the child makes a statement that suggests she had contact with genital secretions, ask her to describe whether she did anything afterward to clean herself, if so what was used (washcloth, shirt) and what she did with those items. There is always the potential that with the details of how she cleaned herself, and if the items were not washed, semen could be identified, corroborating the child's history.

Children will frequently state that an object has been placed "inside" of them, and yet no confirmatory physical findings are present. When this situation occurs this should suggest to the examiner that the child experienced vulvar coitus, even though the child's perception may have been different.

Penile-Vaginal Penetration

Depending on the child's age, penetration of the vagina by a penis may or may not lead to significant findings.[72,98–102] The findings depend on a number of variables that mitigate for or against residua. It is expected that the introduction of an adult penis into a prepubertal child's vagina should produce acute and obvious signs of trauma and result in chronic residua such as transections and healing scar tissue. This is true if the contact is acute and forceful. A transection of the hymen observed in the prepubertal child should remain evident even when

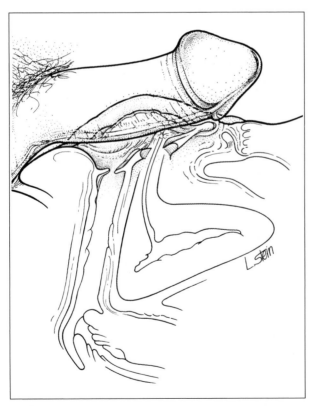

FIGURE 3.18
Penis placed between labia minor penetrating into the vaginal vestibule, demonstrating the anatomical relationship of a penis to genital structures in vulvar coitus.

the membrane becomes estrogenized in puberty. However, rather dramatic acute non-transection injuries may heal with surprisingly little residua.[85,86]

Lubricants, the child's "cooperation," and delayed disclosure of the events all reduce the likelihood of identifying acute residua to sexual contact. In the pubertal patient who experiences vaginal penetration, the potential to identify diagnostic findings is limited, and the historical details are likely to be the most important and available component of the diagnosis. The history may include details to suggest that she experienced pain, dysuria, and/or observed signs of injury/contact with ejaculate. The pubertal child is no more likely to disclose immediately following the contact than the prepubertal child, and thus any superficial genital injuries that occurred will have healed without residua.[85]

Hormonal factors may add to the difficulty in interpreting the residua to suspected sexual abuse. Rising estrogen levels, as described in Huffman's staging, will alter the appearance of the prepubertal child's genitalia. This will lead to progressive changes in the thickness, redundancy, elasticity, and vascular pattern of the hymen and related structures as the child approaches menarche. Redundancy and thickening of the hymen secondary to estrogen effect may alter the appearance of preexisting trauma and make residual findings quite subtle and difficult to identify. The elasticity of the membrane in the pubertal child may afford the intromission of a penis with surprisingly little residua.

Clinical experience suggests that because of the elasticity and distensibility that result from the estrogenization of the hymen, the hymenal orifice can dilate well beyond the diameter of an adult erect penis without diagnostic residua. Clinically, if an adult vaginal speculum can be introduced through the orifice of the adolescent hymen, then the opening is sufficient to have allowed introduction of a foreign body such as a penis. An adult vaginal speculum measures 35 mm in width, which exceeds the average transverse diameter of the adult erect penis.[103] The common perception that women bleed during their first coitus, thus confirming their virginal status, is incorrect. In a review of 100 women questioned regarding the degree of discomfort and the amount of bleeding associated with first intercourse, 44% did not have bleeding, 35% had only mild bleeding, 32% had no pain, and 22% experienced slight pain.[104,105]

Palmer et al[106] found that in adult women who experienced sexual assault, 22% had diagnostic genital trauma and 46% had minor extragenital trauma. White et al[107] compared findings in adolescent virgins and nonvirgins who experienced sexual assault. Virgins experienced overall genital injuries in 53% of the cases with only 32% anticipated to demonstrate chronic residua. In the nonvirgin group, 32% of the adolescent girls had genital trauma. Hymenal trauma was identified in 51% of the virgins and significantly less frequently in nonvirgins (12.4%). Both groups had a similar frequency (51%) of extragenital trauma.[106,107] Kellogg and colleagues[108] found that only 2 of 36 pregnant adolescents had abnormal hymenal findings confirming penetrating trauma.

Intragluteal Coitus

Intragluteal coitus occurs in the male or female victim when the penis is placed between the gluteal folds. The friction of the penis over the surface of the external anal verge tissues between the buttocks may result in edema, contusions, and abrasions involving the natal cleft, perianal, and anal tissues.

In cases where the perpetrator has rubbed his penis on the child, the examiner should assess for the presence of seminal products on the back and buttocks. Pubic hair and other trace elements (eg, fibers) may also be found on the child's body. In any case where the perpetrator has direct genital contact with the child's body or indirect contact through genital secretions, the possibility exists of acquiring STIs.

Penile, Digital, and/or Foreign Body Contact With Anus

The interpretation of residual findings from the introduction of a foreign body such as a penis, digit, or other object into the anus is difficult when the child is examined and has no acute signs of injury. The external anal sphincter has the ability to dilate significantly to pass large stools without any obvious injury to the sphincter or anal canal. Therefore, depending on the age of the child, the size of the object introduced, the degree of force, the cooperativeness of the child, and the use of lubricants, there may or may not be any residual

findings from either the single or repeated introduction of an object into the anus. Because most perpetrators have little intent to harm the child physically while introducing an object into the anorectal canal or on the external anal verge, it is most likely that only superficial and nonspecific signs will be noted if the child presents acutely. Superficial injuries to the anorectal canal may include rectal fissures, chafing, and erythema. Rubbing an object over the anal verge tissues and between the gluteal cleft can result in abrasion or ulcerative-like lesions between the buttocks. More significant acute injuries may include bruising, lacerations, edema, and posttraumatic hemorrhoid-like tags.[82,109] The most serious acute injuries include complete transection of the external anal sphincter, laceration, and perforation of the rectosigmoid. Chronic residua, as seen in the adult population engaging in anal sex, most frequently include the presence of fissures and cryptitis.[110-112] Lacerations that extend onto the perineum should not be thought to have occurred from passing hard stool. Eighteen percent of males following male on male anal sexual assault had acute signs of injury.[113]

Some clinicians have suggested that when an object is introduced repeatedly into the anus, the following may be seen: (a) loss of fine, symmetrical rugal pattern/irregular rugae; (b) anal scars as the healed residua to significant acute injuries; (c) loss of subcutaneous fat; (d) decrease in sphincter tone; (e) venous congestion or dilated veins; and

(f) abnormal response to traction of external anus when rectal ampulla is free of stool. The loss of a fine, symmetrical rugal pattern; the "tyre" effect; funneling; and loss of subcutaneous fat believed to occur following anal penetration are subjective observations from some clinicians.[114] There are no published studies that state the prevalence of or predict the frequency of these presumed posttraumatic findings. The only published study,[110] which looked at 68 adults engaging in consensual anal sex, found that "it was not possible to relate the appearance of the anus to the practice of sodomy; there was no appreciable difference of the anus in those who practiced sodomy frequently and those that practiced it rarely." In addition, "patulous anus, contrary to a commonly held impression was not observed in the patients in the present study." As always, there must be an attempt to correlate any abnormal physical findings with an appropriate history.

No experimental models exist to assess the effect of repeated introduction of a foreign body into the anus of a child. Thus the question of how often and how much force is necessary to cause any changes that may be the residua to repeated anal penetration is difficult to answer.

Just as children who provide histories of vaginal penetration commonly have examination findings to suggest otherwise, genital-anal contact can be perceived as entering the anorectal canal when, in fact, pressure over the external sphincter dilated the anus, creating the sensation of an object entering the canal without actual penetration (Figure 3.19). Children who experience penetration into the anorectal canal may provide a history of pain associated with defecation. Children commonly describe their discomfort with defecation as burning. This burning sensation develops when the mucosal area between the intersphincteric groove and dentate line, which has no secretory glands, is abraded.

Nonspecific findings, such as erythema, perianal excoriation, and pigmentary venous changes, require an appropriate history and must be correlated with the alleged contact to be considered as residual to the alleged contact. Diagnostic findings include serious injuries such as transection of the anus, perianal scarring, perforation of the rectosigmoid colon, and the recovery of seminal products from the anorectal canal, with or without signs of acute or chronic trauma.

Extragenital Trauma

Frequent sites for extragenital trauma include breasts, extremities, neck, buttocks, and oropharynx. Extragenital findings of trauma represent residual to the use of force and restraint. Ligature marks and traction alopecia are additional signs of the use of restraint and force. Extragenital trauma was present in 51% of female adolescents following sexual assault.[107] The health care professional should document all abrasions, lacerations, contusions, and bite marks.[115] Documentation is most complete when diagrams or photographs of the findings are included in

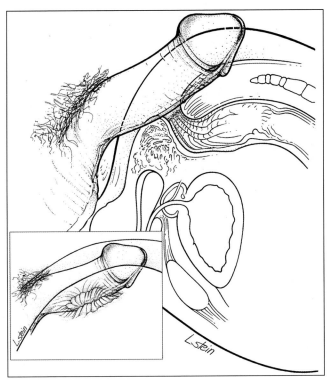

FIGURE 3.19
Placement of penis rubbing between the gluteal cleft with
child on abdomen and buttocks elevated. Insert illustrates
how downward pressures during rubbing can result in
dilation of the anus.

the report.[44] The medical record must
also provide a clear explanation of the
examination findings to support any
photographic documentation. Thus if
photographs fail to develop properly or
are otherwise unsatisfactory, written
documentation remains.

Genital Findings in Males

In the male child, fondling of the
genitals may result in edema or
abrasions on the shaft, glans, and
foreskin of the penis, or on the surface
of the scrotum or perianal area. The
severity of the abrasions usually
depends on the degree of force used.

Occasionally, bite, pinch, or ligature
marks will be evident on the penis.

**Summary of Findings
Following Sexual Contact**

Acute findings of injury, whether noted
in the genital or anal area, include
edema, abrasions, lacerations, and
bruising. As acute injuries heal, they
may leave little or no residual findings,
making the retrospective interpretation
of changes in anogenital anatomy
difficult. Close attention is paid to the
appearance of the edge of the hymenal
membrane when assessing whether
an object has penetrated through the

orifice and into the vagina per se. When a large-diameter object is passed forcefully through a small-diameter orifice, there is the potential for identifying a laceration of the hymen that extends to the posterior vaginal wall. A laceration of the hymen is diagnostic of penetrating trauma when observed in the posterior quadrant of the hymenal membrane. However, a small-diameter object passed through a large-diameter orifice may not tear the membrane or, if it does, the tear may not extend to the vaginal wall. When healed, smaller interruptions in the edge of the hymenal membrane that do not extend to the posterior wall may be difficult to differentiate from congenital clefts.

Penetration injuries most commonly result in changes to the hymenal membrane in the most posterior portion and may include injury to the fossa navicularis and posterior fourchette. Scar tissue may be observed as residual to trauma, affecting any or all of the following structures: (a) labia minora, (b) hymenal membrane, (c) fossa navicularis, (d) posterior fourchette, and (e) anus. When scar tissue is observed, then the examiner must seek a history of trauma significant enough to result in such findings. When vulvar coitus occurs, the pattern of acute injury usually involves the medial aspects of the labia minora, the posterior fourchette, and the periurethral area. On rare occasions, an object introduced into the vagina may perforate the posterior fornix and enter into the peritoneal cavity.

Fondling of the genitalia usually involves a finger or fingers entering the vaginal vestibule from a superior to inferior approach over the mons pubis, rubbing between the labia minora inferior to the clitoral hood. The rubbing that the child experiences most commonly results in superficial abrasions to the periurethral area, the inner aspects of the labia, and the fossa. If examined shortly after the rubbing, there may be localized redness, superficial abrasions, and edema. Superficial abrasions are best observed with magnification and the use of a red-free filter. Under most circumstances, there will not be any chronic residual find-ings to genital fondling, other than a history of post-fondling dysuria that can corroborate the event.

Hymenal Orifice

Controversy existed over the relevance of the size of the hymenal orifice as a diagnostic criterion.[36] With time and experience the importance of a specific diameter has become less relevant. The size of the hymenal opening can vary with the degree of traction placed on the labia majora and the degree of relaxation of the child during the examination. The age and pubertal development of the child may also affect the size of the hymenal opening.[8,116] The diameter of the hymenal orifice alone should not be used as a screening test for the presence of sexual abuse. The hymenal diameter may be helpful in specific cases, but no generalization can be made.

Anal Penetration

See the previous section on anal examination findings for a related discussion.

Accidental Trauma

The most common type of accidental injury involving the genitalia is the straddle injury. Straddle injuries occur when the child's soft tissues are crushed between the pubic bone and a hard object.[80,81] These injuries are typically seen after the child falls on a bicycle crossbar, balance beam, or jungle gym. It is improbable that such an accident could damage the recessed hymenal membrane.[74,75,117] Trauma to the hymenal membrane may result from an accidental impaling injury or from an object directed purposely at the membrane.[79] Clinicians are surprised by the extraordinary explanations that may be provided to account for genital injuries. When a history of accidental injury seems implausible, a scene investigation may provide clarity regarding the mechanism of injury.

At present, there is no scientific evidence to support the common belief that girls injure their hymens during activities such as horseback riding, gymnastics, and tree climbing.[74] Furthermore, little is known about the changes to the genital anatomy that result from masturbation.[118,119] Clinical practice supports the belief that self-inflicted injuries, especially in the context of masturbation, are exceedingly rare unless the child is psychologically impaired.[120]

When they occur, accidental injuries to the anus are most likely to be impaling and present in an emergent manner. The anal verge tissues are protected by the buttocks and are unlikely to be injured accidentally.

Laboratory and Forensic Specimen Collection

The collection of appropriate laboratory specimens for the identification of STIs (Chapter 5) and forensic evidence (Chapter 6) is an important aspect of the clinical evaluation. The physical examination provides an appropriate setting for the health care professional to collect clinical specimens for diagnostic purposes, as well as specimens that may have evidentiary value. Because most children are unlikely to disclose their sexual contact immediately following their experience, the opportunity to identify and collect seminal products or other indications of sexual contact is limited. Although seminal products are found infrequently, when present, they must be collected in a manner that preserves the material appropriately. In most child sexual abuse cases, in contrast to rape, identification of the individual engaging the child in the sexually inappropriate activities is generally not an issue. In rape cases, the recovery of seminal products or trace evidence may be central to confirmation of the assailant. When children disclose sexual abuse, they may be taken to an emergency department where an individual experienced in conducting evidentiary examinations for adult victims of rape might conduct the same on the child. Preferably, children should have only one examination. Every effort should be made to ensure that all diagnostic, treatment, and evidentiary needs are met through that one examination.

Summary

- The medical history provides the greatest insight into what a child might have experienced and assists in predicting the probability of residua.
- Signs and symptoms that follow genital contact reflect the most available "evidence" in sexual abuse of girls and are more frequent than physical examination findings.
- The physical examination in the evaluation of sexual abuse allows for (a) diagnosis of residua from the alleged contact and (b) reassurance of the child's physical well-being.
- Findings of sequelae or residua are not essential to the diagnosis of sexual abuse, and their absence does not negate the child's story. Reasons for the absence of findings should be explained.
- The evaluation of the anogenital structures should occur only within the context of a head-to-toe examination.
- The examiner should describe the appearance of anogenital structures with meticulous detail and note the presence of acute or chronic signs of injury, STIs, and/or trace substances.
- In addition to obtaining cultures for the most common STIs, rape kits are available for the collection of forensic evidence if indicated by the clinical situation.
- The description of all examination findings should be clear and precise, using accepted terminology. Terms such as *intact hymen* and *virginal hymen* are inexact and should not be used in conversation or in the documentation of findings.
- Ideally, the examination should be conducted with enhanced visualization equipment, such as a colposcope or alternative instrument that provides for enhanced visualization.
- All diagnostic findings should be memorialized through both written description and photodocumentation.
- Discrepancies between a child's description of his or her experience and the physical examination findings must be explained.
- The diagnostic conclusions should be descriptive and in narrative form.
- Recommendations for mental health assessment/treatment should be incorporated into all assessments.

The physical examination should be therapeutic for the child, confirming his or her sense of physical intactness and normality. The clinician should discuss with the child and parent the results of the examination in language appropriate for the child's age. A child who incurred injuries can be reassured that his or her injuries will heal or have already healed. Give children the analogy of scraping their knees or elbows, and how their knees and elbows may have hurt and bled but have since healed, and no one can now tell that they were ever hurt. Children with infections can be reassured that medicine can help them get better. Older children may be worried that their experience can affect their ability to have children or sexual relations. Most children can be reassured that there will be no long-term physical consequences of their experience.

The clinician should emphasize the need for mental health services for both the child and the parent. In speaking to young children, the clinician can refer to a psychologist as a "talking doctor" who knows how to help children with their feelings about what has happened. A mental health professional can assist in determining the full impact of the child's experience and make appropriate recommendations regarding assessment and specific treatment approaches. The clinician should also emphasize to child protective services and law enforcement the importance of securing mental health evaluation/treatment services. Documentation of recommendations for mental health evaluation and/or treatment should be noted in the diagnostic assessment. (See Chapter 15.)

References

1. Davies J. Anatomy of the female genital tract. In: Danforth D, ed. *Danforth's Obstetrics and Gynecology.* 6th ed. Philadelphia, PA: Lippincott; 1990

2. Huffman JW. *The Gynecology of Childhood and Adolescence.* Phildelphia, PA: W. B. Saunders; 1969

3. Tanner JM. *Growth at Adolescence.* Oxford, UK: Blackwell Scientific Publications; 1962

4. Gray H. *Anatomy of the Human Body.* Philadelphia, PA: Lea & Febiger; 1985

5. Sloane E. *Biology of Women.* New York, NY: Wiley and Sons; 1985

6. Berenson AB. Normal anogenital anatomy. *Child Abuse Negl.* 1998;22(6):589–596, discussion 597–603

7. McCann J, Voris J, Simon M, Wells R. Perianal findings in prepubertal children selected for nonabuse: a descriptive study. *Child Abuse Negl.* 1989;13(2):179–193

8. McCann J, Voris J, Simon M, Wells R. Comparison of genital examination techniques in prepubertal girls. *Pediatrics.* 1990;85(2):182–187

9. Enos WF, Conrath TB, Byer JC. Forensic evaluation of the sexually abused child. *Pediatrics.* 1986;78(3):385–398

10. Rimsza ME, Niggemann EH. Medical evaluation of sexually abused children: a review of 311 cases. *Pediatrics.* 1982;69(1):8–14

11. White ST, Ingram DL, Lyna PR. Vaginal introital diameter in the evaluation of sexual abuse. *Child Abuse Negl.* 1989;13(2):217–224

12. Emans SJ, Goldstein DP. The gynecologic examination of the prepubertal child with vulvovaginitis: use of the knee-chest position. *Pediatrics.* 1980;65(4):758–760

13. American Professional Society on the Abuse of Children. *Descriptive Terminology in Child Sexual Abuse Medical Examinations.* Chicago, IL: American Professional Society on the Abuse of Children; 1995

14. Mahran M, Saleh AM. The microscopic anatomy of the hymen. *Anat Rec.* 1964;149:313–318

15. Pritchard JA. Anatomy of the reproductive tract of woman. In: Cunningham FG, MacDonald PC, Grant NC, eds. *Williams Obstetrics.* Norwalk, CT: Appleton-Century-Crofts; 1985

16. Gelhorn G. Anatomy, pathology and development of the hymen. *Am J Obstet Dis Women Child.* 1904;50:161

17. Skinner HA. *The Origin of Medical Terms.* Baltimore, MD: Williams & Wilkins; 1948

18. Wile IS. The psychology of the hymen. *J Nerv Ment Dis.* 1935;85:143-156

19. Ahmed S, Morris LL, Atkinson E. Distal mucocolpos and proximal hematocolpos secondary to concurrent imperforate hymen and transverse vaginal septum. *J Pediatr Surg.* 1999;34(10):1555–1556

20. Deuterman JL, Gabby SL. Imperforate hymen. *Ill Med J.* 1942;82:161

21. Schneider K, Hong J, Fong J, Sanders CG. Hematocolpos as an easily overlooked diagnosis. *Curr Opin Pediatr.* 1999;11(3):249–252

22. Berenson A, Heger A, Andrews S. Appearance of the hymen in newborns. *Pediatrics.* 1991;87(4):458–465

23. Berenson AB. A longitudinal study of hymenal morphology in the first 3 years of life. *Pediatrics.* 1995;95(4):490–496

24. Jenny C, Kuhns ML, Arakawa F. Hymens in newborn female infants. *Pediatrics.* 1987;80(3):399–400

25. Berenson AB, Heger AH, Hayes JM, Bailey RK, Emans SJ. Appearance of the hymen in prepubertal girls. *Pediatrics.* 1992;89(3):387–394

26. Goldstein AM, Cook TW. Unusual hymenal perforations appearing as Skene's ducts. *J Urol.* 1977;117(2):264–265

27. Mor N, Merlob P. Configuration of the hymen. *Am J Obstet Gynecol.* 1989;160(5 Pt 1):1253–1264

28. McCann J. Use of the colposcope in childhood sexual abuse examinations. *Pediatr Clin North Am.* 1990;37(4):863–880

29. Merlob P, Bahari C, Liban E, Reisner SH. Cysts of the female external genitalia in the newborn infant. *Am J Obstet Gynecol.* 1978;132(6):607–610

30. Mor N, Merlob P, Reisner SH. Tags and bands of the female external genitalia in the newborn infant. *Clin Pediatr.* 1983;22(2):122–124

31. Mor N, Merlob P, Reisner SH. Types of hymen in the newborn infant. *Eur J Obstet Gynecol Reprod Biol.* 1986;22(4):225–228

32. Pokorny SF. Configuration of the prepubertal hymen. *Am J Obstet Gynecol.* 1987;157(4 Pt 1):950–956

33. Emans SJ, Woods ER, Flagg NT, Freeman A. Genital findings in sexually abused, symptomatic and asymptomatic, girls. *Pediatrics.* 1987;79(5):778–785

34. Gardner JJ. Descriptive study of genital variation in healthy, nonabused premenarchal girls. *J Pediatr.* 1992;120(2 Pt 1):251–257

35. Goff CW, Burke KR, Rickenback C, Buebendorf DP. Vaginal opening measurement in prepubertal girls. *Am J Dis Child.* 1989;143(11):1366–1368

36. Paradise JE. Predictive accuracy and the diagnosis of sexual abuse: a big issue about a little tissue. *Child Abuse Negl.* 1989;13(2):169–176

37. Finkel MA. Medical examination in alleged sexual abuse of children. In: Governor's Task Force on Child Abuse, ed. *Child Abuse: A Professional's Guide to the Identification, Reporting, Investigation and Treatment.* Trenton, NJ: Governor's Task Force on Child Abuse; 1988

38. Britton H. Emotional impact of the medical examination for child sexual abuse. *Child Abuse Negl.* 1998;22(6):573–579

39. Lynch L, Faust J. Reduction of distress in children undergoing sexual abuse medical examination. *J Pediatr.* 1998;133(2):296–299

40. Parker RI, Mahan RA, Giugliano D, Parker MM. Efficacy and safety of intravenous midazolam and ketamine as sedation for therapeutic and diagnostic procedures in children. *Pediatrics.* 1997;99(3):427–431

41. Yaster M, Maxwell LG. The pediatric sedation unit: a mechanism for safe sedation. *Pediatrics.* 1999;103(1):198–199; author reply 200–221

42. Finkel MA. Technical conduct of the child sexual abuse medical examination. *Child Abuse Negl.* 1998;22(6):555–566

43. Ricci LR. Medical forensic photography of the sexually abused child. *Child Abuse Negl.* 1988;12(3):305–310

44. Ricci LR. Photographing the physically abused child. Principles and practice. *Am J Dis Child.* 1991;145(3):275–281

45. Mears CJ, Heflin AH, Finkel MA, Deblinger E, Steer RA. Adolescents' responses to sexual abuse evaluation including the use of video colposcopy. *J Adolesc Health.* 2003;33(1):18–24

46. Sanfilippo JS. The editor's workshop: sexual abuse—to colposcope or not? *Adolesc Pediatr Gynecol.* 1990;3(2):63–64

47. Teixeira WR. Hymenal colposcopic examination in sexual offenses. *Am J Forensic Med Pathol.* 1981;2(3):209–215

48. Woodling BA, Heger A. The use of the colposcope in the diagnosis of sexual abuse in the pediatric age group. *Child Abuse Negl.* 1986;10(1):111–114

49. De Jong AR, Hervada AR, Emmett GA. Epidemiologic variations in childhood sexual abuse. *Child Abuse Negl.* 1983;7(2):155–162

50. Kernbach G, Puschel K, Brinkmann B. Extragenital injuries in rape [in German]. *Geburtshilfe und Frauenheilkunde.* 1984;44(10):643–650

51. Sweet DJ. Bite mark evidence—human bite marks: examination, recovery, and analysis. In: Bowers CM, Bell GL, eds. *Manual of Forensic Odontology.* Colorado Springs, CO: American Society of Forensic Odontology; 1995:118–137

52. Gabby T, Winkleby MA, Boyce WT, Fisher DL, Lancaster A, Sensabaugh GF. Sexual abuse of children. The detection of semen on skin. *Am J Dis Child.* 1992;146(6):700–703

53. Santucci KA, Kennedy KM, Duffy SJ. Wood's lamp utility in the differentiation between semen and commonly applied medicaments. *Pediatrics.* 1998;102:718

54. Santucci KA, Nelson DG, McQuillen KK, Duffy SJ, Linakis JG. Wood's lamp utility in the identification of semen. *Pediatrics.* 1999;104(6):1342–1344

55. American Board of Forensic Odontology. Guidelines for bite mark analysis. *J Am Dental Assoc.* 1986;112(3):383–386

56. American Academy of Pediatrics Committee on Child Abuse and Neglect, American Academy of Pediatric Dentistry Ad Hoc Work Group on Child Abuse and Neglect. Oral and dental aspects of child abuse and neglect. *Pediatrics.* 1999;104(2 Pt 1):348–350

57. Schleisinger SL, Barbotsina J, ONeill L. Petechial hemorrhages of the soft palate secondary to fellatio. *Oral Surg Oral Med Oral Pathol.* 1975;40(3):376–378

58. Atabaki S, Paradise JE. The medical evaluation of the sexually abused child: lessons from a decade of research. *Pediatrics.* 1999;104(1):178

59. Cantwell HB. Vaginal inspection as it relates to child sexual abuse in girls under thirteen. *Child Abuse Negl.* 1981;7:545–546

60. McCann J, Voris J. Perianal injuries resulting from sexual abuse: a longitudinal study. *Pediatrics.* 1993;91(2):390–397

61. Clayden GS. Reflex anal dilatation associated with severe chronic constipation in children. *Arch Dis Child.* 1988;63(7):832–836

62. Hobbs CJ, Wynne JM. Buggery in childhood—a common syndrome of child abuse. *Lancet.* 1986;2(8510):792–796

63. Hobbs CJ, Wynne JM. Sexual abuse of English boys and girls: the importance of anal examination. *Child Abuse Negl.* 1989;13(2):195–210

64. Holmes WC, Slap GB. Sexual abuse of boys: definition, prevalence, correlates, sequelae, and management. *JAMA.* 1998;280(21):1855–1862

65. Stanton A, Sunderland R. Prevalence of reflex anal dilatation in 200 children. *BMJ.* 1989;298(6676):802–803

66. Adams JA, Harper K, Knudson S, Revilla J. Examination findings in legally confirmed child sexual abuse: it's normal to be normal. *Pediatrics.* 1994;94(3):310–317

67. Adams JA, Knudson S. Genital findings in adolescent girls referred for suspected sexual abuse. *Arch Pediatr Adolesc Med.* 1996;150(8):850–857

68. Berkowitz CD. Medical consequences of child sexual abuse. *Child Abuse Negl.* 1998;22(6):541–550; discussion 551–554

69. Kellogg ND, Parra JM, Menard S. Children with anogenital symptoms and signs referred for sexual abuse evaluations. *Arch Pediatr Adolesc Med.* 1998;152(7):634–641

70. Muram D. Child sexual abuse: relationship between sexual acts and genital findings. *Child Abuse Negl.* 1989;13(2):211–216

71. Muram D. Anal and perianal abnormalities in prepubertal victims of sexual abuse. *Am J Obstet Gynecol.* 1989;161(2):278–281

72. Berenson AB, Chacko MR, Wiemann CM, Mishaw CO, Friedrich WN, Grady JJ. A case-control study of anatomic changes resulting from sexual abuse. *Am J Obstet Gynecol.* 2000;182(4):820–831; discussion 831–834

73. Christian CW, Lavelle JM, De Jong AR, Loiselle J, Brenner L, Joffe M. Forensic evidence findings in prepubertal victims of sexual assault. *Pediatrics.* 2000;106(1 Pt 1):100–104

74. Finkel MA. Anogenital trauma in sexually abused children. *Pediatrics.* 1989;84(2):317–322

75. Heppenstall-Heger A, McConnell G, Ticson L, Guerra L, Lister J, Zaragoza T. Healing patterns in anogenital injuries: a longitudinal study of injuries associated with sexual abuse, accidental injuries, or genital surgery in the preadolescent child. *Pediatrics.* 2003;112(4):829–837

76. McCann J, Miyamoto S, Boyle C, Rogers K. Healing of hymenal injuries in prepubertal and adolescent girls: a descriptive study. *Pediatrics.* 2007;119(5):e1094–e1106

77. Baker RB. Seat belt injury masquerading as sexual abuse. *Pediatrics.* 1986;77(3):435

78. Bond GR, Dowd MD, Landsman I, Rimsza M. Unintentional perineal injury in prepubescent girls: a multicenter, prospective report of 56 girls. *Pediatrics.* 1995;95(5):628–631

79. Boos SC. Accidental hymenal injury mimicking sexual trauma. *Pediatrics.* 1999;103(6 Pt 1):1287–1290

80. Dowd MD, Fitzmaurice L, Knapp JF, Mooney D. The interpretation of urogenital findings in children with straddle injuries. *J Pediatr Surg.* 1994;29(1):7–10

81. Greaney H, Ryan J. Straddle injuries—is current practice safe? *Eur J Emerg Med.* 1998;5(4):421–424

82. Kadish HA, Schunk JE, Britton H. Pediatric male rectal and genital trauma: accidental and nonaccidental injuries. *Pediatr Emerg Care.* 1998;14(2):95–98

83. Waltzman ML, Shannon M, Bowen AP, Bailey MC. Monkeybar injuries: complications of play. *Pediatrics.* 1999;103(5):e58

84. Sgroi SM. *Handbook of Clinical Intervention in Child Sexual Abuse.* Lexington, MA: Lexington Books; 1982

85. Finkel MA. The medical evaluation of child sexual abuse. In: Schetky DH, Green AH, eds. *Child Sexual Abuse: A Handbook for Healthcare and Legal Professionals.* New York, NY: Brunner/Mazel; 1988:82–103

86. McCann J. The appearance of acute, healing, and healed anogenital trauma. *Child Abuse Negl.* 1998;22(6):605–615; discussion 617–622

87. McCann J, Voris J, Simon M. Genital injuries resulting from sexual abuse: a longitudinal study. *Pediatrics.* 1992;89(2):307–317

88. Adams JA, Kaplan RA, Starling SP, et al. Guidelines for medical care of children who may have been sexually abused. *J Pediatr Adolesc Gynecol.* 2007;20(3):163–172

89. Myers JEB. *Evidence in Child Abuse and Neglect Cases.* 3rd ed. New York, NY: John Wiley; 1997

90. DeLago C, Deblinger ED, Schroeder C, Finkel MA. Girls who disclose sexual abuse: urogenital symptoms and signs following sexual contact. *Pediatrics.* 2008;122(8):e221–226

91. Finkel MA. "I can tell you because you're a doctor." Commentary on girls who disclose sexual abuse: signs and symptoms following genital contact. The importance of the pediatricians detailed medical history when evaluating suspected child sexual abuse. *Pediatrics.* 2008;122(8):422

92. Klevan JL, De Jong AR. Urinary tract symptoms and urinary tract infection following sexual abuse. *Am J Dis Child.* 1990;144(2):242–244

93. Reinhart MA. Urinary tract infection in sexually abused children. *Clin Pediatr.* 1987;26(9):470–472

94. Damm DD, White DK, Brinker CM. Variations of palatal erythema secondary to fellatio. *Oral Surg Oral Med Oral Pathol.* 1981;52(4):417–421

95. Macklin M. Honeymoon cystitis. *N Engl J Med.* 1978;298(18):1035

96. Olsen AM. The goose, the gander, and honeymoon cystitis. *JAMA.* 1986;256(21):2963

97. Roy JB. Intercourse cystitis. *Hawaii Med J.* 1974;33(11):418–419

98. Adams JA, Ahmad M, Philips P. Anogenital findings and hymenal diameter in children referred for sexual abuse examination. *Adolesc Pediatr Gynecol.* 1988(1):123–127

99. Adams JA, Girardin B, Faugno D. Signs of genital trauma in adolescent rape victims examined acutely. *J Pediatr Adolesc Gynecol.* 2000;13(2):88

100. Biggs M, Stermac LE, Divinsky M. Genital injuries following sexual assault of women with and without prior sexual intercourse experience. *CMAJ.* 1998;159(1):33–37

101. Kerns DL, Ritter ML, Thomas RG. Concave hymenal variations in suspected child sexual abuse victims. *Pediatrics.* 1992;90(2 Pt 1):265–272

102. Slaughter L, Brown CR, Crowley S, Peck R. Patterns of genital injury in female sexual assault victims. *Am J Obstet Gynecol.* 1997;176(3):609–616

103. Paul DM. The medical examination in sexual offences. *Med Sci Law.* 1975;15(3):154–162

104. Weis DL. The experience of pain during women's first sexual intercourse: cultural mythology about female sexual initiation. *Arch Sex Behav.* 1985;14(5):421–438

105. Whitley N. The first coital experience of one hundred women. *JOGN Nurs.* 1978;7(4):41–45

106. Palmer CM, McNulty AM, D'Este C, Donovan B. Genital injuries in women reporting sexual assault. *Sex Health.* 2004;1(1):55–59

107. White C, McLean I. Adolescent complainants of sexual assault; injury patterns in virgin and non-virgin groups. *J Clin Forensic Med.* 2006;13(4):172–180

108. Kellogg ND, Menard SW, Santos A. Genital anatomy in pregnant adolescents: "normal" does not mean "nothing happened." *Pediatrics.* 2004;113(1 Pt 1):e67–e69

109. Donald TG. Pediatric male rectal and genital trauma: accidental and nonaccidental injuries [comment]. *Pediatr Emerg Care.* 1998;14(6):452–453

110. Feigen GM. Proctologic disorders in sex deviants. *Calif Med.* 1954;81(2):79–83

111. Feigen GM, Kilpatrick ZM. Morbidity caused by anal intercourse. *Med Aspects Hum Sex.* 1974;8(6):177–186

112. Paparo GP, Siegel H. Histologic diagnosis of sodomy. *J Forensic Sci.* 1979;24(4):772–774

113. McLean IA, Balding V, White C. Forensic medical aspects of male-on-male rape and sexual assault in greater Manchester. *Med Sci Law.* 2004;44(2):165–169

114. Paul DM. What really did happen to Baby Jane?—the medical aspects of the investigation of alleged sexual abuse of children. *Med Sci Law.* 1986;26(2):85–102

115. Rothwell BR. Bite marks in forensic dentistry: a review of legal, scientific issues. *J Am Dent Assoc.* 1995;126(2):223–232

116. Heger A, Emans SJ. Introital diameter as the criterion for sexual abuse [comment]. *Pediatrics.* 1990;85(2):222–223

117. Boos SC, Rosas AJ, Boyle C, McCann J. Anogenital injuries in child pedestrians run over by low-speed motor vehicles: 4 cases with findings that mimic child sexual abuse. *Pediatrics.* 2003;112(1 Pt 1):e77–e84

118. Finkelstein E, Amichai B, Jaworowski S, Mukamel M. Masturbation in prepubescent children: a case report and review of the literature. *Child Care Health Dev.* 1996;22(5):323–326

119. Schoon DL. Practical pediatrics: readers view on masturbation [letter to the editor]. *Pediatr News.* 1988;22:41

120. Leung AK, Robson WL. Childhood masturbation. *Clin Pediatr.* 1993;32(4):238–241

Appendix

When Sexual Abuse Is Suspected:
Common Concerns About the Medical Examination

The CARES Institute is a specialized facility that provides both medical and mental health examinations and treatment for children suspected of being sexually abused. Our doctors, pediatric nurse practitioner, social worker, and psychologists have specialized expertise to assist children and their parents in addressing the many concerns when abuse is suspected. Examinations are also conducted for children when abuse is not a consideration, but when there are other medical and psychological concerns. The techniques that the institute's professionals use to examine and meet the medical and mental health needs of child victims are state of the art.

The following information will help answer the many questions that parents have regarding the medical evaluation when there is suspected sexual abuse. Institute doctors and our pediatric nurse practitioner are always available to answer any specific concerns that may not be addressed below.

1. Why does my child have to go through one more thing after he/she has been through so much?

   - The medical examination is a very important aspect in evaluating concerns of child sexual abuse. The physical examination can identify both new and old injuries, test for sexually transmitted infections, and collect evidence of sexual contact. Children and adolescents often express worries about their bodies following sexual abuse. This examination is designed to answer all of these questions as well as reassure the child and family regarding the child's well-being.

2. My child just told me about what happened. The last time he/she was touched that way was more than a year ago. Is there still a need for an examination?

   - Yes. Most children tell about the experiences of sexual abuse either accidentally or at some time after the contact, when they feel safe. Many children have worries about their bodies after being touched. These worries can be best addressed through an examination, even if the last contact was a long time ago. Some children have experienced injuries that have healed and that can be seen with the use of special equipment.

3. Will this examination be uncomfortable for my child?

    - Our doctors and pediatric nurse practitioner understand the fears and worries that children of all ages may have when having something new happen to them. We take every effort to explain exactly what will happen as well as answer all of their questions. We want the physical examination to be a positive experience for the child. The examination itself rarely causes any physical discomfort for the child. Some children will need blood work when sexually transmitted infections are suspected. Blood is drawn at a laboratory at a different office within our building.

4. Is this the same as an adult female gynecologic examination with a vaginal speculum and internal?

    - In a child who has not yet had her period, the examination is completed without the use of internal instruments. The examination of a child who has not reached puberty is one that involves the doctor looking at the child's private areas. In the child who has begun her period, the examination may involve the use of a speculum made especially for the young adolescent. Not every adolescent victim of sexual abuse requires a complete pelvic examination.

5. Will the doctor/nurse be able to tell if there was vaginal penetration?

    - This is a very common concern of parents. In a child who has not yet had her period, this examination will be able to tell if there has been penetration into the vagina. Determining whether vaginal penetration has occurred in the adolescent is not always possible.

6. As part of the examination, the doctor uses a special machine called a *colposcope*. Why does this examination need to be done with a colposcope?

    - The colposcope is nothing more than a fancy magnifying glass with a strong light that assists the doctor/nurse in seeing the smallest injuries, whether recent or healed. This machine does not touch the child but illuminates the child's private areas during the examination. A very special part of this light is its connection to a television so both the child and parent can see what is being done. The ability of a child to actually watch the examination and have a sense of participation and control throughout the examination helps to relax the child, making the examination a comfortable one. This machine also allows for the recording of findings, assuring the child that there will be no need to undergo this examination again should anyone question the meaning of examination findings.

        The examination of a child's private parts is only one part of the complete head-to-toe examination. We want the child to know that all parts of his or her body are important, and thus the examination is done with this in mind. The examination not only helps us diagnose and treat any medical problems, but also lets the child know that his or her body can still be OK, no matter what might have happened.

7. How is the examination of a boy different from that of a girl?
   - Boys have many of the same concerns that girls do when touched inappropriately. Boys are examined with the same sensitivity and concern for their well-being. Their examination differs in that they can have injuries to the penis and/or anus. Although anal and penile injuries are unusual, we use the colposcope in the same manner to see fresh and old injuries. Sometimes we need to use a small instrument to look into the anus to see if there are injuries inside. Most of the time, looking inside is not necessary. Boys are examined head to toe as well and tested for sexually transmitted infections if needed.

8. Will I be able to be with my child throughout the physical examination?
   - Yes. We want you to be there to comfort your child. You will have an opportunity to observe all aspects of the examination. Some adolescents prefer privacy and request a female assistant in the room rather than having a parent present. When adolescents express a desire for privacy, we attempt to accommodate their request.

9. Why can't my family physician/pediatrician or gynecologist do the examination? My child knows that physician and is familiar with his/her office.
   - This examination requires knowledge of the ways in which children experience sexual victimization. The examination is best done by someone who has both the experience in caring for children suspected of being abused and the special skills and equipment necessary to conduct the examination. The medical examination of sexually abused children is an area of pediatrics that requires special training. Just as an individual who has a problem with his or her heart seeks a heart doctor, a child suspected of being abused will be best evaluated by a doctor or nurse specifically trained to conduct this assessment.

10. Will they test my child for sexually transmitted infections?
    - Some children who experience sexually inappropriate contact can acquire a sexually transmitted infection. Each child is assessed individually for the need to test for sexually transmitted infections. Some sexually transmitted infections may be seen through a physical examination, some with the use of cultures, and others through blood tests. When a sexually transmitted infection is identified, institute doctors will initiate treatment/referral and follow-up. Fortunately, the likelihood of a child contracting a sexually transmitted infection is quite low.

11. Will the doctor/nurse testify in court if needed?

- Yes. Our doctors/nurse will cooperate fully with all legal proceedings and testify in any civil or criminal matter as required.

12. Will the doctor/nurse need to speak to my child?

- Yes. Children sometimes express concerns about their body when they have experienced inappropriate sexual contact. The doctor/nurse can address these worries and offer information that is often reassuring to children.

13. I am very concerned about my child. Will I be able to talk to the doctor/nurse alone either before or after the examination?

- Yes. The doctor/nurse will speak with you before the examination. We will explain what will happen, answer any immediate questions, review your child's medical history, and hear your understanding of what your child might have experienced of a sexually inappropriate nature. After the examination, the results will be discussed, follow-up recommendations will be made, and you will be allowed to ask any additional questions.

14. Will my child be sedated for the examination?

- No. Most children are very cooperative for the examination because the doctor/nurse explains exactly what will happen to the child and encourages the child to ask questions and express any fears or worries. Our experience suggests that children who fully understand what they will experience, are provided choices, and have a sense of participation throughout the examination readily cooperate for the examination. Some children are emotionally not ready for the examination. In such cases, the examination will be delayed until the child is ready and willing to cooperate. An examination will be done only with a child's consent and cooperation.

15. Who will follow my child if he/she needs treatment for injuries or a sexually transmitted infection?

- If your child needs treatment for a sexually transmitted infection, we will initiate it and provide follow-up as well, except in unusual circumstances in which a pediatric infectious disease expert is appropriate. Any injuries will be seen in follow-up to ensure complete healing.

16. Will the doctor provide a written report to child protective services and law enforcement about his or her findings?

- After seeing your child, a full and detailed report will be completed and provided to the appropriate authorities.

17. What happens after the examination? Can the institute help me deal with my child's mental health needs?

    - Although addressing the medical concerns of your child is very important, it is just as important that your child see a mental health specialist to help him/her address any worries and concerns. The institute has professionals capable of providing both evaluative and treatment services to child and adolescent victims as well as helping parents deal with their child's experience. Evidence-based treatment approaches such as trauma focused-cognitive behavioral therapy have been demonstrated to be very effective in helping children overcome the trauma of sexual abuse.

Colpophotographic Case Studies

The colpophotographic case studies that follow demonstrate the spectrum of normal and abnormal physical findings seen in children being evaluated for possible sexual abuse.

Case studies are used to demonstrate the following:

1. Anatomical variations of the female genital anatomy   Photos 1–29

2. Variations in the appearance of genital tissues
   due to examination position and techniques   Photos 30–36

3. Acute and healed genital trauma cases   Photos 37–46

4. Normal anal examination cases   Photos 47–58

5. Anal trauma: acute and healed   Photos 59–68

6. Male genital trauma cases   Photos 69–72

7. Accidental genital trauma cases   Photos 73–80

8. Extragenital trauma cases   Photos 81–83

All images were obtained using a Cryomedics MM 6000 colposcope with beam splitter and a Nikon camera with a 100ASA Ektachrome.

Anatomical Variations of the Female Genital Anatomy, Photos 1–29

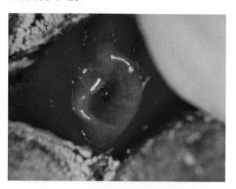

PHOTO 1
Newborn hymen demonstrating estrogen effect.

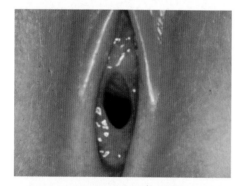

PHOTO 2
Annular, flared, and thickened appearance to hymen of a 15-month-old.

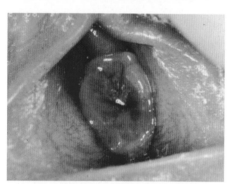

PHOTO 3
Annular configuration to hymenal orifice in an 8-year-old. Note the well-demarcated, uninterrupted edge of the hymen circumferentially. Slight hyperemia in fossa and asymmetry of fourchette are normal findings.

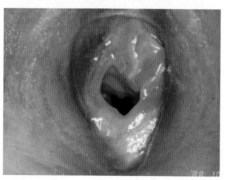

PHOTO 4
Annular hymen with anterior redundant tissue most prominent between 12 and 2 o'clock. The irregular appearance of the edge of the membrane with a slight dip at the 6 o'clock position and a bump at the 7 o'clock position are both normal findings.

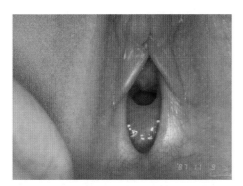

PHOTO 5
Crescentic hymenal orifice in a 4-year-old.

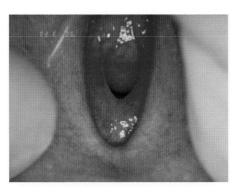

PHOTO 6
Crescentic hymen with anterior flaps creating impression of annular configuration. Note fine, lacy, symmetrical vascular pattern on vestibular aspect of hymen and increased vascularity in the sulci.

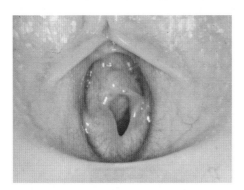

PHOTO 7
Crescentic hymen demonstrating sharp, well-delineated, uninterrupted margins with attachments at 11 and 1 o'clock. The membrane edge is translucent.

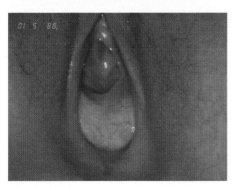

PHOTO 8
Early estrogen effect in a child in sexual maturaty rating (Tanner stage) 2 resulting in decreased vascularity of crescentic hymen. Note small laceration at the fourchette, which is the result of labial separation and traction.

Anatomical Variations of the Female Genital Anatomy, Photos 1–29, continued

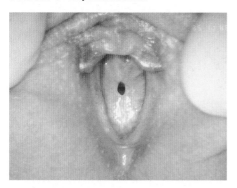

PHOTO 9
Annular hymenal orifice in a 3-year-old. Note that the labia minora have a butterfly appearance and attach to the labia majora at the 11 and 2 o'clock positions.

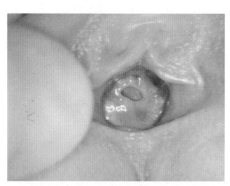

PHOTO 10
Anteriorly placed annular orifice in a 7-year-old. Note translucency of membrane between 4 and 5 o'clock. The hymen may vary considerably in regard to its thickness, and thus translucency, as well as its elasticity.

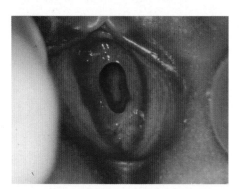

PHOTO 11
Annular hymen with small, slightly raised, ovoid lymphoid follicles in fossa navicularis. Lymphoid follicles are of no clinical significance.

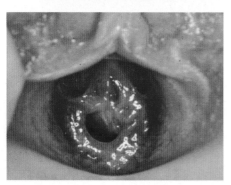

PHOTO 12
Crescentic hymenal orifice in a 5-year-old with redundant tissue in superior quadrants. With traction, pubo-urethral supporting ligaments form the margins of the periurethral pockets noted lateral to the meatus.

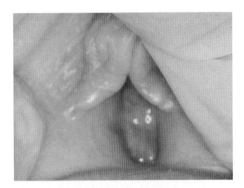

PHOTO 13
An 18-month-old hymen without a visible orifice. Hymen is microperforate. If imperforate, the hymen would bulge secondary to mucocolpos.

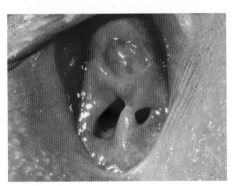

A

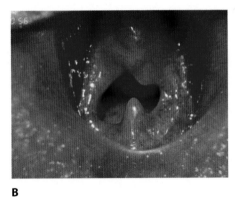

B

PHOTO 14
A. Appearance of "septum" secondary to hymenal projection at the 6 o'clock position adhering to tissue at 1 o'clock. **B.** With persistent traction, cohesive force of moist tissue is broken and prominent projection noted at 6 o'clock

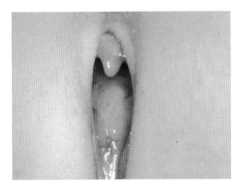

PHOTO 15
Projection of hymenal tissue at the 6 o'clock position. Knee-chest position assists in visualizing projection, which is an extension of a longitudinal column. In the supine position, this projection may appear less prominent when folded into the vagina.

Anatomical Variations of the Female Genital Anatomy, Photos 1–29, continued

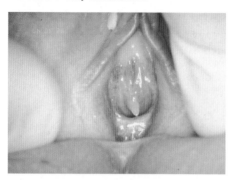

PHOTO 16
Tag projecting from anterior vaginal wall below urethra.

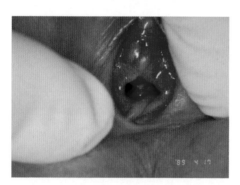

PHOTO 17
Hymenal tag in a 6-year-old prolapsed into the fossa navicularis. Tag originates from a longitudinal intravaginal column.

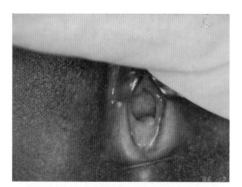

PHOTO 18
Hymenal tag prolapsed over edge of hymen originating as extension of intravaginal column.

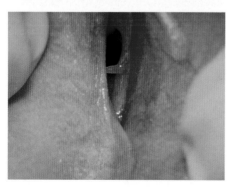

PHOTO 19
Hymenal tags can be found at any location around the edge of the hymen. This tag, noted at the 3 o'clock position, is somewhat unusual because most are found between 5 and 7 o'clock.

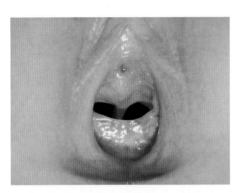

PHOTO 20
Intravaginal septum in this 7-year-old is unusual because most will be attached to the inner aspect of the hymenal membrane.

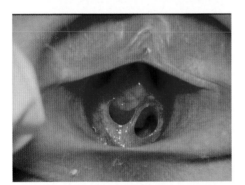

PHOTO 21
Intravaginal septum, which can be associated with an upper tract duplication.

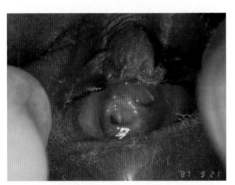

PHOTO 22
Septate hymen secondary to incomplete cannulization of urogenital septum (hymen).

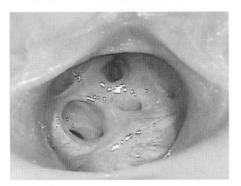

PHOTO 23
Multiple openings as a result of a distal mullerian duct malformation.

Anatomical Variations of the Female Genital Anatomy, Photos 1–29, continued

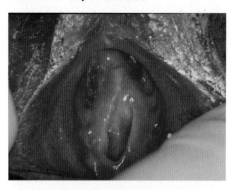

PHOTO 24
Scalloped appearance of pubo-urethral supporting ligaments. Labial traction improves recognition of ligaments. Ligaments should not be interpreted as bands of scar tissue or synechae. Supporting ligaments may also be observed laterally or inferiorly. When so noted, they are referred to as pubo-vaginal and pubo-rectal ligaments, respectively.

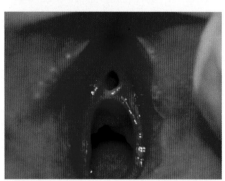

PHOTO 25
Urethral dilation with traction and narrow rim of hymenal tissue circumferentially. The limited amount of hymenal tissue should not be interpreted as attenuated without knowledge of a preexisting condition. Nonspecific erythema is present.

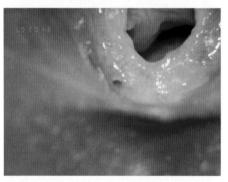

PHOTO 26
Congenital pit of no clinical significance at the 7 o'clock position in a 10-year-old.

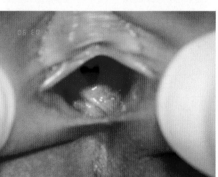

PHOTO 27
External ridge traversing hymen from 8 to 5 o'clock. This is a normal finding and should not be interpreted as a band of scar tissue.

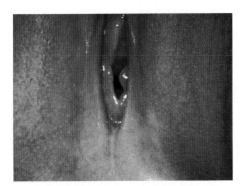

PHOTO 28
Linea vestibularis represents a midline sparing of vascularity. This finding should not be interpreted as scar tissue.

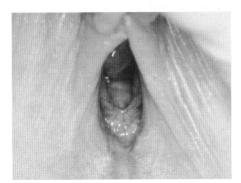

PHOTO 29
Midline blanching of fossa navicularis with labial separation. Avascular area disappears when traction is removed, which differentiates this finding from scar tissue.

**Variations in the Appearance of Genital Tissues
Due to Examination Position and Techniques, Photos 30–36**

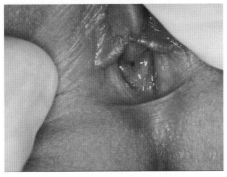

A

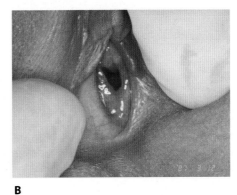

B

PHOTO 30
A. Pinpoint orifice in a 4-year-old during initial phase of examination when child is not relaxed. **B.** With relaxation, there is a significant change in the appearance of the orifice.

Variations in the Appearance of Genital Tissues
Due to Examination Position and Techniques, Photos 30–36, continued

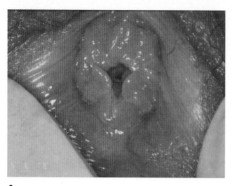 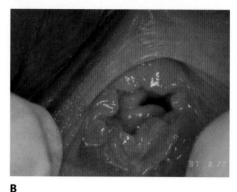

A   B

PHOTO 31
A. Multiple small clefts circumferentially create the fimbriated appearance of this
estrogenized annular hymen. The folded nature of the redundant hymen contributes
to the distensibility of membrane orifice. **B.** With traction and relaxation, the orifice
dilates. The elasticity and distensibility of the estrogenized fimbriated hymen illustrates
the difficulty in determining whether an object has penetrated into the vagina.

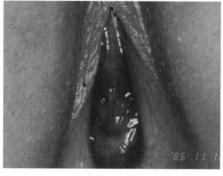 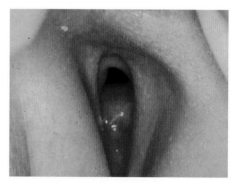

A   B

PHOTO 32
A. Orifice not fully visualized in supine position with the use of labial traction and separation.
Use of knee-chest indicated to visualize membrane edge. **B.** Crescentic appearance to hymen
in knee-chest position differs considerably from appearance in supine position. Whenever
examination is not optimal in the supine position, the knee-chest position should be used.

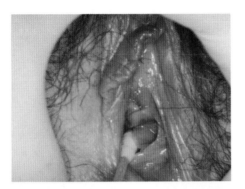

PHOTO 33
A saline-moistened cotton swab in pubertal children can be particularly helpful in defining the edge of a redundant hymenal membrane or an intravaginal structure such as the column noted above.

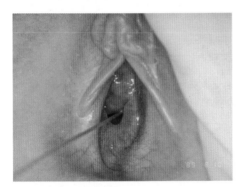

PHOTO 34
A Foley catheter passed through the hymenal orifice, inflated with air, and pulled to lay the hymenal edge on the balloon, is a technique that can be helpful in examining a redundant hymen.

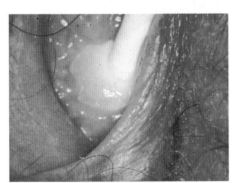

PHOTO 35
Saline-moistened urethral swabs can be readily passed through even the smallest orifice without discomfort to the child in order to obtain culture material.

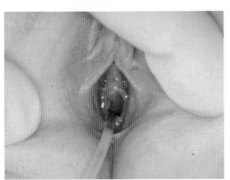

PHOTO 36
A urethral catheter can be easily passed through the orifice and into the posterior portion of the vagina and instilled with non-bacteriostatic saline to obtain washings for culture and slides. This same technique can be used for the irrigation removal of a foreign body, such as toilet paper.

Acute and Healed Genital Trauma Cases, Photos 37–46

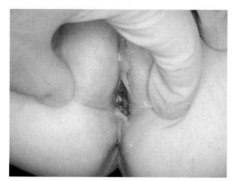

A

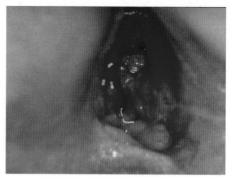

B

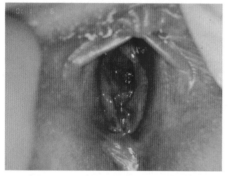

C

PHOTO 37
A. Acute injuries in a 3-year-old at 4x magnification with transection extending onto perineum presenting on day 3 following penetrating trauma by a penis. **B.** At 10x magnification, the significant trauma to the hymen, extending to the base of attachment, fossa, fourchette, and onto the perineum, can be viewed. **C.** Healed injury demonstrates clear interruption in the integrity of the hymen membrane extending to the posterior vaginal wall. The finding is diagnostic of blunt penetrating trauma in the absence of acute examination.

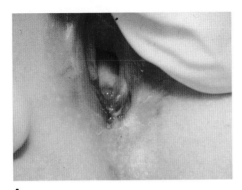
A

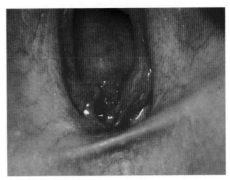
B

PHOTO 38
A. Acute blunt-force penetrating trauma to vaginal floor, hymen, fossa, and fourchette in a 23-month-old. **B.** Two-month follow-up examination demonstrates "keyhole" configuration to healed injuries.

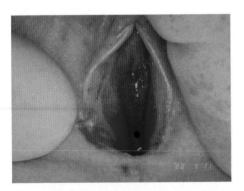

PHOTO 39
Acute injuries to the inner aspects of the labia minora and fourchette are the result of vulvar coitus. Submucosal hemorrhages are noted near fourchette. Although the child perceived the penis as going all the way inside her, the hymenal orifice is atraumatic. The child complained as well of dysuria immediately following the genital-to-genital contact, reflecting superficial trauma to the vestibular structures.

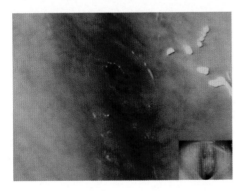

PHOTO 40
Mucosal abrasion in 4-year-old as a result of genital fondling. Red free filter enhances margins of abrasion with 10x magnification. Insert in corner demonstrates location of abrasion barely visible with naked eye.

Acute and Healed Genital Trauma Cases, Photos 37–46, continued

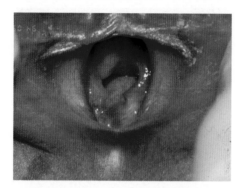

PHOTO 41
Healed transection of hymen with neovascularity in the fossa at the point where the hymen was attached to the posterior vaginal wall.

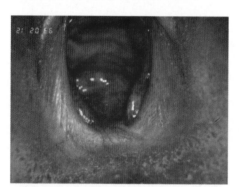

PHOTO 42
Healed transection of hymen with interruption of the hymenal membrane between the 4 and 7 o'clock positions in a 3-year-old.

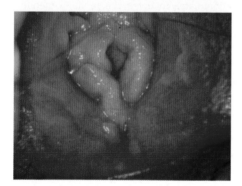

PHOTO 43
Healed transection of estrogenized hymen at 5 and 9 o'clock positions in a pregnant 13-year-old.

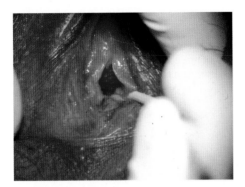

PHOTO 44
Acute transection of the hymen extending to vaginal floor as a result of penile penetration in a 14-year-old.

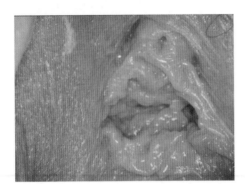

PHOTO 45
Healed transection of hymen at the 9 o'clock position in a 16-year-old severely retarded child.

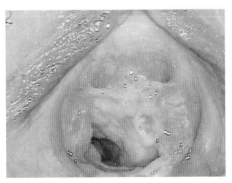

A

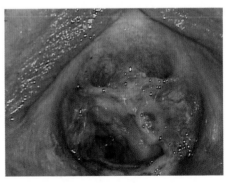

B

PHOTO 46
A. Acute superficial trauma to vaginal and vestibular mucosa. **B.** Note how the use of a red-free filter enhances visualization of injuries.

Normal Anal Examination Cases, Photos 47–58

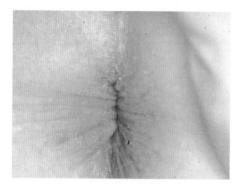

PHOTO 47
Normal anal anatomy with symmetrical radiating folds around orifice. Mild erythema, as noted, is a common non-specific finding.

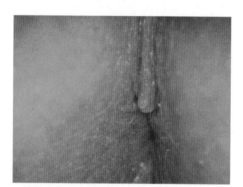

PHOTO 48
Prominent median raphe extending onto the external anal verge tissue interrupting the symmetry of anal rugae.

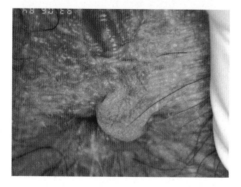

PHOTO 49
Anal tag in an adolescent. Anal tags interrupt the symmetry of the perianal skin folds. Tag present since birth.

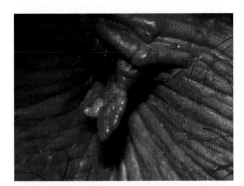

PHOTO 50
Unusual verruciform appearance of a
congenital anal tag in adolescent.

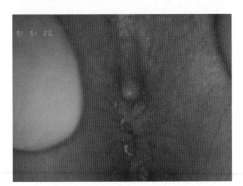

PHOTO 51
Diastasis ani is a congenital defect and is
the result of the crossing of underlying
corrugator ani muscle fibers, creating a
depressed smooth area at either the 6 or
the 12 o'clock position.

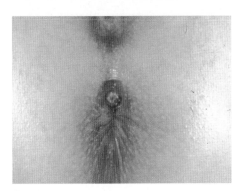

A   **B**

PHOTO 52
A. Congenital midline fusion defect creating concavity at 12 o'clock. **B.** At 10x magnification,
the mucosal nature of the midline fusion defect is more apparent.

Normal Anal Examination Cases, Photos 47–58, continued

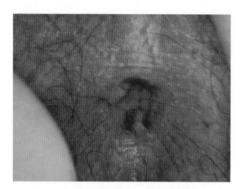

PHOTO 53
Dilated anus provides view of pectinate line, which is the demarcation between the columnar epithelium of the rectum and the stratified epithelium of the anal canal. This line is comblike or scalloped in appearance.

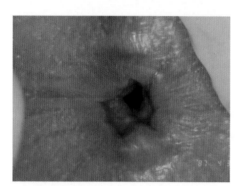

PHOTO 54
Venous pooling around dilated anus can give impression of bruising. With constriction, "bruising" disappears.

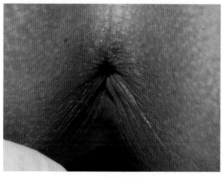

A

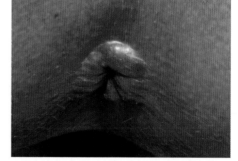

B

PHOTO 55
A. Anal verge tissues during the initial part of the examination. With time, hemorrhoidal veins dilate due to the dependent position of the anus. **B.** Venous distention can be quite prominent and confused with bruising in light-skinned children. With constriction of anus, pooling disappears.

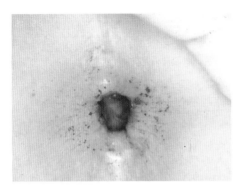

PHOTO 56
Anal dilation in a 3-year-old without stool in ampulla prior to passage of flatus.

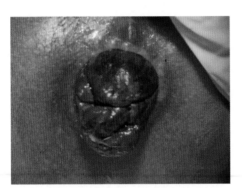

PHOTO 57
Passage of stool requires dilation of the anus. This case illustrates that a 4-year-old child can pass a stool of large diameter without injury to the sphincter. The diameter of the extruded stool is greater than the diameter of an adult male finger.

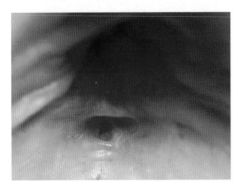

PHOTO 58
Congenital, asymptomatic, perianal pit in a 4-year-old.

Anal Trauma: Acute and Healed, Photos 59–68

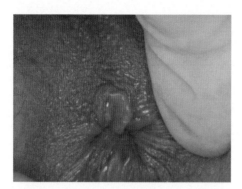

PHOTO 59
Posttraumatic anal tag at 11 o'clock
and healing laceration at 6 o'clock
in a 14-year-old.

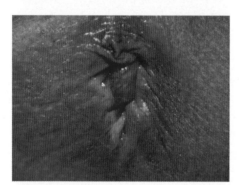

PHOTO 60
Acute lacerations, ecchymosis, and tissue
edema to anal verge and distal anorectal
canal following sodomy in a 6-year-old
female. Anus dilated without separation of
buttocks.

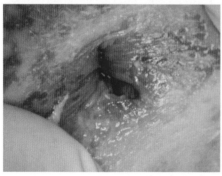

A

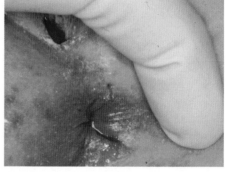

B

PHOTO 61
A. Acute laceration on day 2 following penetration with penis in a 2-year-old. **B.** Laceration
1 week postinjury, with marked decrease in tissue swelling.

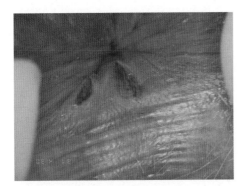

PHOTO 62
Two small lacerations of anal verge in a
12-year-old observed 2 days following
attempted anal penetration.

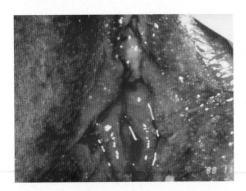

A

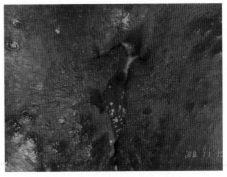

B

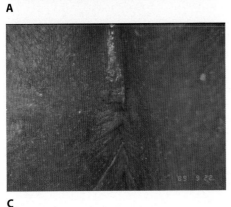

C

PHOTO 63
A. Prolapsed edematous rectal tissue after surgical repair of complete transection of anal
sphincter in a 5-year-old male. **B.** Appearance 6 days postrepair, with markedly reduced tissue
edema and constriction of anal sphincter. **C.** Almost imperceptible scar tissue hidden in rugal
fold at 11 o'clock position almost 1 year following surgical repairs illustrates how difficult it can
be to interpret healed residua retrospectively.

Anal Trauma: Acute and Healed, Photos 59–68, continued

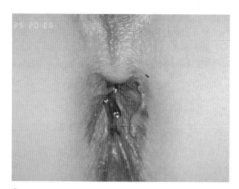
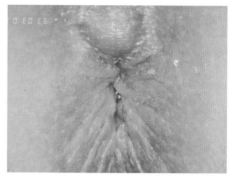

A   B

PHOTO 64
A. Three-year-old male within 24 hours of sodomy, with lacerations of anal verge tissue, bruising, and tissue edema. **B.** Two-month follow-up demonstrates marked decrease in swelling, resorption of bruising, and normalization of anal anatomy with the exception of healed laceration at 6 o'clock.

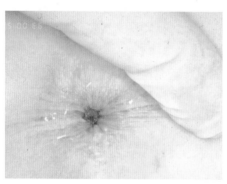
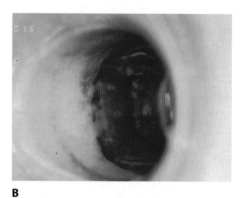

A   B

PHOTO 65
A. A 12-year-old following disclosure of anal penetration 1 day prior to examination. Complaint of blood on stool and burning sensation with passage of stool following sodomy. **B.** Anoscopy demonstrates marked erythema of anorectal canal and superficial mucosal abrasions. During anoscopy, child stated that the feeling of anoscopy was similar to when he was penetrated with a penis.

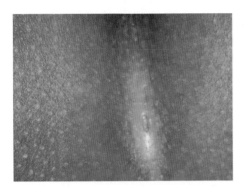

PHOTO 66
Small healing abrasion in gluteal cleft of an 11-year-old male secondary to rubbing from the convex side of the shaft of a penis. Some children refer to this form of sexual contact as "freaking."

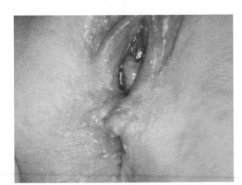

PHOTO 67
Healed laceration extending from fossa through the fourchette, the anal verge tissues, and into the anal canal in a 7-year-old developmentally delayed child unable to provide a history of the acute event.

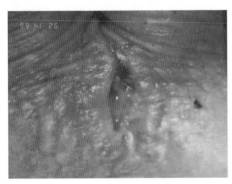

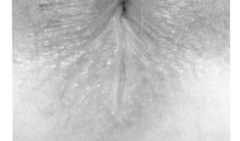

A   **B**

PHOTO 68
A. Acute laceration to anal verge without extension into the canal in a 21-month-old male after witnessed fall onto a sharp edge of a rocking horse. **B.** Laceration 1 week postinjury. Injury healing with formation of linear scar.

Male Genital Trauma Cases, Photos 69–72

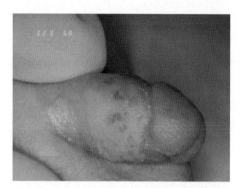

PHOTO 69
Circumferential bite mark impressions with subcutaneous bruising and superficial abrasions. Child complained of dysuria.

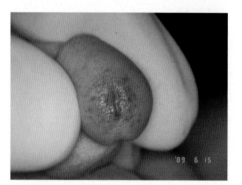

PHOTO 70
Suction petechiae to glans in a 4-year-old.

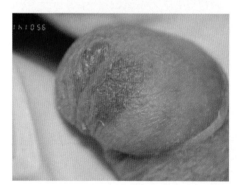

PHOTO 71
Bruising of glans in a 3-year-old due to pinching.

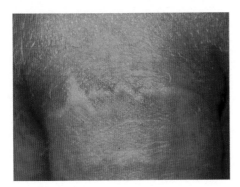

PHOTO 72
An 11-year-old sexually abused boy with healed scar around shaft of penus. Circumferential nature of injury inconsistent with history of accidental injury 4 years prior.

Accidental Genital Trauma Cases, Photos 73–80

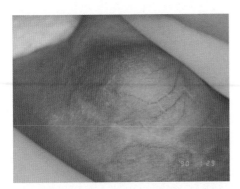

PHOTO 73
Hypopigmented scar to scrotum of a 7-year-old as the result of an accidental injury from attempting to climb over a metal fence.

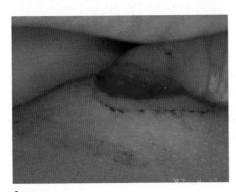

A

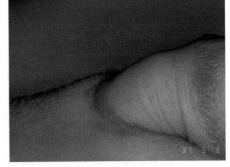

B

PHOTO 74
A. A 3-year-old with an acute laceration of dorsal aspect of penis at base secondary to being hit by a falling toilet seat. **B.** Healed laceration 1 month postinjury continues to demonstrate some neovascularity around wound edge.

Accidental Genital Trauma Cases, Photos 73–80, continued

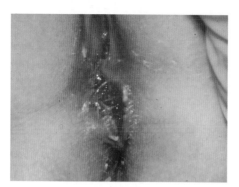

PHOTO 75
Acute accidental trauma in 2½-year-old who fell on a rocking horse. Injury extends from fourchette to just above external anal verge tissue.

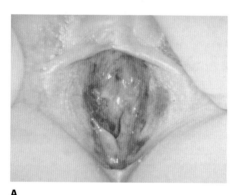

A

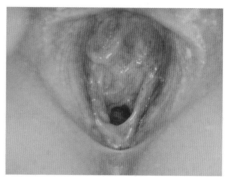

B

PHOTO 76
A. Acute accidental injury in a 3-year-old that occurred while playing slip slide in the bathtub with her twin sister. Injury due to impaling from sister's great toe as she slid down the tub with her sister's legs spread at the drain end of tub. Trauma primarily to inner aspects of labia and external surface of hymen. **B.** One-week follow-up examination shows resorption of edema and mucosal injuries. Hymenal membrane is without any residua.

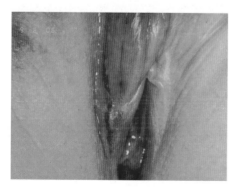

PHOTO 77
Classic unilateral, accidental crush injury to labia and mons pubis area as a result of falling on a monkey bar in school playground.

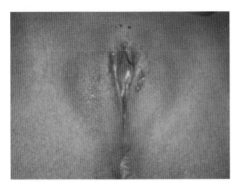

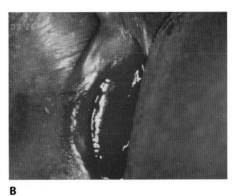

A   **B**

PHOTO 78
A. Vulvar hematoma from accidental penetrating trauma to the inner aspect of right labia minora. **B.** Laceration of inner aspect of labia minora. Hematoma bulges tissue into vestibule, obscuring hymen. With gentle displacement of hematoma, hymen visualized and atraumatic.

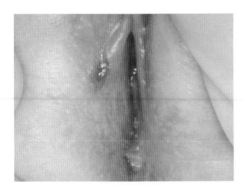

PHOTO 79
Accidental straddle injury from falling on a bicycle crossbar. Note unilateral nature of injury, with small avulsion of labia minora and perineal injury.

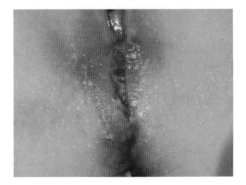

PHOTO 80
A 4-year-old with accidental superficial perineal laceration and ecchymosis incurred when falling on horizontal portion of footboard to bed.

Extragenital Trauma Cases, Photos 81–83

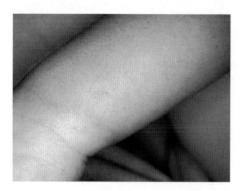

PHOTO 81
Circumferential ligature mark on the wrist of a 3-year-old as a result of being hung in a closet. The use of force and restraint that results in extragenital trauma is unusual.

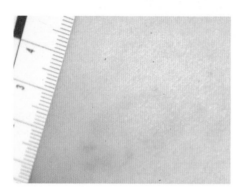

PHOTO 82
Bite mark 24 hours after injury on upper posterior thigh of a 2-year-old. Child stated that that her daddy "bit her heiney and licked her pee pee." A standardized ruler that allows for color correction is used when photographing bite marks.

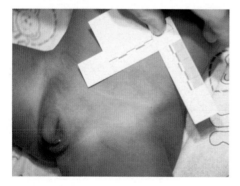

PHOTO 83
Multiple curvilinear whip marks secondary to an electrical cord.

Chapter 4

Documentation of Physical Evidence in Child Sexual Abuse

Lawrence R. Ricci

When a clinician is involved in the provision of diagnostic services to children alleged to have been abused, he or she must anticipate legal inspection and challenge. Meticulous documentation remains the best defense against such a challenge.

Modalities for documenting physical findings include written description, drawing, and photodocumentation. Written descriptions should be detailed and clear, using standardized language such as that found in the terminology guidelines of the American Professional Society on the Abuse of Children.[1] Likewise, drawings, if used, should be based on commonly accepted formats.[2,3]

Although a written description of physical findings remains an important aspect of documentation, it is incumbent on the medical provider to obtain adequate photographic documentation of visible lesions. Photodocumentation, whether still or video, provides the clearest demonstration that the findings that the examiner reports as present are, indeed, present. Some states require that reasonable efforts be made by providers "to take or cause to be taken" color photographs of any areas of visible trauma on a child.[4,5]

The advantages of photodocumentation include the following:

1. Photographs allow the clinician to obtain a second opinion of unclear findings. Absent a high-quality photograph or video, the ability to provide such an opinion is severely compromised.
2. Peer review is increasingly important in the field of child abuse diagnosis as a mechanism of education and accountability. As with a second opinion, such review is limited, if not impossible, without high-quality still or video documentation.
3. Imaging during a first visit can be compared with findings during a

repeat visit should the child evidence healing of acute lesions or should new allegations arise. However, this is not to say that all examinations must be photodocumented. Certainly all abnormal examinations should be photographed, but a number of experienced examiners are no longer photographing all normal examinations. However, some examiners will still photograph a normal examination if there is reason to believe that the child might be at risk, to establish a baseline reference if concerns arise in the future.

4. Photographic imaging can provide a record for an opposing expert to review, rather than require reexamination of the child.

5. Images provide an excellent tool to teach normal and abnormal anatomy.

6. Still photographs and videos are useful in court to demonstrate significant findings to the judge and jury. However, sexual abuse images, given their subtlety to a lay observer, are probably less useful than physical abuse images.

Photodocumentation

The traditional format for documentation of visible lesions is 35-mm still photography. Camera systems recommended for photographing the sexually abused child range from 35-mm close-up systems[6,7] to colposcope-based still and video cameras.[8–12]

Since the first edition of this text, which described 35-mm film as the standard for photodocumentation, a revolution has occurred in digital still and video imaging such that newer modalities of digital video and digital still imaging have virtually replaced 35-mm slide and print photography for image documentation. Digital video and the digital still cameras provide more than adequate or, in some cases such as video, superior documentation. Video, for example, provides a moving image that clearly reveals changes during the examination, whereas the value of a still photograph is contingent on whether the picture was taken at an appropriate moment for adequately revealing important findings (Figure 4.1). The remainder of the discussion in this chapter will touch on older modalities of still imaging using film media but will focus more on the newer digital technologies.

The newer point and shoot digital still cameras are simple and easy to use. They are relatively inexpensive and fully automatic. They incorporate telephoto and limited macro or close-up (up to ×0.25 magnification) capability, built-in integrated flash, and autofocus. Digital single lens reflex (SLR) cameras combined with a ×1 macro lens and ring flash compare favorably to, and are significantly less expensive than, colposcopic cameras for photographing the sexually abused child[7] (Figure 4.2).

Digital still cameras typically save the image in JPEG format. When setting the camera up for operation it is important to set the resolution at the highest setting and the compression at the lowest. There is really no reason given the price of modern memory cards to record at anything but the highest resolution and lowest compression.

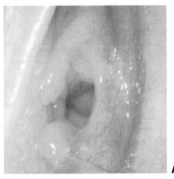
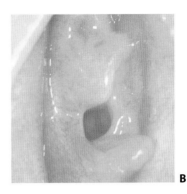

A   B

FIGURE 4.1
Two 35-mm colposcopic photographs taken at slightly different moments during the hymenal examination of a prepubertal child. The first image **(A)** appears to show a hymenal notch at 9 o'clock. However, the second image **(B)** shows the now moved tag at 6 o'clock and bump at 10 o'clock, and the newly revealed intact hymenal border at 9 o'clock. If B had not been captured, there could have been confusion about interpreting the findings.

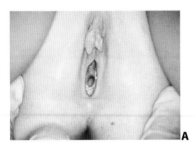
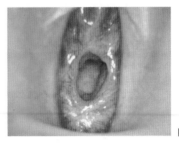

A   B

FIGURE 4.2
Close-up and distant 35-mm photographic views of a hymenal examination of a prepubertal girl. Both pictures were taken with a 35-mm camera with ×1 macro lens and ring flash. **A.** A distant view at approximately ×.25 magnification that reveals neighboring anatomy. It is best for documenting surrounding pathology, such as bruising. **B.** A close-up view at ×1 macro reveals hymenal anatomy with excellent detail.

The size of lesions may be documented on the photograph by positioning a measuring device, such as an adhesive metric scale, directly above or below the injury.[4,5,9,13]

Color slides, if used, are relatively inexpensive, quickly developed, and easy to file, and they can be converted into satisfactory color prints if necessary. After the film is developed, each image should be reviewed for both technique and content. However, no photograph, even a poor one, should be discarded. This action could be misconstrued as destruction of evidence.[13,14] Likewise, no video should ever be discarded. However, with the use of digital still technologies and the ability to immediately review images during the examination, some examiners have suggested that a very poor image such as one completely out of focus or blurred because of movement can be deleted in the camera before printing. Deleting poor images from the camera during shooting or afterward remains a controversial issue and should be resolved at the local level with legal assistance.

In contrast to color slides, self-processing Polaroid film is expensive, difficult to reproduce, and difficult to store. Polaroid and 35-mm film can be mechanically damaged and can deteriorate, especially if exposed to light, and are no longer options that make sense for photodocumentation in light of the new technology. Videotape, both analog and digital, can be affected by magnets, and the iron oxide matrix that makes up the tape has been known to deteriorate over time. Computer floppy disks seem to have a fairly long shelf life if not exposed to a magnetic field. Compact disks (CDs) and digital video disks (DVDs) store data using optical laser technology (as opposed to magnetic floppy disks or chemical film). Images can be stored on CD or DVD using a read-write drive and can then be read by any other drive. However, caution should be exercised when saving to rewritable CDs or DVDs because many older CD drives may not be able to read the disks. CDs and DVDs will not deteriorate, but they can be damaged mechanically.

Whatever storage medium is used—whether 35-mm prints or slides, Polaroid film, videotape, or CD/DVD—images should be stored and released according to specific institutional policies. Guidelines such as those developed by the American Professional Society on the Abuse of Children[15] for photographing the abused child should be consulted.

Problems in Photodocumentation

A common problem in photodocumentation is blurring of the still or video image. With newer autofocus cameras, this is less of a problem. However, an out-of-focus image can still occur when the examiner moves the camera closer than the closest focusing distance allowed by the camera in the hope of obtaining more magnification.

When photographs are obtained while simultaneously using a video or still camera attached to a colposcope, there should be no difficulty in obtaining images that are in focus as long as the image on the monitor is crisp. When a colposcope is equipped with a beam splitter, it is possible to obtain both still and video images as well as view an image on a monitor screen simultaneously. As long as the image is in focus on the monitor, the image will be in focus on either still or video images that are obtained. Colposcopes have a fixed focal length and the focused image on the monitor is best obtained by simply moving the scope either closer or farther away from the patient until the image is in focus, with no need to view through the oculars. If colposcopic still or video images are obtained without the use of a video monitor and are out of focus, it is usually because the examiner failed to appropriately compensate for his or her own visual correction through adjustment of the scope's ocular. If possible, visualization through the ocular should be conducted while wearing glasses with the ocular settings on zero. If the examiner does not have 20/20 vision and is not wearing glasses or contact lenses, then ensuring focus can be problematic unless a reference object is used, such as an American Board of Forensic Odontology (ABFO) ruler. If the examiner is using a colposcope equipped with a beam splitter and wants to conduct the examination through the binoculars, then he or she should first focus the image on the monitor (if only a still camera is used, through the eyepiece of the still camera) and then look through the ocular and adjust the eyepieces into focus. Once the eyepieces are in focus, any movement of the scope, if visually in focus for the examiner, will be focused on either the film plane or the monitor. Because of movement of the focusing rings on the eyepiece, this refocusing should be done daily.

Colpophotography

The colposcope is a binocular viewing device with an attached light source. As mentioned in Chapter 3, it was originally developed for the study of cervical pathology and was first used to study sexual assault–related genital injuries.[10] Subsequently, Woodling and Heger,[11] Finkel,[16] McCann et al,[17] and others applied the colposcope to the study of genital and rectal anatomy in children. Colposcopy enhances the ability to examine genitalia with excellent magnification and lighting in a noninvasive manner. Perhaps most important, it allows for close-up photographic documentation of findings. This high-quality documentation supports the development of a common anatomical language, peer consultation, consensus building, and research.

Typically, to provide a permanent record of a colposcopic examination, a standard 35-mm camera body, whether film or digital, is attached to the colposcope and still images are obtained at key points during the examination. Still photography of genital and rectal findings may be difficult through the colposcope, however, because of rapid changes in genital and rectal shape, child movement, excessive magnification (narrow angle of view), and narrow depth of field.[18] Video photography through the colposcope is a versatile tool to obtain visual documentation.[8]

Colposcopes can differ significantly from one manufacturer to another in quality, accessories, and cost. Ease of use, quality of optics and light source, magnification, and photographic capabilities are important features. Equally important is manufacturer/distributor support, available attachments, and expansion capability, particularly in the area of telemedicine. Any system chosen must be tested thoroughly by the examiner before clinical use.

Recently, alternatives to colposcopes have been introduced[19] (Figure 4.3). In general, these alternatives incorporate a close-up video camera attached to a stand with the image projected onto a monitor and saved on videotape. These systems are less expensive than colposcopes, provide the same quality of video documentation, and allow viewing of the findings on a monitor rather than through the eyepiece of the colposcope. An even simpler solution to

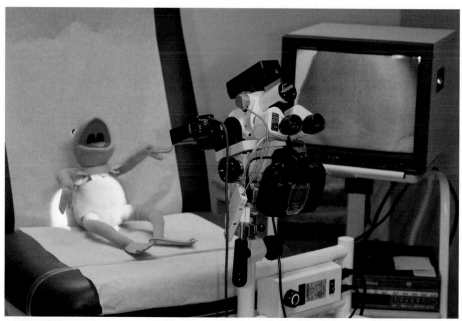

FIGURE 4.3
An example of equipment dedicated to video documentation of the physical examination. This image shows a camera attached to a stand and accompanying monitor. A super VHS video recorder and video printer are often included with such systems.

video documentation is to use a hand-held video camera. These cameras will often allow close-up viewing, although without the advantage of the ring lighting of dedicated systems (Figure 4.4).

Even more recently inexpensive systems using digital video cameras mounted on a wheeled tripod have been shown to produce comparable image documentation to more expensive colposcopic systems (Figure 4.5 and 4.6). As with any photodocumentation, but perhaps even more so with equipment that *looks* like a camera, care should be taken to ensure that the child and parents are comfortable with the documentation process by informing the child and parent about the reasons for documentation and how the confidentiality of images will be

protected. One clear benefit of image documentation to the child and parent is that there will be no need for a re-examination if, in the future, a defense expert challenges the diagnosis. If this occurs the defense can be supplied with the image documentation for review demonstrating the diagnostic finding. Children who have been involved in the creation of pornography may have special concerns that will need to be addressed before obtaining image documentation.

Video and Digital Imaging

Obtaining a photograph that adequately represents genital and rectal findings can be challenging given both the inherent dynamic variability of these

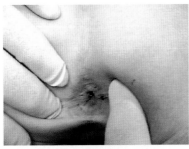
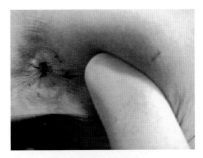
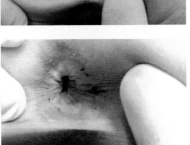
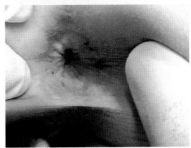

FIGURE 4.4
Series of stills captured from a handheld Hi-8-mm video camera of the anal examination of a boy. The images reveal a wide linear scar extending from 7 o'clock to 8 o'clock just outside the anal verge. The scar was from an inflicted match burn.

structures and motion by the child.[8] This problem has led to the use of video photographic techniques for both documentation and teaching.[8,20]

Video provides a number of advantages over still photography.

1. The dynamic variability of anogenital anatomy can be studied with greater ease.
2. Viewing the findings on a television or computer monitor, rather than through an eyepiece on the scope, allows the examiner to maintain visual contact with the child and quickly respond to changes in demeanor.
3. An unanticipated advantage of the monitor is a reduction in anxiety for many children, who are able to view the examination along with the examiner.
4. The examination can be recorded in its entirety for future reference.
5. Video recordings can be made available for opposing expert review, thus saving the child from a repeat examination.

The older consumer format for videotape was VHS. The 8-mm format allowed use of a smaller sized tape and, hence, a smaller camera. Eight millimeter is comparable in quality to standard VHS and is easier to store. Hi-8 and

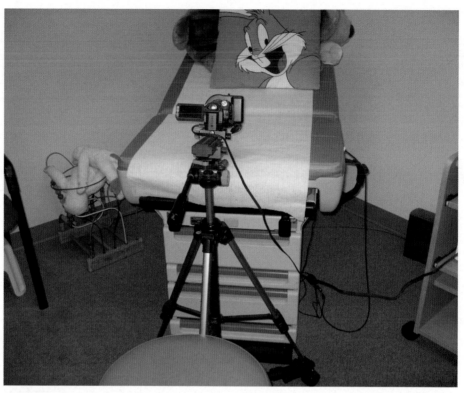

FIGURE 4.5

Digital video camera setup for sexual abuse examination. The camera is on a tripod, which should have a leveling device and either built in or attached wheels. The camera also has an LED ring light, which is very useful for correct lighting. Auto focus can be used, as can variable zoom. A macro focusing slide is attached to the tripod to allow extension over the examination table. The camera can be easily removed to document other visible findings. Advantages of such a system include cost, ease of use, high-quality state-of-the-art video, excellent stills from incorporated still camera and/or captured stills from video, and portability. This system is good for sexual and physical abuse both in the office as well as in the hospital.

super VHS (S-VHS) video cameras offer a significant improvement in image quality or resolution over 8 mm and VHS. Digital video cameras and recorders are better still. VHS and 8-mm video record approximately 200 lines of resolution, whereas S-VHS and Hi-8 record 400 lines and digital video records 500 lines.[20] The newer high definition (HD) digital video cameras further boost the resolution of the video image and allow even higher resolution still capture. For example, current HD cameras allow 720 lines or, depending on the format, up to 1,080 lines of horizontal resolution. Although lines of resolution, a video construct, is not directly translatable to pixels, one can see that increasing the number of lines of horizontal resolution by as much as 100% over standard digital video should not only increase the resolution of the video but should significantly increase the resolution of a still later grabbed from the video.

A drawback of older video documentation systems such as VHS and S-VHS has been the lack of a high-quality image for publication, courtroom use, or teaching. This problem can be solved simultaneously, albeit perhaps awkwardly, by recording the examination with a video camera and a still camera. However, with digital processing techniques, a video image can be converted to a digital image and then into a photograph of quite reasonable quality. Newer HD video cameras with upwards of 6 megapixel still capability have virtually solved that problem.

Digitized images—whether digitized primarily by using a digital still camera or digital video camera, or secondarily by scanning a slide, negative, or print or by capturing a frame from a video—can be transmitted via the Internet (encrypted, of course) or direct computer-to-computer connection to colleagues for discussion. The use of telemedicine communication techniques has emerged as a powerful tool in child abuse consultation and education.[20]

The newer 5 megapixel or higher digital still cameras challenge traditional 35-mm still cameras in image quality. Such megapixel cameras can produce an 8- by 10-inch photograph that rivals 35 mm (Figure 4.7). Megapixel digital still cameras require a large flash memory card and superior batteries, such as lithium or nickel metal hydride.

Photographing Children

When photographing a child, it is important to explain what is going to

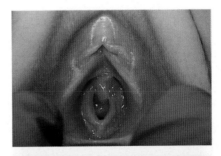
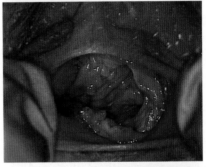
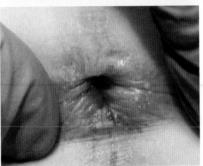

FIGURE 4.6
Examples of stills captured from videos taken with the camera setup in Figure 4.5 using proprietary video editing software.

happen in language that the child will understand.[21-23] A significant benefit of videocolposcopy over simple still photography is that the child can actually watch the examination on the video monitor. The ability to observe what the examiner is doing may demystify the experience for the child, reduce his or her anxiety, and increase his or her cooperation. After explaining to the child the equipment that will be used as

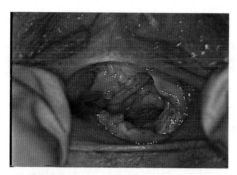

FIGURE 4.7
Digital still image of a hymenal examination
using a 6 megapixel digital camera.

a part of the examination procedure,
allow the child to assume a position of
comfort for the examination. It is better
to have a cooperative child who is
somewhat out of optimal photographic
position yet not moving, than an uncooperative, moving child. It is useful to
allow the child to have a trusted support person of their choice in the examination room. Infants and toddlers may
be photographed more easily if they
are held in the lap of a guardian or
assistant.[24] Adolescents may prefer not
having their parent or guardian in the
room during the examination and
should be allowed to make the decision
as to who will accompany them for the
examination.[25]

At all times, the examiner must be cognizant of the potential effect of photographing an abused child, with regard
to both the photographic process itself
and the use of the photographs/video-
tape in court. Some children may refuse
photographic documentation, despite
the examiner's best efforts. This refusal
should be respected.[26] If pornography
has been a component of the child's

experience, then photographing the
child in the context of documentation
of findings may have an adverse effect.
Similarly, the adverse effects of photographing children, particularly sexually
abused children, should not be underes-
timated. The clinician should openly
and sympathetically address this issue
both before and after obtaining any
visual documentation.

Legal Issues

Medical photographs must show injuries as realistically as possible and
should not be used to enhance or exaggerate trauma. From a medicolegal perspective, photographs of abused
children should convey a fair and accurate representation of the findings. For
courtroom use, photographs must be
properly verified and relevant.[27] Relevance is a judicial decision.[28] Photographs may have evidentiary value yet
be deemed prejudicial to the defendant.
Whether the probative value outweighs
the prejudicial danger remains a decision for the trial judge. However, photographs are generally considered
admissible if they shed light on the
issue, enable a witness to better describe
the objects portrayed, permit the jury to
better understand the testimony, or corroborate testimony. Courts generally
permit medical providers to explain
and illustrate their testimony with a
photograph. A simple explanation by
the provider that the images are needed
to adequately describe the complexity
and extent of the injuries is all that is
usually necessary. Verification rests
with the examiner, who can testify in
court whether the images accurately

reflect the findings.[4,5] To help verify that the photographs are actually of a particular child, an identifying sign may be placed in front of the patient for each picture or at the beginning of the film cassette or tape. The inclusion of such signs or labels in each photograph, however, is time-consuming and distracting[29] and may not be necessary. In the end it is the examiner who must verify that a photograph or video is of a particular child.

When copying stills and video for legal purposes it is important to create as exact a copy as possible. This means that with regard to stills the image should not be modified or cropped and if it is converted to a print, that print should be on high-quality photographic paper using a high-quality color printer. Black and white copies on plain ink jet or laser paper are virtually worthless. When copying video, the copy (and for that matter the original) should be made using the highest quality media at the best recording and copying setting (in the case of VHS video this means using standard play rather than extended play for recording and copying).

Although many child abuse laws state that permission is not needed if photographs are obtained as a part of a child abuse evaluation, going through the process of obtaining consent can establish an alliance with the family. A variety of consent forms are available, including a model form drafted by the American Medical Association.[6,29,30] Each institution should have a policy for the handling and release of photographs.[4,5]

A particular legal concern about digital photographs is that there is the potential for images to be digitally manipulated and hence might not be accepted in court. To date there have been no legal precedents set excluding the use of digitally obtained images. Changing traditional 35-mm slides and negatives via color, contrast, or brightness manipulation has always been possible. The concern over digital image alteration seems to be based on both the ease with which such changes can be made and the possibility of drastic, substantive change, such as selectively enhancing one element of the image over another. Original images for courtroom use should, of course, never be altered. If a copy is altered to improve viewing, such as by enlargement or brightening, these changes should be noted clearly. Ultimately, however, photographs are useful only as demonstration aids for the examiner to explain the findings. As such, they should be as fair and accurate a representation of the findings as possible. Capturing a digital camera image on disk and then printing it on a computer printer is really no different from capturing a 35-mm camera image on silver-based film and then printing in a darkroom.[20] Ultimately, it is the examiner who must tell the court if a particular image represents what he or she originally saw.

Conclusion

Visualization and documentation technology and equipment have evolved alongside our understanding of the pathophysiology of child sexual abuse. Early magnification tools, such as otoscopes and eye loops, have given way to colposcopes and close-up video cameras attached to high-resolution monitors. The earliest documentation techniques included words and drawings. Fortunately, the ready availability of still and video documentation formats affords clinicians the opportunity to use visual documentation to obtain a second opinion, participate in peer review, and facilitate teaching. Currently accepted documentation techniques include still and video photography, which should be augmented with thorough written descriptions of findings. The colposcope has been a valuable tool for enhancing visualization through magnification and offers the ability to obtain digital video and stills images effortlessly. Less expensive alternatives to a colposcope are now available. For many, a decision whether to use a colposcope or another form of imaging equipment is based on a number of issues including cost, ease of use, compatibility with existing systems, and availability of technical assistance.[31–36] Regardless of the method of obtaining images, photodocumentation of significant findings must be considered a standard of care for any clinician providing diagnostic and treatment services to children alleged to have been sexually abused.

References

1. American Professional Society on the Abuse of Children. *Descriptive Terminology in Child Sexual Abuse Medical Evaluations*. Chicago, IL: American Professional Society on the Abuse of Children; 1995

2. De Jong AR, Finkel MA. Sexual abuse of children. *Curr Probl Pediatr*. 1990;20:489–567

3. Heger A, Emans SJ. *Evaluation of the Sexually Abused Child*. New York, NY: Oxford University Press; 1992

4. Ford RJ, Smistek BS. Photography of the maltreated child. In: Ellerstein NS, ed. *Child Abuse and Neglect: A Medical Reference*. New York, NY: John Wiley; 1981:315–325

5. Smistek S. Photography of the abused and neglected child. In: Ludwig S, Kornberg AE, eds. *Child Abuse: A Medical Reference*. New York, NY: Churchill Livingstone; 1992:467–477

6. Cordell W, Zollman W, Karlson H. A photographic system for the emergency department. *Ann Emerg Medicine*. 1980;9:210–214

7. Ricci LR. Medical forensic photography of the sexually abused child. *Child Abuse Negl*. 1988;12:305–310

8. McCann J. Use of the colposcope in childhood sexual abuse examinations. *Pediatr Clin North Am*. 1990;37:863–880

9. Soderstrom RM. Colposcopic documentation: an objective approach to assessing sexual abuse of girls. *J Reprod Med*. 1994;39:6–8

10. Teixeira WR. Hymenal colposcopic examination in sexual offenses. *Am J Forensic Med Pathol*. 1981;2:209–215

11. Woodling BA, Heger A. The use of the colposcope in the diagnosis of sexual abuse in the pediatric age group. *Child Abuse Negl*. 1986;10:111–114

12. Woodling BA, Kossoris P. Sexual misuse: rape, molestation and incest. *Pediatr Clin North Am*. 1981;28:481–499

13. Spring GE. Evidence photography: an overview. *J Biol Photogr*. 1987;55:129–132

14. Gilmore J, Miller W. Clinical photography utilizing office staff: methods to achieve consistency and reproducibility. *J Dermatol Surg Oncol*. 1988;14:281–286

15. American Professional Society on the Abuse of Children. *Guidelines for the Photographic Documentation of Child Abuse*. Chicago, IL: American Professional Society on the Abuse of Children;1995

16. Finkel MA. Anogenital trauma in sexually abused children. *Pediatrics*. 1989;84:317–322

17. McCann J, Wells R, Simon M, Voris J. Genital findings in prepubertal girls selected for nonabuse: a descriptive study. *Pediatrics*. 1990;86:428–439

18. Adams JA, Phillips P, Ahmad M. The usefulness of colposcopic photographs in the evaluation of suspected child sexual abuse. *Adolesc Pediatr Gynecol*. 1990;3:75–82

19. Siegel RM, Hill TD, Henderson VA, Daniels K. Comparison of an intraoral camera with colposcopy in sexually abused children. *Clin Pediatr*. 1999;38:375–376

20. Finkel MA, Ricci LR. Documentation and preservation of visual evidence in child abuse. *Child Maltreat*. 1997;2:322–330

21. Ricci LR. Photographing the physically abused child: principles and practice. *Am J Dis Child*. 1991;145:275–281

22. Ricci LR. Photodocumentation of the abused child. In: Reece RM, ed. *Child Abuse: Medical Diagnosis and Management*. Philadelphia, PA: Lea & Febiger; 1994:248–264

23. Steward MS, Schmitz M, Steward DS, Joye NR, Reinhart M. Children's anticipation of and response to colposcopic examination. *Child Abuse Negl*. 1995;19:997–1005

24. Reeves C. Paediatric photography. *J Audiov Media Medicine*. 1986;9:131–134

25. Mears CJ, Heflin AH, Finkel MA, Deblinger E, Steer RA. Adolescents' responses to sexual abuse evaluation including the use of video colposcopy. *J Adolesc Health*. 2003;33:18–34

26. Muram D, Aiken MM, Strong C. Children's refusal of gynecologic examinations for suspected sexual abuse. *J Clin Ethics*. 1997;8:158–164

27. Flower MS. Photographs in the courtroom: getting it straight between you and your professional photographer. *North Ky State Law Forum*. 1974;2:184–211

28. Myers JEB. *Legal Issues in Child Abuse and Neglect*. Newbury Park, CA: Sage Publications; 1992

29. Sebben JE. Office photography from the surgical viewpoint. *J Dermatol Surg Oncol*. 1983;9:763–768

30. Weiss CH. Dermatologic photography of nail pathologies. *Dermatol Clin*. 1985;3:543–556

31. Atabaki S, Paradise JE. The medical evaluation of the sexually abused child: lessons from a decade of research. *Pediatrics*. 1999;104:178–186

32. Brayden RM, Altemeier WA, Yeager T, Muram D. Interpretations of colposcopic photographs: evidence of competence in assessing sexual abuse? *Child Abuse Negl*. 1991;15:69–76

33. Muram D, Elias S. Child sexual abuse— genital tract findings in prepubertal girls. II. Comparison of colposcopic and unaided examinations. *Am J Obstet Gynecol*. 1989;160:333–335

34. Muram D, Arheart KL, Jennings SG. Diagnostic accuracy of colposcopic photographs in child sexual abuse evaluations. *Pediatr Adolesc Gynecol*. 1999;12:58–61

35. Norvell MK, Benrubi GI, Thompson RJ. Investigation of microtrauma after sexual intercourse. *J Reprod Med*. 1984;29:269–271

36. Sinal SH, Lawless MR, Rainey DY, et al. Clinician agreement on physical findings in child sexual abuse cases. *Arch Pediatr Adolesc Med*. 1997;151:497–501

Sexually Transmitted Infections in Child and Adolescent Sexual Assault and Abuse

Deborah C. Stewart

Overview

A sexually transmitted infection (STI) can be the presenting symptom of unsuspected sexual assault or abuse, an asymptomatic infection found in routine screening during a sexual abuse examination or, particularly in adolescents, a reason to seek medical care following a previously unreported assault. The presence of such an infection following sexual assault or abuse of a child or adolescent has profound medical, legal, social, and psychological implications. Sexually transmitted infections are found in approximately 1% to 5% of prepubertal victims examined for sexual abuse.[1] In adolescents, it has been more difficult to determine the acquisition rate of new infections arising from sexual assault because there may be a preexisting STI in previously sexually active teens. The true incidence of STIs in child and adolescent sexual abuse and assault is unknown because much remains unreported.

In cases of suspected child and adolescent sexual assault and abuse, decisions about which children and adolescents should receive testing for STIs should be individualized. The American Academy of Pediatrics (AAP) and the Centers for Disease Control and Prevention (CDC) have published guidelines regarding factors to consider when making such decisions (Box 5.1).

As noted in Box 5.1, the specific circumstances of a case must be considered in totality when making a decision to test for an STI. The routine testing for STIs when children present with allegations of sexual abuse is not warranted. For example, if based on the history there is no indication that the child had the potential to have contact with infected genital secretions, testing is not warranted unless an examination finding suggests otherwise. It is the medical history that will provide the best insight into a child's experience and, when combined with

BOX 5.1
Factors to Consider When Testing for Sexually Transmitted Infections (STIs) in Suspected Sexual Abuse of Assault

1. Age of the child
2. Types of sexual contact
3. Time lapse from the last sexual contact
4. Signs and symptoms suggestive of an STI
5. Family member or sibling with an STI
6. Abuser with risk factor for an STI
7. Request/concerns of child or family
8. Prevalence of STIs in the community
9. Presence of other examination findings
10. Patient/parent support for testing

Adapted from Kellogg N, American Academy of Pediatrics Committee on Child Abuse and Neglect. The evaluation of sexual abuse in children. *Pediatrics.* 2005;116:506–512.

an examination, will determine the need for testing. When the decision is made to perform STI testing, the examiner should keep in mind the forensic as well as the medical significance of any results, either positive or negative, particularly in the low prevalence population of the prepubertal child (Table 5.1). Thus it is very important that

1. Chain of custody procedures should be followed for STI testing as for any other evidence collection procedures.
2. An examiner skilled in the evaluation for child and adolescent sexual assault needs to perform testing for STIs using forensically defensible methods available prior to treating the patient.
3. The examiner must have an up-to-date knowledge of the epidemiology

and pathophysiology of the common STIs in the prepubertal child and adolescent.

4. Specimens for suspected sexual abuse cases should always be sent to an experienced reference laboratory. Examiners should be familiar with the laboratory's procedures for testing including confirmatory testing. Key laboratory personnel should be familiar with and comfortable with forensic and courtroom procedure.
5. It is important to be vigilant about the use of appropriate transport media and procedures when obtaining specimens for STIs.
6. Particularly in the evaluation of the prepubertal child, if the initial sexual assault exposure was recent, the amount of infectious material present may not have reached sufficient quantities to produce positive test results. In such cases, a 2-week follow-up visit after the most recent sexual exposure with a repeat physical examination and collection of specimens for possible STIs would be important to optimize the chances of recovering a positive specimen. Conversely, if the abuse was ongoing, and the last episode was significantly prior to the examination, such a follow-up visit would not be necessary (Boxes 5.2 and 5.3).

Over the past 10 years there have been significant changes in recommendations for the evaluation and treatment of STIs in sexually abused children and adolescents (Box 5.4). This chapter will review the (1) biology, (2) incidence and epidemiology, (3) clinical presentation, (4) laboratory diagnosis methods including the newest methods, and (5) current treatment recommendations, in general, of the most common STIs seen in the prepubertal and the adolescent sexual abuse and assault population.

The Organisms

Gonorrhea

Biology

Neisseria gonorrhoeae is a gram-negative intracellular oxidase-positive diplococcus bacterial organism that infects only mucous membranes that are lined by columnar or cuboidal, non-cornified epithelial cells. This epithelial structure is typical of that found in the urethra, the estrogenized endocervix, the conjunctivae, and the prepubertal vagina. It is extremely sensitive to drying and temperature changes and requires strict environmental conditions for growth and infectivity.

Epidemiology

The transmission of *N gonorrhoeae* requires intimate contact with epithelial or mucous secreting cells. *N gonorrhoeae* is communicable as long as a person harbors the organism. The incubation period is 2 to 7 days.

In all prepubertal children beyond the newborn period and in all non–sexually active adolescents, a gonococcal infection is usually diagnostic of sexual abuse. Studies of routine screening in pediatric sexual assault victims have shown the usual prevalence of *N gonorrhoeae* in most studies to be about 0.8% to 1.4%.[2,3] Studies of sexual assault victims have found *N gonorrhoeae* in 2.4% to 12% of initial evaluations, and in 2.6% to 4% of follow-up

TABLE 5.1
Implications of Commonly Encountered Sexually Transmitted Infections (STIs)[a]

STI Confirmed	Sexual Abuse	Suggested Action
Gonorrhea[b]	Diagnostic[c]	Report
Syphilis[b]	Diagnostic	Report
Human immunodeficiency virus infection[d]	Diagnostic	Report
Chlamydia trachomatis infection[b]	Diagnostic[c]	Report
Trichomonas vaginalis infection	Highly suspicious	Report
Condylomata acuminata infection[b,e] (anogenital warts)	Suspicious	Report
Herpes simplex (genital location)	Suspicious	Report[f]
Bacterial vaginosis	Inconclusive	Medical follow-up

[a] Adapted from Kellogg N, American Academy of Pediatrics Committee on Child Abuse and Neglect. The evaluation of sexual abuse in children. *Pediatrics.* 2005;116:506–512.
[b] If not perinatally acquired and rare nonsexual vertical transmission is excluded.
[c] Although the culture technique is the gold standard, current studies are investigating the use of nucleic acid amplification tests as an alternative diagnostic method in children.
[d] If not acquired perinatally or by transfusion.
[e] Outside of the neonatal period.
[f] Unless there is a clear history of autoinoculation.

BOX 5.2
Laboratory Evaluation in Suspected Sexually Abused Prepubertal Children[a]

Initial and 2-Week Follow-Up Examination

If indicated, they should include

- Visual inspection of the genital, perianal, and oral areas for genital discharge, odor, bleeding, irritation, warts, and vesicular or ulcerative genital or perianal lesions. Appropriate diagnostic specimens should be obtained when warranted.

- Specimen collection for culture for *Neisseria gonorrhoeae* from the pharynx and anus in both boys and girls, the vagina in girls, and the urethra in boys. Cervical specimens are not recommended for prepubertal girls. For boys with a urethral discharge, a meatal specimen discharge is adequate. Isolates should be preserved.

- Cultures for *Chlamydia trachomatis* from specimens collected from the anus in both boys and girls and from the vagina in girls. If urethral discharge is present in boys, a meatal specimen should be obtained. Pharyngeal specimens should not be obtained. Isolates should be preserved. Only standard culture systems for the isolation of *C trachomatis* should be used. Data are insufficient to adequately assess the utility of nucleic acid amplification tests (NAATs) in the evaluation of children who might have been sexually abused, but these tests might be an alternative if confirmation is available and culture systems for *C trachomatis* are unavailable. Confirmation should consist of a second US Food and Drug Administration–cleared NAAT that targets a different sequence from the initial test.

- Culture and wet mount of a vaginal swab specimen for *Trichomonas vaginalis* infection and bacterial vaginosis when symptoms indicate.

- Collection of serum samples to be evaluated immediately, preserved for subsequent analysis, and used as a baseline for comparison with follow-up serologic test. These include *Treponema pallidum,* human immunodeficiency virus (HIV), and hepatitis B virus.

- HIV infection has been reported in children whose only risk factor was sexual abuse. The decision to test for HIV infection and to offer postexposure prophylaxis should be made on a case-by-case basis.

Follow-Up Examination After Assault

In circumstances in which transmission of syphilis, HIV, or hepatitis B is a concern, but baseline tests are negative, an examination approximately 6 weeks, 3 months, and 6 months after the last suspected sexual exposure is recommended to allow time for antibodies to infectious agents to develop. Decisions regarding testing should be made on an individual basis.

[a]Adapted from Centers for Disease Control and Prevention. Sexually transmitted diseases treatment guidelines 2006. *MMWR Recommend Rep.* 2006;55[RR11]1–94.

BOX 5.3
Laboratory Evaluation of Sexually Transmitted Infections (STIs)
in Adolescent Sexual Abuse or Assault[a]

Initial Examination

An initial examination should include

- Testing for *Neisseria gonorrhoeae* and *Chlamydia trachomatis* from specimens collected from any sites of penetration or attempted penetration using culture or US Food and Drug Administration–cleared nucleic acid amplification tests for either *N gonorrhoeae* or *C trachomatis*.

- Wet mount and culture of a vaginal swab specimen for *Trichomonas vaginalis* infection. If malodor, vaginal discharge, or pruritis is present, the wet mount should also be examined for bacterial vaginosis and candidiasis.

- Collection of a serum sample for immediate evaluation for human immunodeficiency virus (HIV), hepatitis B, and syphilis.

Follow-Up Examination

Examination for STIs should be repeated within 1 to 2 weeks post-assault. Because organisms acquired through the assault might not have had sufficient time to multiply to produce sufficient concentrations to result in positive test results at the initial examination, testing should be repeated at the follow-up visit, unless prophylactic treatment was provided. If treatment was provided, symptomatic patients should be tested. Serology for syphilis and HIV should be repeated in 6 weeks, 3 months, and 6 months post-assault if initial tests were negative and infection in the assailant could not be ruled out.

[a]Adapted from Centers for Disease Control and Prevention. Sexually transmitted diseases treatment guidelines 2006. *MMWR Recommend Rep.* 2006;55[RR11]1–94.

evaluations.[4,5] In sexually assaulted adolescents, the true incidence of new infection resulting from the sexual assault can be difficult to differentiate from preexisting infection from consensual sexual activity. In addition, the presence of *N gonorrhoeae* at the initial evaluation may not represent preexisting infections because it is possible that a culture could be positive as a result of the culture of remaining male ejaculate. The diagnosis of gonococcal disease in a child must prompt an immediate evaluation for the source of infection, and the evaluation should include testing of other children who may have been exposed to the same source.

Clinical Presentations

N gonorrhoeae in the newborn may present with ophthalmia, scalp abscess, and disseminated infections. In the prepubertal child, vaginitis in females is the most common manifestation of infection and is almost always symptomatic, including discharge, itching, and dysuria. Lack of endocervical glands on the ectocervix in prepubertal children makes ascending infection and cervical infection extremely unlikely. Urethritis is uncommon in boys. Anorectal and pharyngeal infections can occur in prepubertal boys and girls and may be asymptomatic.[6]

Genital gonococcal infections in adolescent females, as in adults, may be asymptomatic. Potential infections include vaginitis, endocervitis, urethritis, and salpingitis, and infection in more than one site is common. In females, both vaginal and rectal cultures will often test positive. In males, infection is usually symptomatic, causing urethritis. Other potential sites of infection include proctitis, epididymitis, and pharyngitis. Rectal and pharyngeal infections are often asymptomatic.

Bacteremic spread to secondary sites in adolescents and adults can cause arthritis, myocarditis, perihepatitis, dermatitis, meningitis, or endocarditis. Coinfection with *Chlamydia trachomatis* is extremely common in adolescents.

Laboratory Diagnosis
The gold standard for the diagnosis of gonococcal infection remains the culture in prepubertal and adolescent sexual abuse/assault cases. Swabs should be inoculated and incubated immediately onto modified Thayer-Martin media or appropriate transport media. The organism is fastidious, requiring incubation at 35°C to 37°C as well as a carbon dioxide–enriched medium. Thus media for incubation must be pre-warmed. Positive cultures must be confirmed by 2 of the following methods: carbohydrate utilization, direct fluorescent antibody testing, or enzyme substrate testing, which differentiates *N gonorrhoeae* from organisms such as *Neisseria meningitidis, Neisseria lactamica,* and *Neisseria cinerea,* which may be normal flora. Isolates should be preserved in case additional or repeat testing is needed. A recent paper has described the use of pulsed-field gel electrophoresis and neisserial lipoprotein gene sequencing in the evaluation of possible perpetrators against a 3-year-old child found to be infected with genital *N gonorrhoeae.*[7]

Much interest has been generated in the use of nucleic acid amplification tests (NAATs) to diagnose *N gonorrhoeae,* which in general require less sample and may be done using urine. Test methods include transcription-mediated amplification, strand-displacement assays, and polymerase chain reaction (PCR.) They are highly sensitive and specific when used on urethral (males) discharges, endocervical specimens, and urine specimens. False-positives may result from other *Neisseria* species or gram-negative cocci in the female genital tract. Nucleic acid amplification tests are not recommended for pharyngeal or rectal swabs. Thus these methods are not recommended for medical forensic work. In prepubertal children and adolescents, if culture is unavailable, there is some support for the use of NAAT on vaginal swabs if a second NAAT targeting a different portion of the DNA than the first NAAT can be used for confirmation of a positive result.[8,9] Some centers have used NAAT for screening and a second NAAT along with a culture for confirmation in cases of gonococcal infection in prepubertal children.

A confirmed positive test for gonorrhea must be reported to authorities for investigation, even if there is no prior history of sexual abuse and the child or adolescent does not disclose sexual contact. Whenever possible, cultures or NAAT with confirmatory cultures should be obtained from all people having contact with the child suspected of having been sexually abused. Chil-dren or adolescents with positive tests for *N gonorrhoeae* should be tested for other STIs, particularly *C trachomatis*.

Treatment (Box 5.4)

For more information, consult guidelines from the CDC (Sexually transmitted diseases treatment guidelines 2006. *MMWR Recommend Rep.* 2006;55[RR11]1–94) and the AAP (*Red Book: 2006 Report of the Committee on Infectious Diseases*, 27th ed).

Chlamydia Trachomatis

Biology

C trachomatis is an obligate intracellular bacterial agent with multiple serotypes. It is difficult to grow in culture requiring live tissue culture. It has a very complex life cycle with distinct infectious and reproductive forms, which lead to the ability to cause prolonged, often subclinical infections. *C trachomatis* is also the causative agent of trachoma and lymphogranuloma venereum (LGV).

In adolescents and adults, *C trachomatis* infects the transitional epithelium of the endocervix, and rates of infection in adolescents can be as high as 15% to 20%.[10]

Epidemiology

Genital *C trachomatis* infection is recognized as the world's most common reportable STI. The prevalence of *C trachomatis* in sexually abused prepubertal children routinely tested for STIs is between 1% and 6%.[2] The prevalence of *C trachomatis* in sexually assaulted pubertal adolescents has been estimated to be between 4% and 17%, although this rate may also include baseline infection.[11] The true risk of acquiring *C trachomatis* after an adolescent or adult sexual assault may be closer to 2%.[4]

The incubation period for infection is 7 to 14 days. Infections are commonly asymptomatic and may persist up to 3 years in postpubertally infected prepubertal girls.[1]

Transmission of *C trachomatis* occurs via direct contact with infective material. In children this may occur via sexual contact or via perinatal acquisition. Pregnant women who have cervical *C trachomatis* infection are usually asymptomatic and can

BOX 5.4
Sexually Transmitted Infection (STI) Prophylaxis in Child and Adolescent Sexual Assault[a]

Prepubertal Child

The risk of a child acquiring an STI as a result of sexual abuse or assault is not well understood. Routine presumptive treatment for children who have been victims of sexual abuse or assault is not recommended for multiple reasons.

1) The incidence of acquisition of STIs in this population is believed to be very low.

2) Prepubertal girls are at much lower risk for ascending infection than pubertal women.

3) It is more likely that follow-up of these children can be ensured if cultures are positive. If the parents, patients, or providers are particularly concerned in a specific situation, presumptive treatment may be considered after all relevant specimens are obtained.

Adolescent

Many specialists working with adolescents recommend routine preventive therapy after a sexual assault because of the difficulty in ensuring follow-up care.

The following regimen is suggested for STI prevention.

Hepatitis B	Hepatitis B vaccination for those not previously vaccinated
	Follow-up vaccination at 1–2 and 4–6 months
Chlamydia	Ceftriaxone 125 mg intramuscularly in a single dose
Gonorrhea	PLUS
Trichomonas	Metronidazole 2 g orally in a single dose
	PLUS
Bacterial vaginosis	Azithromycin 1 g orally in a single dose
	OR
	Doxycycline 100 mg orally twice daily for 7 days
	Alternative regimens are available.

Emergency contraception	– Provider should also provide emergency contraception (EC) should pregnancy be a possibility from the assault.
	– Because the regimen could cause nausea, particularly in combination with EC, an antiemetic such as Meclizine 25–50 mg should also be prescribed.
	– Side effects and alternatives should be discussed with the patient. Post-pubertal females should be tested for pregnancy before antimicrobial treatment or EC is given.

---

[a]Adapted from Centers for Disease Control and Prevention. Sexually transmitted diseases treatment guidelines 2006. *MMWR Recommend Rep.* 2006;55[RR11]1–94.

transmit the infection to their infants during vaginal delivery. The risk of perinatal transmission is 50% to 75%.[12] Colonization can occur at one or more anatomical sites including the conjunctiva, nasopharynx, rectum, and vagina. Infection after cesarean section is rare and usually occurs after early rupture of the amniotic membrane. There is no evidence to support nonsexual postnatal transmission from household contacts or family members. Sexual abuse is highly likely to be the cause of anogenital *Chlamydia* infection in the prepubertal child outside of the perinatal transmission period. Perinatally transmitted *C trachomatis* infection of the nasopharynx, urogenital tract, and rectum may persist for more than 1 year. Nasopharyngeal carriage has been documented for up to 28 months, vaginal and rectal carriage for 29 months in a few cases.[13]

Clinical Presentation

In newborns, *C trachomatis* infections affect the conjunctiva, nasopharynx, rectum, and vagina, with conjunctivitis being the most common clinical presentation. Infants born to infected mothers may develop pneumonia.

Prepubertal children may present with vaginitis, though most infections are asymptomatic in this age group and are found in routine screening for sexual abuse.

C trachomatis may cause a spectrum of disease in adolescents including mucopurulent cervicitis and urethritis, bartholinitis, endometritis, salpingitis, perihepatitis, and subsequent ectopic pregnancy and infertility. Adolescent males may present with urethritis, proctitis, prostatitis, and Reiter syndrome. Lymphogranuloma venereum is typified by the presence of genital or rectal papules or ulcerations followed by the development of unilateral or bilateral fluctuant inguinal lymphadenopathy. Coinfection with *N gonorrhoeae* is extremely common in adolescents and has been noted in 60% of students screened for gonorrhea and chlamydia genital infections in a recent large school-based study.[14]

Laboratory Diagnosis

In prepubertal children, standard cultures using McCoy media systems should be obtained. Specimens should be collected from the anus in both boys and girls and from the vagina in girls. Because *Chlamydia* is intracellular, the swab used must be inserted into the vagina and rolled against the wall to collect cells. Culturing the vaginal discharge, if present, does not give adequate results because there is not adequate cellular material present. If urethral discharge is present in boys, a meatal sample should be obtained. Pharyngeal specimens for *C trachomatis* are not recommended for children of either sex because the yield is low, perinatally acquired infection might persist beyond infancy, and culture systems in some laboratories do not distinguish between *C trachomatis* and *Chlamydia pneumoniae.* The isolation of *C trachomatis* should be confirmed by microscopic identification of inclusions by staining with fluorescein-conjugated monoclonal antibody specific for *C trachomatis*. Enzyme immunoassays (EIAs) are not acceptable confirmatory methods. Isolates should be preserved. Non-culture tests for chlamydia (eg, non-amplified probes, EIAs, and direct fluorescent antibody testsare not sufficiently specific for use in circumstances involving possible child abuse or assault. Insufficient data exist to adequately assess the utility of NAATs in the evaluation of children who might have been sexually abused, but these tests might be an alternative if confirmation is available and culture systems for *C trachomatis* are unavailable. If NAATs are used for screening, confirmation tests should consist of a second US Food and Drug Administration (FDA)-cleared NAAT that targets a different sequence from the initial test.[15]

Adolescents may be screened for *C trachomatis* from specimens collected from any sites of penetration or attempted penetration using culture or FDA-cleared NAATs for *C trachomatis*. Nucleic acid amplification tests offer the advantage of increased sensitivity in the detection of *C trachomatis*. As with children, confirmation tests should consist of a second FDA-cleared NAAT that targets a different sequence from the initial test.

Treatment (Box 5.4)
For more information, consult guidelines from the CDC (Sexually transmitted diseases treatment guidelines 2006. *MMWR Recommend Rep.* 2006;55[RR11]1–94) and the AAP

(*Red Book: 2006 Report of the Committee on Infectious Diseases,* 27th ed).

Trichomonas vaginalis

Biology
Trichomonas vaginalis is a motile flagellated parasitic protozoan found in the human genitourinary tract. It is related to *Trichomonas hominis* (found in the gastrointestinal [GI] tract) and is differentiated by the fact that *T hominis* has a much longer undulating membrane.

Epidemiology
T vaginalis is transmitted almost exclusively by sexual intercourse/direct sexual contact. There has been no proven fomite transmission, though fomite transmission has been postulated because survival for several hours has been documented in urine and wet towels.

In most postpubertal populations, women are often coinfected with other organisms such as mycoplasmas and *Gardnerella vaginalis*. *Trichomonas* facilitates the growth of other anaerobic organisms. The incubation period is 4 to 28 days with an average of 7 days. Although trichomoniasis has been one of the most frequently diagnosed infections following sexual assault in adolescents and adults, very limited data are available about the risk of acquiring trichomoniasis after sexual abuse in children. Most studies evaluated only symptomatic children, performing only wet mounts of vaginal discharge.

Between 2% and 17% of female infants born of infected women develop evidence of infection.[16] The neonatal vaginal epithelium resembles the adult epithelium because of the presence of maternal estrogens, and thus is susceptible to infection by *T vaginalis*. Typical infections are asymptomatic. Metabolism of maternal estrogens occurs by 3 to 4 weeks of age, at which time the vaginal epithelium assumes a prepubescent state and the epithelium becomes relatively resistant to *T vaginalis* infection. Presence of *T vaginalis* in young girls beyond the perinatal period is considered highly suspicious for sexual abuse.

Clinical Presentation

T vaginalis often presents in prepubertal female children as urethritis and may be found in spun urine specimens. In peripubertal children and adolescents, it presents with a frothy, malodorous yellow or white vaginal discharge, which may cause itching, dysuria, bleeding, or pain. It may be asymptomatic in 50% of women and be found on routine testing. *T vaginalis* may infect the vagina, urethra, and Skene and Bartholin glands. Up to 90% of infected men are asymptomatic but may have urethritis. If untreated, they may reinfect the female. Perinatally acquired infections may persist in infant urine samples up to 1 year.[17]

On examination, the vulva may be excoriated and erythematous with a visible discharge, which is most often gray or white. Classic descriptions of a yellow-green (20%–35% of cases) frothy (10%) discharge may also be seen in bacterial vaginosis. Strawberry cervix (punctuate hemorrhage with swollen papillae) can be seen grossly in 2% but in 15% by magnification using colposcopy. When present, this finding is very sensitive for *Trichomonas* (99%).

Laboratory Diagnosis

Trichomonas is most commonly diagnosed via wet mount microscopy, but the sensitivity of 60% to 70% is problematic. It requires immediate evaluation of wet prep for optimum results. An experienced laboratory technician can differentiate *T hominis,* which can be found as a commensal parasite in the GI tract characterized by its longer undulating membrane.

Testing by culture for suspected *Trichomonas* is positive in more than 80% of cases and should be used for confirmation of *Trichomonas* infection. Nucleic acid–based testing, which is FDA approved, has high detection rates, has 97% to 98% specificity in vaginal samples, is commercially available, and is being used in clinical settings, but there are potential issues with false-positives in low-prevalence populations.

Treatment

Treatment is with metronidazole or tinidazole. Metronidazole-resistant strains have been reported.

Bacterial Vaginosis (BV)

Biology

Bacterial vaginosis is a polymicrobial clinical syndrome resulting from the alteration of the microbial flora of the vagina. It results from a decreased concentration of peroxide-producing lactobacillus and an overgrowth of *G vaginalis, Mycoplasma hominis,* and anaerobic organisms such as *Prevotella* and *Mobiluncus* species. This overgrowth results in an elevated vaginal pH and production of characteristic fishy malodorous amines. The cause of the microbial alteration is not fully understood.

Epidemiology

Bacterial vaginosis is associated with having multiple sex partners, a new sex partner, douching, and lack of vaginal lactobacilli; whether BV results from acquisition of a sexually transmitted pathogen is unclear. Women who have never been sexually active are rarely affected. Treatment of male sex partners has not been beneficial in preventing the recurrence of BV. Although *G vaginalis* is closely associated with BV, it is not the sole cause of BV and is not an appropriate marker for sexual activity.

Bacterial vaginosis is one of the most common transmissible infections after sexual assault and has been found in 5% to 20% of postpubertal assault victims at follow-up. One large study found BV in 34% of postpubertal rape victims at baseline and 19% at follow-up.[5] Data on prepubertal children are conflicting, but BV has been noted following sexual assault in children. The condition is uncommon in sexually inexperienced females. The presence of BV in prepubertal girls raises concern about but does not prove sexual abuse. The incubation period for BV is unknown.

Clinical Manifestations

Bacterial vaginosis is the most prevalent cause of vaginal infections of malodor in sexually active adolescents; however, more than 50% of women with BV are asymptomatic. Symptoms include foul-smelling thin yellow, white, or gray, noninflammatory vaginal discharge. Abdominal pain and irregular or prolonged menses can be accompanying symptoms, but are uncommon. Vaginitis and vulvitis in prepubertal children usually have other causes and rarely are manifestations of BV.

Laboratory Diagnosis

Three of 4 criteria can make the diagnosis in pubertal adolescents.

- A homogeneous, white, noninflammatory discharge that smoothly coats the vaginal vault
- The presence of clue cells (epithelial cells studded with small bacteria) on microscopic examination (at least 20% of the vaginal epithelial population)
- A pH of vaginal fluid greater than 4.5 (This criterion is inappropriate for diagnostic use in prepubertal children whose vaginal pH is physiologically alkaline [pH 6.5–7.5].)
- A fishy odor of vaginal discharge before or after addition of 10% KOH

A gram stain of the discharge demonstrating the lack of lactobacilli (≤4 lactobacilli per oil immersion field) and the presence of *Gardnerella* morphologic types plus one or more other bacterial morphologic types (gram-negative or gram-variable coccobacilli) is a sensitive test but may overdiagnose BV in a low-prevalence population.

Treatment (Box 5.4)

For more information, consult guidelines from the CDC (Sexually transmitted diseases treatment guidelines 2006. MMRW *Recommend Rep.* 2006;55[RR11]1-94) and the AAP (*Red Book: 2006 Report of the Committee on Infectious Diseases,* 27th ed)

Human Papillomavirus (HPV)

Biology

Human papillomaviruses are small, double-stranded DNA viruses that infect and preferentially replicate in specific epithelia in specific anatomical sites. They are subdivided into cutaneous and mucosal types, with types 1 through 5 and type 7 referred to as cutaneous and types 6, 8, and upward as mucosal. Mucosal types can be found in the genital tract and the respiratory and digestive tracts. More than 2,000 genotypes have been identified, more than 30 of which are genital. Human papillomavirus genital subtypes can be further divided into low risk and high risk based on their association with the risk of cervical cancer. High-risk groups include most commonly types 16, 18, 31, and 45. Types 6 and 11 are most common types associated with condyloma acuminatum.

Epidemiology

Anogenital warts are one of the most commonly diagnosed STIs in the United States, occurring in more than 40% of sexually active adolescent females. Recent data suggest a marked increase in symptomatic and asymptomatic infection with anogenital strains of HPV in this country. Anogenital warts have been reported in 0.3% to 2% of children who have been sexually abused.[18]

Human papillomavirus infections are transmitted from person to person through close contact. Nongenital warts are acquired through minor injuries through the skin. Anogenital HPV transmission is accepted to be sexual in adults. Anogenital HPV infections in children may be acquired perinatally or through sexual abuse. In general, the older the child, the more likely the possibility of acquisition through sexual abuse. Acquisition of HPV in children via any other mode such as autoinoculation, heteroinoculation, and fomite transmission remains controversial but may occur. The perinatal transmission rate of infected mothers may be less than 3% and may be transient due to the loss of maternal estrogen mucosal effects as the newborn ages.[18] Vertical transmission of HPV has been reported to be responsible for at least 20% of anogenital warts in younger children and occurs by contamination of the newborn descending through the birth canal, by viral ascent through the membranes in utero, or by the hematogenous transplacental transmission. Sequelae of vertical transmission of HPV in infants are uncommon, but have been documented in the respiratory tract as well as in vulvar and anal condyloma.

Development of vulvar condylomata due to vertical HPV transmission has been felt to be uncommon after age 3 or 4 and should raise concern for sexual abuse. A recent retrospective epidemiological study of 124 children younger than 13 years with anogenital and respiratory tract HPV infections concluded that children acquired anogenital HPV from nonsexual contact as well as sexual contact, with increasing concern for sexual abuse with increasing age.[19] The positive predictive value of the presence of genital HPV lesions for sexual abuse in children 2 to 12 years of age was 37%. It increased to 70% when the age group of 8 to 12 was considered.[20] The most common HPVs reported in anogenital warts of neonates and infants have been types 16, 18, 6, and 11. Types 6 and 11 are most commonly reported in sexually abused children (vs types 16 and 18).

Studies on the prevalence of HPV in prepubertal children note that a history of or findings consistent with sexual abuse are frequently associated with the presence of anogenital warts and/or the presence of HPV DNA.

All children with anogenital HPV lesions should undergo a complete medical evaluation for child sexual abuse to include

a. A detailed history from the child and family, a thorough medical examination for cutaneous warts, and consideration of referral of family members for examination
b. Examination of the child including the anogenital area for signs of physical injury, including a close visual examination for the presence of genital warts to differentiate them from normal findings such as micropapillomatosis labialis in females or pearly penile papules in males, and testing for the presence of other STIs (Consideration could be given to the use of a NAAT as a first screen with a second NAAT if the first was positive.)
c. Behavior and social assessment by trained professionals
d. Reporting of any suspicion of child sexual abuse to authorities
e. Appropriate emotional support and follow-up

The incubation period for HPV infection is unknown but may range from 3 months to several years.

Clinical Manifestations

Genital HPV usually manifests as soft, sessile, irregular growths on anogenital surfaces ranging from flat to exophytic, cauliflower-like lesions. These surfaces can include labial, vaginal, perianal, rectal, penile, scrotal, cervical, and perineal. In patients who have had receptive anal intercourse, lesions can be internal and require anoscopy. Lesions can be inapparent on the cervix and perineum. Secondary infection with maceration and ulceration can occur, especially in younger children, and make visual diagnosis more challenging. The differential diagnosis of HPV includes epithelial papillae, pink pearly penile papules, molluscum contagiosum, and condylomata lata.

Laboratory Diagnosis

Most anogenital HPV is diagnosed clinically through visual inspection. Diagnosis can be enhanced in some cases using colposcopy or by applying 3% to 5% acetic acid, which turns the HPV lesions white. Human papillomavirus cannot be cultured. If confirmation of the presence is required for forensic purposes, suspected tissue may be biopsied and analyzed for the presence of HPV DNA. The use of other nucleic acid–based methods such as PCR to detect HPV DNA anogenital lesions in populations of children suspected of sexual abuse is currently under investigation, has been used in some centers, and shows promise.

Treatment

Treatment of anogenital warts is controversial because spontaneous remission occurs in up to 67% of children. Many experts recommend leaving the lesions untreated if they are not significantly symptomatic. Treatment options are based on location and extent of the disease and include burning, refreezing, surgery, and laser and chemical treatments. Topical therapy includes podofilox 0.5% solution or gel, imiquimod 5% cream, podophyllin resin 10% to 25%, or trichloroacetic acid or bichloracetic acid 80% to 90%. Intralesional interferon has also been used. In general, warts located on moist surfaces or intertriginous areas respond best to topical treatment compared with warts on drier surfaces. Most warts respond within 3 months to the treatment modalities.

Herpes Simplex Virus (HSV)

Biology

Herpesviruses are enveloped, double-stranded DNA viruses with 2 subtypes: herpes simplex virus type 1 and type 2 (HSV-1 and HSV-2).

Epidemiology

Herpes simplex virus type 1 infections usually involve the mucocutaneous areas of the oral mucosa, face, and skin above the waist, but can involve genital sites.

Herpes simplex virus type 2 infections usually involve the mucocutaneous areas of the genitalia, perineum, and skin below the waist, but can involve oral sites in 25% of cases.

The risk of acquiring HSV after a sexual assault is unknown.[16] In studies of prepubertal children being evaluated for sexual abuse, genital herpes was very uncommon.[21]

Herpesviruses are transmitted via close contact with infected secretions or lesions. The organism is readily inactivated at room temperature and by drying. Although the greatest concentration of HSV is shed during symptomatic infection, most HSV is transmitted as a consequence of asymptomatic shedding. Oral HSV-1 is primarily transmitted via nongenital person-to-person contact. In adults and adolescents, genital HSV is solely sexually transmitted. In children, genital infection with HSV-1 can result from autoinoculation of the virus from the mouth or from sexual abuse.[22] Herpes simplex virus type 2 isolated from any site in the prepubertal child should warrant an evaluation for possible sexual abuse because infections with HSV-2 usually result from direct contact with infected genital secretions or lesions through sexual activity.

Fifty percent to 85% of first infections of genital herpes are caused by HSV-2. Infections can be classified as primary (first-time infections with no antibody to HSV-1 or HSV-2), non-primary first episodes (patient does have antibody to one type, commonly infected with type 2 with antibodies to type 1), and recurrent infections. After the first episode, 14% of patients with genital HSV-1 and 60% of patients with genital HSV-2 will have a recurrence. Asymptomatic shedding is not unusual, and cultures may be positive in the absence of characteristic lesions.

The incubation period is 2 to 14 days.

Clinical Manifestations
The characteristic anogenital lesions are tender, painful grouped vesicles or pustules, which erupt on the labia, vestibule, vagina and/or cervix, penis, scrotum, rectum, and anus. One to 3 days later, they rupture, leaving the characteristic painful yellowish ulcer. During this time, the patient experiences local burning, pain, irritation, and dysuria, which may be severe. Inguinal adenopathy may be present. Systemic symptoms may be present such as headache, fever, myalgia, and malaise, or symptoms suggesting aseptic meningitis. The patient may experience urinary retention, sacral anesthesia, and constipation for

up to 4 to 8 weeks. Anorectal symptoms may include discharge (may be bloody), pain, and tenesmus, and fever in severe cases. Extragenital sites include buttocks, groin, thighs, pharynx, fingers, and conjunctivae. Positive cultures may persist 8 to 10 days. Symptoms may last 10 to 21 days in primary infections. Recurrence of genital HSV usually manifests with milder symptoms, less shedding, and less severe vesicular lesions.

Atypical lesions include fissures, furuncles, excoriations, and nonspecific vulvar erythema. Herpes simplex may occur in 5% of women with dysuria and frequency.

The differential diagnosis of genital ulcers includes the following[23]:

1) Sexually transmitted
   a) Chancroid
   b) Granuloma inguinale
   c) LGV
   d) Syphilis
2) Non–sexually transmitted
   a) Behçet disease
   b) Epstein-Barr virus/infectious mononucleosis
   c) Trauma
   d) Contact or allergic dermatitis
   e) Viral infections such as influenza, coxsackie, varicella-zoster
   f) *Staphylococcus aureus* infections
   g) Aphthous ulcers

Laboratory Diagnosis
Isolation of herpesvirus via cell culture is the preferred method of diagnosis if lesions are present: best results in vesicles (94% positive rate); ulcers much less likely to yield a positive culture

(70% positive rate); crusted lesions (24% positive rate).[1] The examiner should unroof the vesicle and rub a swab vigorously over the base. Several lesions may be sampled using several swabs and placed into specific appropriate transport media, placed on ice, and sent immediately. Methods of culture confirmation include fluorescent antibody staining and EIAs. This method then allows for viral typing, which can be helpful in cases where the perpetrator is identified as having herpes.

As an adjunctive technique to culture, NAAT/PCR is a very sensitive tool for identifying HSV DNA. Polymerase chain reaction can differentiate between HSV-1 and HSV-2.

Rapid diagnostic techniques including direct fluorescent antibody staining of vesicle scrapings and EIA testing are not sufficiently sensitive nor specific for medical forensic application in low-prevalence populations such as seen in child and adolescent sexual abuse populations.

Recent glycoprotein G–based type-specific assays have been FDA approved, which have high specificities but may also have false-positives and are not appropriate for use in the medicolegal setting.[24]

It is important to recognize that lack of HSV detection via culture or other methods does not indicate a lack of HSV infection because viral shedding may be intermittent.

Type-specific herpes serology is available. Type 1- and 2-specific antibodies form early after disease and are detectable after several weeks. A rise in titer indicates a recent or recurrent infection. However, HSV infections, which may have occurred as a result of sexual abuse, should be diagnosed by culture or PCR, not by serology. No test for antibodies to HSV-1 or HSV-2 can be considered to be completely accurate because every serologic test has a potential for false-positive or false-negative results, and the use of type-specific serology to link the victim with possible perpetrators in abuse or assault cases is not recommended because even the most accurate test cannot reveal when and by whom the victim became infected.[25]

Treatment

Oral acyclovir, or famciclovir* or valacyclovir* (*approved for adults). For more information, consult guidelines from the CDC (Sexually transmitted diseases treatment guidelines 2006. MMRW *Recommend Rep.* 2006;55[RR11]1-94) and the AAP (*Red Book: 2006 Report of the Committee on Infectious Diseases,* 27th ed).

Syphilis

Biology

Syphilis is a systemic disease caused by a spirochete *Treponema pallidum.*

Epidemiology

Rarely seen in children, the incidence of acquired syphilis is about 0% to 1.8% in published studies.[16]

The organism may be transmitted in utero or through direct contact with moist mucosal or cutaneous lesions via abuse from an infected individual. The rate of acquisition from an infected person is estimated at about 30%.[25]

The primary lesion of syphilis, the painless ulcer known as a *chancre,* occurs 10 to 90 days postexposure, may not be easily visible especially in girls, and heals spontaneously in a few weeks. Primary lesions in nongenital sites, particularly anal sites, may have non-characteristic appearances. Lesions of secondary syphilis result from hematogenous spread and appear 4 to 10 weeks after the initial appearance of primary lesions, with some overlap in some patients. Secondary syphilis is characterized by an initial diffuse macular rash followed by a diffuse popular eruption, which is generally scaly and characteristically includes the palms and soles. Systemic manifestations are protean and include alopecia, generalized symptoms, hepatitis, nephritis, neurologic symptoms, arthritis, and iritis. Tertiary syphilis involves neurologic, cardiac, ophthalmologic, audiologic, and gummatous lesions, among others.

Condylomata lata have been described in child victims of sexual abuse and are large, raised, whitish or gray lesions found in warm, moist areas of the body including the axilla, groin, perineum, and anus. They are found in areas adjacent to the primary chancre and are now thought to be an intermediate stage of the infection.

Diagnosis

The observation of treponemes on darkfield examination or DFA tests of material taken from lesions of primary or secondary syphilis are the only tests that definitively establish the diagnosis of primary syphilis, but this is often not readily available in many non-referral laboratories and can be difficult to perform. Nontreponemal tests (Venereal Disease Research Laboratories and rapid plasma reagin) and treponemal tests (FTA-ABS and TP-PA) are usually used for presumptive diagnoses. Nontreponemal tests require at least a 4-fold change in titer for significance and usually become nonreactive with time after treatment; however, some antibodies persist at a low titer, and there may be false-positives associated with medical conditions unrelated to syphilis. Most patients with reactive treponemal tests will have reactive tests throughout their lives.

Treatment

Children outside the newborn period with syphilis should have a cerebrospinal fluid examination for asymptomatic neurosyphilis. Treatment is with benzathine penicillin G 50,000 U/kg intramuscularly up to 2.4 million units intramuscularly in a single dose. Patients should be reexamined clinically and serologically 6 months and 12 months after treatment or more frequently if follow-up is uncertain.

For more information, consult guidelines from the CDC (Sexually transmitted diseases treatment guidelines 2006. MMRW *Recommend Rep.* 2006;55[RR11]1-94) and the AAP (*Red Book: 2006 Report of the Committee on Infectious Diseases,* 27th ed).

Human Immunodeficiency Virus (HIV)

Biology

Infection is caused by the human RNA retrovirus HIV-1 and, less commonly, HIV-2.

Epidemiology

The virus has been demonstrated to be transmissible from blood, semen, cervical secretions, and human milk.

The median age of onset of symptoms of untreated perinatally infected children is 12 to 18 months in the United States, but some children have remained asymptomatic more than 5 years.

The established routes of transmission of HIV in the United States include (a) sexual contact (vaginal, anal, orogenital), (b) percutaneous or mucous membrane exposure to contaminated blood/body fluids, (c) vertical (prenatal/perinatal), and (d) breastfeeding. The estimated risk of HIV transmission for receptive penile-vaginal exposure is 10 per 10,000 exposures; for receptive penile-anal exposure is 50 per 10,000 exposures.

A few cases of HIV infection in children have resulted from sexual abuse by an HIV-seropositive person. The actual risk to a child or adolescent from a single act of sexual abuse from an infected assailant is unknown.

The rate of acquisition of HIV during adolescence continues to increase, and approximately 50% of HIV acquisition in the United States is estimated to occur among people 13 to 24 years of age. Most HIV-infected adolescents are asymptomatic, and without testing they remain unaware that they are infected. The rate of acquisition of HIV from sexual assault in adolescents is completely unknown.

Clinical Manifestations

Infection with HIV produces a spectrum of disease, which ranges from asymptomatic HIV infection to an immunocompromised host with multiple organ system involvement. Common clinical manifestations in children include lymphadenopathy, hepatosplenomegaly, recurrent diarrhea, persistent or recurrent respiratory infections, recurrent bacterial infections, and progressive neurologic deterioration.

Incubation period from infection with HIV to disease state (AIDS) is a few months to 17 years (median 10 years).

The clinician should be familiar with the early symptoms of infection, particularly in adolescents. Termed the *acute retroviral syndrome,* it is characterized by fever, malaise, lymphadenopathy, and skin rash and occurs within the first few weeks after HIV infection before antibody test results become positive (but nucleic acid tests are positive.)

Human immunodeficiency virus in children and adolescents causes a broad clinical spectrum of disease with AIDS at the most severe end of the spectrum.

Laboratory Diagnosis

Enzyme immunoassay for serum HIV antibody is an initial screening test, with Western blot confirmation. Additional testing includes HIV DNA PCR, culture, and viral load.

Treatment

Careful consideration for postexposure prophylaxis (PEP) for HIV should be given in each case of child or adolescent sexual assault. Multiple factors must be considered prior to offering PEP (Table 5.2).

Whenever possible, serologic testing for the alleged perpetrator should be attempted, although it is usually quite difficult to attain shortly after the abuse. Counseling of the child and family needs to be provided to include risks and benefits of PEP, risks of HIV transmission from the assault, toxicity, and unknown efficacy of PEP. The examiner should work closely with an infectious disease specialist experienced in treating HIV-infected children if PEP is considered. The child or adolescent should have HIV testing at the time of the examination, and then 6 weeks, 3 months, and 6 months later.

Conclusion

The evaluation of the child or adolescent for the presence of an STI is a critical element of the examination when sexual abuse or sexual assault is suspected. The examiner must have knowledge of the biology and a current understanding of the literature on the epidemiology of each infection as well as the clinical manifestations of the organism in the prepubertal as well as the adolescent population. The examiner must be familiar with the appropriate tests for screening and diagnosis of these infections in a medical setting. It is particularly important for each examiner to have access to a highly qualified reference laboratory with well-established chain of evidence procedures. Current prophylaxis and treatment guidelines for STIs in the prepubertal and adolescent populations are published periodically by the CDC (Sexually Transmitted Disease Treatment Guidelines) and professional agencies such as the AAP (*Red Book: Report of the Committee on Infectious Diseases*) and should be referred to to obtain the latest guidelines because they may change from year to year.

When STIs are confirmed they represent only one piece of the diagnostic puzzle of suspected sexual abuse. The clinician must not only diagnose and treat STIs but also try to understand as comprehensively as possible how and under what circumstances the child acquired the infection. Understanding the circumstances that surround the transmission of the infection may be quite challenging, particularly in young children. Adolescents may misrepresent their experiences out of privacy needs or based on fears of consequences. Physicians may require the collective insights of child protection and law enforcement professionals to fully understand a child's experience, which then becomes the first step to protection, intervention, and treatment.

TABLE 5.2
Factors to Consider in Offering Postexposure Prophylaxis in Child/Adolescent Sexual Assault[a]

Treatment/Prevention	
Timing: Within 72 h of assault	
Age of patient	• Age ≥12, makes own decision • Age <12, parents/legal guardian decides

Consideration of acts of assault	• Acts with measurable risk
	  – Anal/vaginal penetration
	  – Injection with a contaminated needle
	• Acts with possible risk
	  – Oral penetration with ejaculation
	  – Unknown act
	  – Contact with other mucous membrane
	  – Victim biting or getting bit with bloody mouth
	• Acts with no risk
	  – Kissing
	  – Ejaculation onto intact skin
	  – Digital/object penetration of vagina/mouth/anus

Consideration of assailant's human immunodeficiency virus (HIV) status	• Known positive HIV assailant • Past/present intravenous drug user • Commercial sex worker • Men who have sex with men • Individuals who have multiple sex partners • Individuals with prior convictions for sexual assault or incarceration • Unknown assailant or with unknown risk factors
Other factors of the assault	• Presence of blood • Survivor or assailant with sexually transmitted infection with inflammation • Significant physical trauma to survivor (more likely with children) • Ejaculation by assailant • Multiple assailants • Multiple penetrations by assailant

[a]Adapted from Centers for Disease Control and Prevention. Sexually transmitted diseases treatment guidelines 2006. *MMWR Recommend Rep.* 2006;55[RR11]1–94.

References

1. Muram D, Stewart DC. Sexually transmitted diseases In: Heger A, Emans SJ, Muram D, eds. *Evaluation of the Sexually Abused Child: A Medical Textbook and Photographic Atlas.* 2nd ed. New York, NY: Oxford University Press; 2000:187–224

2. Groothuis J, Bischoff MC, Jauregui LE. Pharyngeal gonorrhea in young children. *Pediatr Infect Dis.* 1983;2(2):99–101

3. Simmons KJ, Hicks DJ. Child sexual abuse examination: is there a need for routine screening for *N gonorrhoeae* and *C trachomatis*? *J Pediatr Adolesc Gynecol.* 2005;18(5):343–345

4. Muram D, Speck PM, Dockter M. Child sexual abuse examination: is there a need for routine screening for *N gonorrhoeae*? *J Pediatr Adolesc Gynecol.* 1996;9(2):79–80

5. Jenny C, Hooton TM, Bowers A, et al. Sexually transmitted diseases in victims of rape. *N Engl J Med.* 1990;322(11):713–716

6. Beck-Sague CM, Jenny C. Sexual assault and STD. In: Holmes KK, Mardh PA, Sparling PF, et al, eds. *Sexually Transmitted Diseases.* 3rd ed. New York, NY: McGraw-Hill; 1999:1433–1440

7. DeMattia A, Kornblum JS, Hoffman-Rosenfeld J, et al. The use of combination subtyping in the forensic evaluation of a three-year-old girl with gonorrhea. *Pediatr Infect Dis J.* 2006;25(5):461–463

8. Palusci VJ, Reeves MJ. Testing for genital gonorrhea infections in prepubertal girls with suspected sexual abuse. *Pediatr Infect Dis J.* 2003;22(7):618–623

9. Schachter J, Chernesky MA, Willis DE, et al. Vaginal swabs are the specimens of choice when screening for *Chlamydia trachomatis* and *Neisseria gonorrhoeae*: results from a multicenter evaluation of the APTIMA assays for both infections. *Sex Transm Dis.* 2005;32(12):725–728

10. Shrier L. Bacterial sexually transmitted infections: gonorrhea, chlamydia, pelvic inflammatory disease and syphilis. In: Emans SJ, Laufer MR, Goldstein DP, eds. *Pediatric and Adolescent Gynecology.* 5th ed. Philadelphia, PA: Lippincott Williams-Wilkins; 2005:565–614

11. Asbel LE, Newbern EC, Salmon M, et al. School-based screening for *Chlamydia trachomatis* and *Neisseria gonorrhoeae* among Philadelphia public high school students. *Sex Transm Dis.* 2006;33(10):614–620

12. Schwarcz S, Whittington W. Sexual assault and sexually transmitted diseases: detection and management in adults and children. *Rev Infect Dis.* 1990;12(6):S682–S690

13. Hammerschlag MR. Chlamydial infections in infants and children. In: Holmes KK, Mardh PA, Sparling PF, et al, eds. *Sexually Transmitted Diseases.* 3rd ed. New York, NY: McGraw Hill; 1999

14. Bell TA, Stamm WE, Wang SP, et al. Chronic *Chlamydia trachomatis* infections in infants. *JAMA.* 1992;267(3):400–402

15. Centers for Disease Control and Prevention. 2006 sexually transmitted disease treatment guidelines. *MMWR Morb Mortal Wkly Rep.* 2006;55:1–94

16. al-Salihi FL, Curran JP, Wang J. Neonatal *Trichomonas vaginalis*: report of three cases and review of the literature. *Pediatrics.* 1974;53(2):196–200

17. Hammerschlag MR. Sexually transmitted diseases in sexually abused children: medical and legal implications. *Sex Transm Infect.* 1998;74:167–174

18. Watts DH, Koutsky LA, Holmes KK, et al. Low risk of perinatal transmission of human papillomavirus: results from a prospective cohort study. *Am J Obstet Gynecol.* 1998;178(2):365–373

19. Sinclair KA, Woods CR, Kirse DJ, et al. Anogenital and respiratory tract human papillomavirus infections among children: age, gender, and potential transmission through sexual abuse. *Pediatrics.* 2005;116(4);815–825

20. Jayasinghe Y, Garland SM. Genital warts in children: what do they mean? *Arch Dis Child.* 2006;91(8):696–700

21. Reading R, Rannan-Eliya Y. Evidence for sexual transmission of genital herpes in children. *Arch Dis Child.* 2007;92(7): 608–613

22. Miller RG, Whittington WL, Coleman RM, Nigida SM Jr. Acquisition of concomitant oral and genital infection with herpes simplex virus type 2. *Sex Transm Dis.* 1987;14:41–43

23. Fischer GO. Vulval disease in prepubertal girls. *Australas J Dermatol.* 2001;42:225–236

24. Ashley RL. Sorting out the new HSV type specific antibody tests. *Sex Transm Infect.* 2001;77:232–237

25. Sparling PF. Natural history of syphilis. In: Holmes KK, Mardh PA, Sparling PF, et al, eds. *Sexually Transmitted Diseases.* 3rd ed. New York, NY: McGraw-Hill; 1999

Chapter 6

Forensic Evidence in Child Sexual Abuse

Vincent J. Palusci

Cindy W. Christian

Introduction

Forensic trace evidence plays a valuable role in a small but important number of child sexual abuse cases. A medical examination of the sexually abused child is primarily important for diagnosis and treatment but can also be helpful for forensic puposes. This chapter provides the examining physician information about the nature and approach to identifying and preserving evidence that may have forensic value. This chapter first addresses definitions and general issues related to the types of materials that may be collected, such as sperm, components of seminal fluid, genetic markers, and hair. The chapter then discusses the collection and analysis of each type of specimen before concluding with a brief discussion of how to handle specimens in a manner that maintains a chain of evidence that is important for its eventual admission in a court of law. The health care provider need not become a legal expert with regard to forensic evidence, but it is essential that he or she become proficient in identifying and collecting appropriate specimens in cases where sexual abuse or assault is alleged.

Definitions

Forensic Evidence

The purpose of a medical examination after a sexual assault is to assess the patient for physical injuries, treat and prevent disease, and collect evidence for potential forensic evaluation and legal proceedings.[1,2] Evidentiary collection is the responsibility of the examining clinician but not the primary purpose of conducting this examination. Forensic evidence refers to evidence that pertains to or is used in courts of law and is therefore subject to the scrutiny of the legal system. While all statements made by the child and family and any physical examination and laboratory findings can be potentially used as evidence in the courts, forensic evidence generally refers to physical materials taken from the patient, their clothing, or the crime scene that may be used in a criminal investigation as confirmation of the sexual assault and to identify the perpetrator and the nature of the acts committed.

Rape

Rape is a legal term defined by state statute that refers to forced engagement in a sexual act that includes penetration by the penis into a bodily orifice (most often the vulva or vagina, although the mouth and anus are possibilities as well).[3] Rape is typically a violent act and implies either the use of actual physical force or the threat of such force to the degree that victims feel that their lives are in danger.[4] Various types of rape have been identified.

- Stranger rape—a violent attack by an unknown assailant(s)
- Peer or date rape—an attack by someone known to the victim and with whom the initial contact is consensual but progresses to a point that an element of force is imposed against the other's will
- Domestic rape—a violent sexual attack against one's intimate partner
- Gang rape—a forcible sexual attack on the victim by multiple assailants in a public manner

Sexual Assault

Sexual assault is most broadly defined as coerced sexual contact that is unwanted by the victim. It includes a wide variety of sexual activities, such as fondling; oral sex; and genital penetration by objects, fingers, and the perpetrator's penis. A known or unknown assailant may commit sexual assault, and the coercion may be threat of force, manipulation, or actual application of physical force in a violent attack (eg, rape). The forensic evidence that has been identified in these scenarios depends on the circumstances of each type of contact and the amount of time passed since the act.[1,2]

Sexual Abuse

Sexual abuse refers to the involvement of children in activities of a sexual nature that are inappropriate to their developmental level (emotional, maturational, or cognitive) by someone in a more dominant position by virtue of their age, size, cognitive level, or authority/power over the child.[1] The child cannot give consent to the contact, and the perpetrator coerces the child either directly, with threats or force, or by coercive manipulation (eg, implying to the child that if the perpetrator is discovered, the friendship between the child and perpetrator will come to an end). Sexual abuse usually occurs over extended periods and progresses from noncontact, to fondling, to more invasive types of sexual contact. Disclosure of the abuse may be immediate but is typically delayed. Physical injuries are uncommon after child sexual abuse, and the abusive contact may come to light months or even years after the initial contact (Table 6.1). The most available form of evidence in sexual abuse cases is the medical history obtained from

TABLE 6.1
Description of Sexually Abusive Activities

Activity	Description
Nudity, disrobing, and genital exposure	The perpetrator finds situations to cause the child or adolescent to see the perpetrator's body and genitals in a manner that is beyond what is culturally acceptable. With genital exposure, the perpetrator directs the child's or adolescent's attention to the perpetrator's genitals specifically.
Observation of the child	The perpetrator watches the child or adolescent during donning or doffing of clothing, bathing, and toileting in a manner beyond cultural norms.
Kissing	The perpetrator kisses the child or adolescent in a prolonged and intimate manner mimicking the pattern of sexualized kissing appropriate for adult romantic relationships.
Fondling	The perpetrator inappropriately touches the child's or adolescent's breasts, abdomen, genital area (vulva, penis, associated genital structures), inner thighs, buttocks, or perianal area. The perpetrator may also cause the child or adolescent to fondle the perpetrator's body area.
Masturbation	The perpetrator involves the child or adolescent in any range of behavior around masturbating, such as (a) the perpetrator causing the child to observe the perpetrator masturbating, (b) the perpetrator observing the child or adolescent masturbating, (c) the perpetrator and child or adolescent observing each other masturbating, or (d) the perpetrator and child or adolescent mutually masturbating each other.
Anogenital/oral contact	The perpetrator engages the child or adolescent in various forms of oral contact, such as (a) the perpetrator causing the child or adolescent to place his or her mouth in contact with the perpetrator's anogenital area or (b) the perpetrator placing his or her mouth in contact with the child's or adolescent's anogenital area.
Digital or foreign body penetration of the child's or adolescent's anus	The perpetrator inserts his or her fingers into the child's or adolescent's anus and/or may insert inanimate objects into the child's anal opening.
Digital or foreign body penetration of the child's or adolescent's vagina	The perpetrator inserts his or her fingers into the child's or adolescent's vagina and/or may insert inanimate objects into the vagina.

the child because "forensic" evidence is uncommon in great part due to delayed disclosures.

Forensic Evidence and Legal Outcomes

In general, most criminal cases do not involve the use of any physical evidence, and such evidence, even when available, is seldom seen by the investigators as having important value in the case. Despite popular notions about its use in court,[5] investigators generally use physical evidence to strengthen a position that is usually squarely based on witness and perpetrator statements. Physical evidence has been shown to improve convictions in burglary and robbery cases, but it is particularly important when the alleged perpetrator has not been identified or there is conflicting or potentially challengeable statements available from witnesses.[6] In a review of a large number of cases, evidence of trauma was found in 202 adult and child victims of sexual assault, and spermatozoa were found microscopically at the time of the forensic medical examination in 31% of the cases in which a suspect was identified.[7] Attempting to identify prostate-specific antigen could increase this identification up to 50%. Overall conviction rates of 75% were obtained among those who were charged, and charges were 3 times more likely to be filed when forensic specimens were obtained.[8]

There may be differences between adults and children in the association of legal outcomes and forensic evidence. In general, medical assessment plays an important role in the overall community response after child sexual abuse, and physical findings are associated with findings of guilt.[9] The presence of forensic evidence in reported series varies from approximately 3% to 25%, depending on the population studied and laboratory methods used.[10-13] In a 16-year study of 162 child cases, 15 had positive laboratory tests for sperm, 2 for acid phosphatase, 11 for both, and 1 for trichomonas and sperm.[10] Because adolescents and children assaulted by strangers are brought for medical attention earlier than are young victims of intrafamilial sexual abuse, the likelihood of identifying forensic evidence may be greater in these populations. For example, Dahlke et al[11] reported sperm detec-tion in 3% of children younger than 11 years who were raped, compared with 36% of 11- to 14-year-olds who were similarly victimized. In another series of 115 children, physical evidence was present in 23% of all cases that resulted in felony convictions, but there was a higher proportion of convictions in the absence of physical evidence (79%) than when such evidence was present (67%).[12] Cases involving the youngest victims had a significantly lower conviction rate despite a high frequency of physical evidence, and physical evidence was neither predictive nor essential for conviction (which was thought to depend more heavily on verbal evidence).

In a retrospective analysis of forensic evidence collected in Philadelphia, some form of forensic evidence was identified in 24.9% of 273 prepubertal children, all of whom were examined within 44 hours of their assault.[10] Most (64%) of the forensic evidence was found on clothing and linens, yet only 35% had such evidence collected. Genital injury and a history of ejaculation were associated with an increased likelihood of identifying forensic evidence, but some children had evidence found that was not anticipated by the history provided. In a series of 190 children younger than age 13 years seen at a child advocacy center in Grand Rapids, MI, only 9% were found to have physical evidence identified, and female children older than 10 years who reported ejaculation by the perpetrator or genital contact had the highest likelihood of having physical evidence identified if they had not bathed after the assault.[14] In Arkansas, 16 of 80 children younger than 12 years had positive findings for semen, and 13 of these were adolescents.[15] None of the children younger than 10 years in those studies had semen recovered from any body site 24 hours after the alleged assault.

Incorporating Evidence Collection Into Medical Evaluations

A variety of protocols have been developed to assist physicians and nurse examiners in collecting physical evidence, and many states have issued state-specific guidelines.[16–18] These protocols guide the examiner in obtaining crucial medical history and physical examination findings in addition to collecting specimens for forensic evidence. While physical evidence is often collected in adult victims 72 or more hours after sexual assault, forensic evidence collection in child sexual abuse cases is indicated less often than it is in adult cases. Unlike stranger rape, the child victim often identifies the perpetrator. The type of contact may leave little in the way of potential evidence (eg, fondling). Delayed disclosure limits the role of forensic evidence collection because seminal products do not remain on the body for more than a few days, and evidence on clothing and bed linens can be laundered away.

In dealing with children and adolescents who may have been sexually maltreated, health care providers have both medical and legal responsibilities that are governed in part by state statutory requirements and generally accepted clinical practice standards. The sooner the child or adolescent presents for care after an inappropriate sexual contact, the more immediate the need to pursue the collection of forensic evidence. Guidelines for collecting forensic evidence in child sexual abuse have been extrapolated largely from adult practices related to rape and other forms of sexual assault, and little data specific to young children have been published. Because of the dynamics of child sexual abuse described earlier (ie, the frequent delay in disclosure and subsequent medical evaluation), there is a growing awareness of the low likelihood of identifying forensic evidence in such cases.

Standard guidelines for the evaluation of sexual abuse, including those by the American Academy of Pediatrics,[1] recommend forensic evidence collection when sexual abuse has occurred within the last 72 hours or when there is bleeding or acute injury. This recommendation is based in part on the length of time that sperm can be identified in the vagina after sexual intercourse or adult assault.[11,19] As noted previously, recent data suggest that these guidelines might not be well suited for prepubertal victims of sexual assault.[10,14,15] These findings emphasize the need for further research regarding indications for forensic evidence collection in child and adolescent sexual abuse cases. Until further data are available, clinical judgment and relevant state statutes will continue to guide the decision to collect forensic evidence, although it is prudent to err on the side of caution. All health care providers must remember that the temporal events of child sexual abuse can be vague and, although unlikely, the finding of physical evidence can have a significant influence on the legal investigations and the protection of the child from further abuse.

Evidence Identification and Analysis

The forensic scientist will generally follow one or more protocols based on the current practices of the laboratory, direction from law enforcement officers, and resources available for analysis. Specimens are stored for future analysis and are later analyzed in an order that often depends on the forensic needs of the investigation and the severity of injury to the victim. During analysis, different types of sample will be

analyzed in different parts of the laboratory, by scientists with different expertise. For the assessment of possible semen, acid phosphatase is first sought using a color change reagent in a sample. If positive, smears are taken for staining and evaluation by microscopy. If negative, a sample is tested qualitatively for P-30 antigen. If this is positive, samples are taken for DNA analysis. If it does not appear that genetic markers or DNA evidence is present, hair, fibers, or other trace evidence provided will be analyzed for comparison to known or suspected perpetrators (J. Nye, personal communication, 2007).

Spermatozoa

The identification of spermatozoa by microscopy is considered diagnostic of sexual contact when identified by trained personnel. Sperm can be identified by wet mount preparation, but recovery is enhanced by use of Gram stain, Christmas tree stain, or Pap smear. The length of time that sperm is recoverable after ejaculation varies considerably, primarily by location sampled (Tables 6.2. and 6.3).[19-21] Sperm motility decreases rapidly, and the detection of motile sperm is the best indicator of recent ejaculation. Specimens obtained from the cervical os are slightly more sensitive than those obtained from the vaginal pool. Despite its usefulness in timing an assault, routine examination for motile sperm in the hospital setting is not generally recommended unless the health care provider has extensive experience in searching for sperm, which requires being able to identify

TABLE 6.2
Guidelines for the Estimated Number of Days
Within Which Sexual Intercourse Is Likely to Have Occurred[19-21]

Sample	Sperm Count				
	Few	+	++	+++	++++
Internal vaginal	7	7	3	1.5	1.5
External vaginal	7	3	2-3	2	1
Internal anal	2-3	2-3	2	1	1
External anal	3	3	2	2	1
Oral/saliva	2	2	2	2	NA

TABLE 6.3
Survivability of Specimens, by Location and Test[19-21]

Specimen	Vagina	Cervix	Rectum	Mouth	Skin	Dried Secretions/ Clothing
Motile sperm	3–24 h	2–7 d	Several hours	(na.)?	(na.)?	(na.)?
Nonmotile sperm	12–24 h (max 72+ h)	1+ weeks	2–3 days	? h	24+ h.	12+ mo if dry
Acid Phosphatase	18–36 h (max 72 h)	?	?	?	24+ h	Years
P-30 antigen	<48	?	?	?	28+ h	?

the proper head to tail ratio and density and width of the head. Myxosporidia, a flagellated parasite, has been misidentified as sperm in cases and publications (M. Finkel, personal communication, 1999).

Motile Sperm

Motile sperm are detected by examining a saline wet mount of a freshly collected specimen. The presence of motile sperm in the vagina decreases rapidly. Motile sperm are found 3 hours after consensual intercourse in only 50% of women, although duration may range from 30 minutes to 8 hours.[20,22] In the favorable environment of cervical mucus, motility may be preserved for a number of days. For this reason, separate swabs should be taken from the vagina and cervix in adolescent patients. Lack of cervical mucus decreases sperm survival in prepubertal girls. Motile sperm are less frequently identified in the rectum and, because of the action of salivary enzymes, may persist 30 minutes to 6 hours in the mouth. Because of drying, motile sperm persist less than 30 minutes on clothing.[19]

Nonmotile Sperm

The average time for loss of sperm motility in half of adult cases is 2 to 3 hours, and by 24 hours after intercourse, 50% of vaginal specimens will have no detectable sperm, although sperm can last up to 72 hours in the vagina and more than 1 week in cervical mucus. Sperm identified in the rectum are generally less than 48 hours old, and in the mouth, generally less than 24 hours old. In a controlled study by Gabby et al,[21] more than 50% of semen secretions placed on the skin showed no microscopic evidence of sperm at 28 hours. Sperm is stable in dried secretions and can be detected in clothing stains or on bedding for many months.

Seminal Fluid Analysis

Although the presence of spermatozoa on the body of a child or adolescent disclosing sexual abuse or sexual assault confirms sexual contact, health care providers should be aware that seminal products may be present without the presence or identification of sperm cells. A number of techniques are used to identify seminal products.

Acid Phosphatase

Acid phosphatase is an enzyme secreted by the prostate gland and found in seminal products. Although acid phosphatase is also found in vaginal fluid and urine of women, it is found in much higher concentrations in semen (130–1,800 IU/L) than in vaginal fluid

(<50 IU/L). Acid phosphatase is found in normal levels in vasectomized men. The presence of acid phosphatase is a less specific and less sensitive marker of ejaculate than is sperm, but acid phosphatase has been noted to persist longer than sperm after sexual assault.[23] Elevated acid phosphatase levels are not always found in patients who have sperm identified, and acid phosphatase levels return to normal between 18 and 24 hours after ejaculation (Table 6.3). Acid phosphatase can be identified on the skin more than 24 hours later, but an average decay of 9 hours has been reported. Acid phosphatase is stable in dried secretions and clothing, and in some instances it can be detected after months or even years.

P-30 Antigen

P-30 (prostate-specific protein, prostate-specific antigen) is a semen glycoprotein found in greatest concentration in seminal fluid and in low concentrations in adult male urine. It is absent in the urine of prepubertal boys, all other male body fluids, and all female body fluids and tissues. The detection of P-30 by enzyme-linked immunosorbent assay (ELISA) is a more specific and sensitive marker for ejaculate than is acid phosphatase, but it is not universally assayed in forensic laboratories.[24] P-30 follows a regular pattern of postcoital decline and is undetectable in the vagina after 48 hours. No data are available on pharyngeal or rectal sites.[19] P-30 ELISA is 100% sensitive in detecting the presence of semen on the skin, and it remains positive at 28 hours in 91% of samples.[21]

Genetic Markers

Genetic markers identify variance among homologous chromosomes. Examples of genetic markers that are important in forensic analysis are blood group antigens and DNA sequences.

Blood Group Antigens

Approximately 80% of the general population secretes blood group antigens in all body fluids, including semen and saliva. The amount of blood group antigen in semen is significantly greater than that in saliva. A comparison of genetic marker subtypes between a sample and the victim can be used to determine whether the sample came from the victim. Red blood cell surface antigens that have been used include ABO, Rh, Kell, Kid, Duffy, Sutter, Lewis-Secretor, and Xg.24. A variety of red cell enzymes and proteins can also be used, especially for paternity testing. Serum proteins and white cell antigens have also been used, but with the advent of DNA analysis (which is more specific), blood group substance testing is used less frequently as a forensic technique.

DNA Sequences

The human genome contains regions that consist of tandemly repeated nucleotide sequences in base pairs, all of which have a common core sequence. Only 1 in 1,000 base pairs differs between individuals, but the number and therefore length of repeated units varies. With more than 6 billion nucleotides within the average human cell, the term *DNA fingerprint* was coined by Jeffreys because DNA analysis revealed patterns unique to

a very small number of individuals based on the individuality of their genetic makeup.[25] Although DNA cannot determine a motive for a crime or when a crime was committed, DNA evidence may be able to place a particular individual at a crime scene.[26] DNA analysis is a forensic tool remarkable in its ability to convict or exonerate a suspect. When properly performed, DNA analysis is both valid and reliable.[27]

DNA analysis provides the most specific information available regarding perpetrator identification.[28] Several major classes of DNA sequence-based genetic markers exist, such as restriction fragment length polymorphism, variable number of tandem repeats, and short tandem repeats. Analysis can be done on blood, sperm, saliva, hair root, or other tissue from the perpetrator found on the victim's body. Restriction fragment length polymorphism analysis requires high molecular weight, high-quality DNA that is later cleaved into smaller fragments. Small amounts of semen (50 μL) can yield sufficient DNA material (50 ng) for this sequencing.[29] Using polymerase chain reaction (PCR), partially degraded and/or very small amounts of DNA can be amplified to allow for additional analysis.[30] Polymerase chain reaction of short-tandem repeat segments (STR) can be used with 1 ng or less of material. The standard Federal Bureau of Investigation laboratory analysis of DNA involves examination of a DNA strand at 13 specific locations or loci.[26] Profiles are generated for comparison to samples from the victim and potential perpetrators. If a match occurs, a statistic is generated that reflects how often one would expect to find this particular DNA in the general population. DNA information, as allowed by state and federal laws, can also be entered into a national database (Combined DNA Index System, CODIS) to allow comparison with a large number (3 million) of potential perpetrators. In Michigan as of this writing, for example, 10 of 13 markers can be entered into a database that currently holds information on 250,000 individuals (J. Nye, personal communication, 2007). In optimal circumstances, sufficient DNA is present to allow definitive inclusion or exclusion of a potential offender.

In cases with a male offender, analyses of the DNA from the Y chromosome have been helpful in further reducing the amount of DNA needed for adequate analysis. Fluorescent in situ hybridization (FISH) uses a Y chromosome–specific DNA probe to identify male cells in sample smears. The technique is relatively easy and has a high sensitivity and specificity in detecting human chromosomes. Fluorescent in situ hybridization can identify both Y chromosome sperm and non-sperm cells. In one study, FISH identified sperm and/or non-sperm cells in 83% of cases where sperm were identified by cytology. Using STR analysis of Y chromosome DNA (Y-STR), Y-STR could detect DNA in 24 of 26 specimens in which regular STR could not.[31] Current research involves the potential use of mitochondrial DNA from hair shafts

and other tissues and the development of less expensive and more sensitive methods with potentially broader applications (J. Nye, personal communication, 2007).

Hair and Fibers

Hair is durable and can be discovered as single hairs, tufts, or mixed with fluids or stuck to bodies, clothes, and other materials. When hairs foreign to the victim are transferred to the victim's body, they are valuable in establishing proximity of an alleged perpetrator and possibly the acts performed. Microscopic hair analysis compares morphologic characteristics of hair samples (root, shaft, and tip) to determine human or animal source with further comparison to hair from the victim to determine the general hair characteristics of a perpetrator.[32] Scalp hair is more useful than axillary, pubic, or body hair.[25] Microscopic hair analysis is useful in determination of race but has limited specificity. When present, dyes and other treatments can be very useful to determine a source. With the ability to perform DNA analysis, there will be additional future potential uses. Because root hairs contribute important morphologic characteristics to the analysis, past recommendations were to pluck, not cut, samples from the victim. However, under optimal controlled collection conditions, hair transfer during intercourse has been found less than 20% of the time and in less than 5% of sexual assaults.[33,34] Routinely plucking hairs from the victim is therefore no longer recommended.

Textile fibers can be exchanged between individuals and objects, but the value of their identification depends on several factors, including type of fiber, color or variation in color, and the number of different fibers at the scene or in the clothing of the victim.[32] Whether a fiber is transferred depends on the nature and duration of any contact between the perpetrator and victim and its persistence thereafter. Fiber analysis includes identification of natural and man-made fibers and fabrics. Transferred fibers are lost rather quickly after sexual assault, but the presence of a fiber from the alleged perpetrator on the victim's genitals is strong presumptive evidence of contact, particularly with nonfamilial perpetrators. Once transferred, fibers can be easily further transferred from nongenital to genital sites in the victim, so their final location is not necessarily indicative of the location of initial contact. Furthermore, the large volume of fabric produced commercially potentially reduces the significance of any fiber association discovered in a criminal case.

Bite Marks and Saliva

A bite mark is a pattern injury that remains as the remnant of biting pressure applied to the skin, often during sexual assault.[25] It may have central or peripheral ecchymoses, contusions, abrasions, or even lacerations that can correspond to the characteristics of the alleged perpetrator's dental arch and teeth. Shape can be affected by the presence of clothing, and a bite may also be confused with trauma caused by other objects, postmortem decay, or insect activity and other causes. A full explanation of bite mark analysis is beyond the scope of this chapter, and forensic dentists are often required for a complete analysis, which includes examination of the size and configuration of any lesions, test bites, overlays, and comparison to known dentition in the victim and alleged perpetrator. A bite mark should be photographed using an American Board of Forensic Odontology[35] (ABFO) or similar ruler so an odontologist can take measurements for potential bite mark identification. Special photography and imaging can be required. If a lesion is indeed a bite, it must be first determined whether it was caused by a human or an animal.[36] If human, adult or child is an important distinction. If the suspect cannot be excluded by comparison, the specificity of the similarities detected needs to be assessed.

Perhaps more important than the configuration of the bite itself is the potential to collect genetic evidence from saliva residue remaining in the area of the bite mark. Approximately 80% of persons are known as secretors, with ABO blood group antigens being more concentrated in their saliva than in their blood. Other DNA can also be isolated. Analysis of saliva blood group antigens and DNA requires rapid collection of trace saliva soon after the alleged assault because saliva may be rapidly lost from living victims.[35] Using PCR, saliva was successfully recovered up to 48 hours later in cadavers.[30]

Alternative Light Sources

The visualization of semen on the skin of children is critical to direct sampling. It has been estimated that semen stains greater than a dime in diameter (18 mm) are preferable for successful DNA analysis. Skin with semen demonstrates spots that are shiny initially, but they become flaky within hours and clear within a day. Skin with urine applied to it appears clear throughout a 24-hour period.[22] To assist the examiner in locating and collecting suspicious material, several alternative light sources (ALS) have been proposed to aid in its visualization. *Alternative light source* is a generic term used to describe instruments that output specific bands or wavelengths of light that are useful in locating physical evidence. An ALS system consists of a powerful light (usually a xenon gas bulb or an argon laser) that can be tuned to output narrow wavelengths of visible light, between about 415 nm (violet light) and 700 nm (red light), depending on the model. Most ALS systems also have long-wave ultraviolet (UV) (365 nm) capabilities, and some have infrared capabilities. Each of these bands of light is used for locating specific types of evidence, including biological fluids, hairs, and fibers. For example, many biological fluids—semen, urine, saliva, and vaginal fluid—fluoresce around 450 nm. At 450 nm, the instrument operator must wear orange-colored barrier filter goggles to block the blue light while allowing light from the previously unseen evidence, which is visible as a brightly glowing area, to pass through the goggles. The evidence can be photographed with either a film or digital camera that is fitted with an appropriate filter.

The most basic ALS is a 365-nm UV light source is commonly called a Wood lamp. While used primarily for dermatophytes, many hairs and fibers and biological fluids are visible under this wavelength. Many companies sell this type of light source, with prices beginning around $50. Advantages include low cost and high portability. The major disadvantage is that these sources lack the flexibility to allow the operator to change to other wavelengths of light, thus fewer types of evidence can be located. The Wood lamp produces a UV light that has been routinely touted as an important aid for identifying seminal products, particularly when large surfaces at the scene need to be inspected. The Wood lamp has also been used to assist in the photography of bruises.[37] When exposed to the Wood lamp, semen is thought to emit light by fluorescence, which is visible to the human eye[38]; however, the ability of examiners to see such light and routinely identify semen is limited.[21,39] This occurs because substances other than semen fluoresce in colors, textures, and patterns that are hard to differentiate from semen using light sources routinely available to medical personnel. These include milk, cocoa, petroleum and lubricating jelly, lotions, and contraceptive foam and cream. Urine and infant formula also fluoresce. Semen tends to fluoresce irregularly, whereas urine fluoresces homogeneously.

A comparison of semen, urine, and other common household products were photographed using room and Wood lamp lighting in Figure 6.1. While zinc oxide and shaving cream appeared white in room lighting and fluoresce well, semen is barely visible. In a study undertaken to determine if pediatric emergency medicine physicians, using a Wood lamp, could correctly differentiate between semen applied to skin and a variety of topical substances that may be found on a child's perineal skin, Santucci et al[39] found that physicians had difficulty differentiating semen spots from lubricating jelly and ointments used for diaper rash prevention and treatment. This finding only serves to highlight the need for careful evidence collection and analysis in cases of possible sexual abuse.

Alternative light sources with wider ranges, such as the Bluemaxx 500, have been used to better identify semen, blood, saliva, and fingerprints. The BlueMaxx is essentially a powerful flashlight that is fitted with a high-quality excitation filter that only allows blue light to pass, and the BlueMaxx is used in conjunction with an orange barrier filter to allow only the fluorescent evidence to be visible. BlueMaxx models starts at about $150; other models provide wavelengths over a wide range (390–500 nm) and identification is further enhanced by orange filter goggles worn by the examiner.[38,39] Forensic laboratories and police agencies generally use ALS systems such as the Polilite that are highly tunable and portable, making them ideal for locating evidence in the

FIGURE 6.1
Comparison of semen, urine, and other materials using incandescent lighting (room lighting, top) and Wood lamps (365 nm florescent, bottom) on dark cloth background.

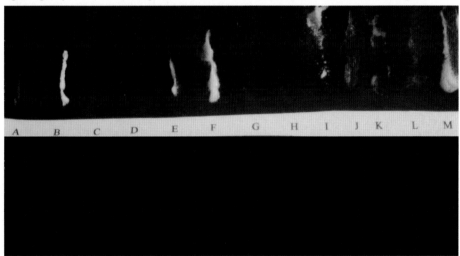

A, urine; **B,** zinc oxide ointment; **C,** antibiotic ointment; **D,** margarine; **E,** petroleum jelly; **F,** moisturizer; **G,** semen; **H,** hand lotion; **I,** mayonnaise; **J,** toothpaste; **K,** hydrocortisone cream; **L,** cosmetics; **M,** shaving cream.

crime laboratory or in the field. These units cost several thousand dollars. No matter what the cost, however, all ALSs remain a tool to identify potential areas for sampling while not being diagnostic in the identification of specimens.[39]

Rape Kits

Standardized sexual assault evidence kits, commonly referred to as *rape kits,* are available from a variety of sources. In some municipalities police departments supply the kits, and commercial kits are also available. The contents of the kits are fairly standard and typically contain the following items:

- Authorization for collection and release of evidence and information form
- History, physical examination, and specimen collection checklists, which give the forensic scientists information regarding the indications for the rape kit and the type of specimens contained within the sealed kit (Figure 6.2)
- Paper bags (Plastic bags may create an airtight seal that can maintain high humidity, which can contribute to the degradation of the evidence collected.)
- Envelopes for hair, nail scrapings
- A large paper envelope or bindle, prefolded, to hold debris, nail scrapings, or clothing
- Envelopes and/or tubes to hold secretions
- Cotton swabs for specimen collection
- Glass slides (some forensic laboratories request that slides not be made outside the laboratory)

- Orange sticks for fingernail scraping
- Combs for collection of pubic and scalp hair
- Gauze square, filter paper, swabs for saliva sample
- Oral scraper for buccal cell collection
- Tamper-proof seals
- Routing form and label for signatures of specimen handlers

Evidence Collection

The collection of evidence should be guided by the history of the disclosure, the child's physical examination, the experience and training of the health care provider, standard protocols, and a measure of clinical judgment and common sense. A medical examination and evidence collection should begin as soon as is feasible after sexual assault, once immediate safety and other health needs can be met. Although evidence technicians may be able to collect fingerprints and other valuable evidence from the crime scene, evidence that may be inside or on a victim's body should only be collected by a physician or properly trained sexual assault nurse examiner.[1] Examiners should always wear gloves when collecting and handling specimens to avoid contamination. Specimens are obtained from the external genitals, anus, mouth, and other parts of the body that may have come into contact with the alleged perpetrator or his or her bodily fluids. Fingernail scrapings and loose hair and fibers are also collected. The victim's clothing, especially undergarments, are also collected if they were worn at the time of the assault or subsequently worn

FIGURE 6.2
Forensic Laboratory Specimens

Patient's Name:	

Address:

Date: ___ /___ /___	Time: _____ AM _____ PM

Swabs for sperm
- ☐ Vulva   ☐ Anal   ☐ Other (Specify) _____
- ☐ Vagina   ☐ Oral   ☐ Other (Specify) _____
- ☐ Cervix   ☐ Other (Specify) _____

Swabs for seminal components
- ☐ Vulva   ☐ Anal   ☐ Other (Specify) _____
- ☐ Vagina   ☐ Oral   ☐ Other (Specify) _____
- ☐ Cervix   ☐ Other (Specify) _____

Victim's DNA
- ☐ Buccal
- ☐ Saliva

Pubic hair (in envelope)
- ☐ Site (Specify)_____
- ☐ Site (Specify) _____

Nail scraping
- ☐ Site (Specify)_____

Clothing in paper bag
- ☐ Site (Specify)_____

Other specimens
- ☐ Site (Specify)_____

because evidence may have transferred to them. When possible, victims should handle their own clothing to prevent cross-contamination. While buccal swabs are obtained for the victim's DNA sample; victim hairs are not routinely collected unless potentially foreign hairs are collected as well. If available, a properly configured drying apparatus may be used to dry swabs and slides, but care must be taken to not confuse specimens before labeling. Cultures testing for sexually transmitted infections and serologies for hepatitis, syphilis, and human immunodeficiency virus are not part of the forensic evidence collection kit and instead are clinical specimens that should be sent to the appropriate laboratory. For legal purposes, each person who handles the completed evidence kit is identified and their name recorded, maintaining a chain of evidence. A sample chain of evidence form is provided in Figure 6.3.

General Guidelines

It is important to obtain consent for the evidentiary examination from the victim and/or guardian so that they understand the process and how steps will be taken to minimize discomfort, and to empower them. However, in child sexual abuse cases, consent from the parent is not required. Ensure that the adolescent understands that this is not a routine examination, and if they refuse, generally it should not be done. Know what your laboratory wants and understand how to obtain specimens before attempting to collect them. Do not assume that something is not or will not be needed as evidence. Use specific

collection checklists and protocols and standardized collection kits when possible. Wear gloves to differentiate the examination from the assault, to protect the examiner and victim from infectious diseases, and to protect against contamination of specimens. Swab all sites (not just the obvious ones), limit the number of personnel involved in handling specimens, and maintain the chain of evidence.

In general, it is best to follow any specimen collection protocols provided with a kit, but general information about specific sampling techniques follows.

Collection of Sperm and Seminal Products

- Consult with your local forensic laboratory regarding its preference for sample preparation. Some forensic laboratories request a dry smear of each secretion sample on a microscopic slide; other laboratories prefer to make their own slides from submitted swabs.
- Obtain at least 2 to 3 swabs from each site sampled.
- Use dry swabs for wet secretions; using moistened swabs can dilute the specimen.
- If obtaining a sample from dried secretions, use a wet swab to facilitate transfer.
- Collect rectal swabs before vaginal swabs to prevent rectal contamination. Insert each swab at least ½ to 1 inch beyond the anus.
- Obtain separate swabs from the vagina and then the cervix from adolescent patients.

FIGURE 6.3
Sample chain of custody documentation for evidence collection kit

EVIDENCE COLLECTION KIT		
For Victims of Assault		
Victim's Name:	Victim's ID No.:	
Hospital:		
Medical Examiner:		
Chain of Custody		
Sealed by:	Date:	Time:
Received by:	Date:	Time:
Received by:	Date:	Time:
Received by:	Date:	Time:
Received by:	Date:	Time:
Opened by:	Date:	Time:

- Obtain mouth samples by swabbing the buccal mucosa and under the tongue.

Preparation of Slides

- Wipe the swab on a clean slide that has been labeled with the source of the secretion.
- Spray the slide with fixative and allow it to dry.

Assessment for Motile Sperm

- Roll the swab sample back and forth on a drop of saline or Hepes media (which preserves sperm motility).
- Place a cover slip on the slide.
- Examine immediately under 400× magnification for the number of motile and nonmotile sperm per high-powered field. Sperm motility should be assessed within 30 minutes of obtaining a sample.

Air-Drying of Swabs

- All swabs must be completely air-dried, and slides should be sprayed with fixative and air-dried. This can be facilitated by the use of any of the commercially available drying units.
- Allow swabs to sit in a rack for 1 hour.
- Do not allow the swabs to cross-contaminate.
- After drying, immediately place the labeled swab in a tube or envelope.

Collection of Clothing

- Wet clothing should be laid out to dry, if possible. If this is not possible, the clothes should be placed in an open brown paper bag.
- Do not cut through any existing holes, rips, or stains in the victim's clothing.
- Do not shake out clothing.
- Place each item of clothing in a separate paper bag. Do not place clothing into plastic bags; plastic bags are not appropriate because they may lock in moisture, which may lead to the degradation of the evidence collected.

Collection of Debris

- Place foreign matter in the center of a clean piece of paper, fold the paper to retain the collected material, and place the paper in an envelope. Do not lick the envelope; use water to close it or a self-adhesive envelope.
- If the victim was wearing a tampon, pad, or diaper at the time of or after the assault, save it for analysis by placing it in a paper bag.

Collection of Fingernail Scrapings

- Take 2 folded paper sheets, unfold one of them, and place it on a flat surface.
- Hold the victim's left hand over the paper and, using the plastic fingernail scraper, scrape under all 5 fingernails, allowing any debris present to fall onto the paper.
- Refold the paper to retain the debris, then mark the folded paper "left hand."
- Repeat for the right hand.

Collection of Hair

Routine plucking of pubic and head hair samples is no longer recom-mended. Any suspicious hair found on a prepubertal child should be secured by placing the hair in an envelope or tube and labeling the envelope or tube with the specimen location. Because pulled hair samples are needed only to provide an oppor-tunity for comparison if foreign hairs are discovered, it is generally recom-mended that hair be collected only by the combing method. Samples can be pulled from the victim at a later time if necessary.

Collection of Blood

- If dried blood is present, attempt to scrape it onto a clean piece of paper with the back of a clean scalpel blade, tongue depressor, or applicator tip. The paper should then be folded.
- If the blood cannot be scraped, rub a slightly moistened swab onto the dried blood. Allow the swab to air-dry completely, and place the swab into an envelope or tube.

Collection of a Saliva Sample

- To collect a sample from the skin, such as from a bite mark, the examiner should use the double swab technique, which has been shown to increase the amount of DNA recovered.[29] Immerse a sterile cotton swab in sterile distilled water and wash the saliva from the skin. Take a second, dry sterile cotton swab and rub it over the area to absorb the water left behind by the initial swab. Air-dry the swabs and submit both of them for analysis.

- To collect a control sample, have the patient chew on a 2 × 2-inch gauze pad or piece of filter paper until moistened. Have the patient place the moistened gauze in an envelope labeled "saliva sample." Allow the envelope to sit open through the remainder of the examination to partially dry. Do not lick the envelope to seal it; instead, use water or self-adhesive labels.

Collection of Victim DNA

While blood has been used in the past, most laboratories now use oral fibroblasts to harvest the victim's DNA for analysis. A variety of commercial kits are available that are designed for use by nonmedical personnel for the collection of DNA (both adult and minor). This specimen is separate from a saliva sample. Using the collectors provided, simply swab the inside of the victim's cheek and gum line, which will result in the transfer of buccal cells onto the cotton bulbs of the swabs. Place the swabs in the container provided and place the container in the kit after proper labeling.

Chain of Evidence

Chain of evidence refers to legal practices governing the collection, disposition, and transfer of forensic specimens.[29] This chain begins with the actual collection and placement in the rape kit, which is then sealed to prevent tampering. Each specimen placed in the kit constitutes a separate piece of evidence, and care must be taken to not confuse samples, sites, or patients. Do not combine patients within a single kit. After the kit is completed and sealed, there must be an unbroken, transparent record of who handled, transported, and deposited the kit, ending at the forensics laboratory, where additional procedures are undertaken during analysis to ensure proper specimen identification. If the chain is "broken," it is possible that specimens were altered or substituted, potentially significantly reducing their value in court. To facilitate a proper chain of evidence, it is important for the examiner to make sure that everything is labeled carefully and correctly: each paper bag, envelope, and kit is marked with the victim's name, contents of bag or envelope, date and time collected, and the collector's name and signature. In practice, the examiner seals the kit and records the victim's name, the date and time of the evidence collection, the examiner's name, and the location of the examination. All hospital personnel who handle the evidence should maintain the chain of evidence and sign the log provided (Figure 6.3).

Common errors made in rape kit completion include (1) failing to complete the kit at all because it is believed there will be no evidence or that it is not needed, (2) mixing up swabs and specimens, (3) not using the proper envelopes, (4) not allowing specimens to dry properly, and (5) not getting training on using the kit. After completion, the sealed kit and any bags are handed directly to a law enforcement officer or evidence technician who signs for them and indicates the date and time they were received. Alternatively, the hospital or child advocacy center can have a policy related to proper storage in a locked cabinet until transport to the forensic laboratory.

Conclusions

Forensic evidence is just one piece of the puzzle of trying to understanding child sexual abuse, confirm a particular type of sexual contact, identify a perpetrator, and protect the child. Forensic evidence plays a valuable role in a small but important number of child sexual abuse cases. Most important for the health and welfare of the child is a comphrensive medical evaluation, realizing that best available "evidence" in most cases comes from what the child has to say rather than the forensic laboratory. The health care provider need not become a legal expert with regard to forensic evidence, but it is essential that he or she becomes proficient in the identification and collection of appropriate specimens and avoids common pitfalls in cases where sexual abuse or assault is alleged.

Acknowledgment

The authors wish to thank Jeff Nye from the Michigan State Police Forensic Science Division for his assistance in reviewing current practices employed in physical evidence identification.

References

1. Kellogg N, American Academy of Pediatrics Committee on Child Abuse and Neglect. The evaluation of sexual abuse in children. *Pediatrics*. 2005;116:506–512
2. American Academy of Pediatrics Committee on Adolescence. Care of the adolescent sexual assault victim. *Pediatrics*. 2001;107:1476–1479
3. Giardin B, Faugno D, Seneski P, Slaughter L, Whelan M. *The Color Atlas of Sexual Assault*. St Louis, MO: Mosby; 1997
4. Burgess A, Groth A, Holmstrom L, Sgroi S, eds. *Sexual Assault of Children and Adolescents*. Lexington, MA: Lexington Books; 1978
5. Toobin J. The CSI effect: the truth about forensic science. *The New Yorker*. 2007; May 7:30–35
6. Horvath F, Meesig R. The criminal investigation process and the role of forensic evidence: a review of empirical findings. *J Forensic Sci*. 1996;41:700–702
7. Santucci KA, Hsiao AL. Advances in clinical forensic medicine. *Curr Opin Pediatr*. 2003;15:304–308
8. Gray-Eurom K, Seaberg DC, Wears RL. The prosecution of sexual assault cases: correlation with forensic evidence. *Ann Emerg Med*. 2002;39:39–46
9. Palusci VJ, Cox EO, Cyrus TA, Heartwell SW, Vandervort FE, Pott ES. Medical assessment and legal outcome in child sexual abuse. *Arch Pediatr Adolesc Med*. 1999;153:388–392
10. Christian CW, Lavelle JM, DeJong AR, Loiselle J, Brenner L, Joffe M. Forensic evidence findings in prepubertal vctims of sexual assault. *Pediatrics*. 2000;106:100–104
11. Dahlke MB, Cooke C, Cunnane M, Chawla P, Lau P. Identification of semen in 500 patients seen because of rape. *Am J Clin Pathol*.1977;68:740–746

12. DeJong AR, Rose M. Legal proof of child sexual abuse in the absence of physical evidence. *Pediatrics.* 1991;88:506–511

13. Enos WF, Conrath TB, Byer JC. Forensic evaluation of the sexually abused child. *Pediatrics.* 1986;78:385–398

14. Palusci VJ, Cox EO, Shatz EM, Schultze JM. Urgent medical assessment after child sexual abuse. *Child Abuse Negl.* 2006;30:367–380

15. Young KL, Jones JG, Worthington T, Simpson P, Casey PH. Forensic laboratory evidence in sexually abused children and adolescents. *Arch Pediatr Adolesc Med.* 2006;160:585–588

16. Howitt J, Rogers D. Adult sexual offenses and related matters. In: McLay WDS, ed. *Clinical Forensic Medicine.* 2nd ed. London, UK: Greenwich Medical Media; 1996:193–218

17. Office of Violence Against Women, US Department of Justice. *President's DNA Initiative. A National Protocol for Sexual Assault Medical Forensic Examination: Adults/Adolescents.* Washington, DC: US Department of Justice; 2004. NCJ 206554

18. Committee on Child Abuse and Neglect of the Ohio Chapter of the American Academy of Pediatrics, Ohio Department of Health, Ohio Attorney General's. *Ohio Pediatric Sexual Abuse Protocol 2000.* http://www.cincinnatichildrens.org/svc/alpha/c/child-abuse/tools/contributions.htm. Accessed May 30, 2008

19. Silverman EM, Silverman AG. Persistence of spermatozoa in the lower genital tracts of women. *JAMA.* 1978;240:1875–1877

20. Willott GM, Allard JE. Spermatazoa—their persistence after sexual intercourse. *Forensic Sci Int.* 1982;19:135–154

21. Gabby T, Winkleby MA, Boyce T, Fisher DL, Lancaster A, Sensabaugh GF. Sexual abuse of children. The detection of semen on skin. *Am J Dis Child.* 1992;146:700–703

22. Finkel M, DeJong AR. Medical findings in child sexual abuse. In: Reece RM, ed. *Child Abuse and Neglect: Medical Diagnosis and Management.* Philadelphia, PA: Lea & Febiger; 1994

23. Soules MR, Pollard AA, Brown KM, Verma M. The forensic laboratory evaluation of evidence in alleged rape. *Am J Obstet Gynecol.* 1978;130:142–147

24. Graves HCB, Sensabaugh GF, Blake ET. Post-coital detection of a male-specific semen protein: application to the investigation of rape. *N Engl J Med.* 1985;312:338–343

25. Spitz WU, ed. *Medicolegal Investigation of Death: Guidelines for the Application of Pathology to Crime Investigation.* 3rd ed. Springfield, IL: Charles C. Thomas; 1993:107–117

26. National Institute of Justice, Office for Victims of Crime. *Understanding DNA Evidence: A Guide for Victim Service Providers.* Washington, DC: National Institute of Justice; 2001

27. Nishimi RY. Forensic DNA analysis: scientific, legal, and social issues. *Cancer Invest.* 1992;10(6):553–563

28. Annas GJ. Setting standards for the use of DNA-typing results in the courtroom—the state of the art. *N Engl J Med.* 1992;326:1641–1644

29. McCabe ERB. Applications of DNA fingerprinting in pediatric practice. *J Pediatr.* 1992;120:499–509

30. Sweet D, Lorente JA, Valenzuela A, Lorente M, Villanueva E. PCR-based DNA typing of saliva stains recovered from human skin. *J Forensic Sci.* 1997;42(3):447–451

31. Delfin FC, Madrid BJ, Tan MP, DeUngria MCA. Y-STR analysis for detection and objective confirmation of child sexual abuse. *Int J Legal Med.* 2005;119:158–163

32. Deedrick DW. Hairs, fibers, crime, and evidence. *Forensic Sci Commun.* 2000;2(3). http://www.fbi.gov/hq/lab/fsc/backissu/july2000/deedrick.htm. Accessed May 10, 2007

33. Exline DL, Smith FP, Drexler SG. Frequency of pubic hair transfer during sexual intercourse. *J Forensic Sci.* 1998;43(3):505–508

34. Young WW, Bracken AC, Goddard MA, Matheson S. Sexual assault: review of a national model protocol for forensic and medical evaluation. New Hampshire Sexual Assault Medical Examination Protocol Project Committee. *Obstet Gynecol.* 1992;80:878–883

35. American Board of Forensic Odontology. *Diplomate's Manual.* http://www.abfo.org. Accessed October 15, 2007

36. Johnson CF. Bites in the night: determining the etiology of bite marks in an infant. *Pediatr Emerg Care.* 1994;10:281

37. Vogeley E, Pierce MC, Bertocci G. Experience with Wood lamp illumination and digital photography in the documentation of bruises on human skin. *Arch Pediatr Adolesc Med.* 2002;156(3):265–268

38. BenYosef N, Almog J, Frank A, Springer E, Cantu AA. Short UV luminescence for forensic applications: design of a real-time observation system for detection of latent fingerprints and body fluids. *J Forensic Sci.* 1998;43:299–304

39. Santucci KA, Nelson DG, McQuillen KK, Duffy SJ, Linakis JG. Wood's lamp utility in the identification of semen. *Pediatrics.* 1999;104:1342–1344

Chapter 7

Adolescent Issues in Sexual Assault

Ann S. Botash

Introduction

Adolescents are frequent victims of sexual assault and rape and, although reported more commonly by females, both males and females can be at risk. Depending on the year of data collection, at least half or more of all rape victims are younger than 18 years.[1-3] Like prepubertal children, teens may experience intrafamilial abuse and be abused by their own parents, other caregivers, siblings, or other relatives. Adolescents are also at risk for abuse by friends, acquaintances, or strangers.[4] Unlike prepubertal children, teens may experience interpersonal violence with a partner or ex-partner similar to that seen in adults, which results in rape, date rape, or sexual assault. Although state statutes vary regarding age of consent and criminal acts, sexual relationships of teens with older adults are considered to be crimes in the United States, and these crimes are commonly referred to as *statutory rape*. Statutory rape is defined as a consensual sexual act with someone who is not old enough to legally consent.[5] *Acquaintance rape* or *date rape* refers to the situation where both the victim and perpetrator are known to each other and where nonconsensual sexual activity occurred.[3]

An adolescent may present for medical care for sexual abuse in one of the following ways: abduction by a stranger or known kidnapper, date rape, suspicion of intrafamilial sexual abuse, genitourinary concerns, symptoms of sexually transmitted infections (STIs), or pregnancy or pregnancy fears. The adolescent may or may not disclose voluntary or forced sexual acts. Other presentations may raise suspicion as well, such as teen suicide or suicide attempts, mental health symptoms, self-mutilation, runaway or promiscuous behavior, substance or alcohol abuse, or a history of juvenile offenses of sexual abuse. In some cases, there may be no disclosure by the teen and the parent has brought the adolescent for an examination due to suspicious behaviors. Identification of certain health concerns may alert the physician to the possibility of sexual abuse or assault. Any STI may be the result of abuse and not necessarily from consensual, same-age adolescent sexual activity. Pregnancy may result from incest or abuse. Adolescents who are physically abused or injured during an assault may not complain of their injuries and may attempt to hide them due to shame.

When an adolescent is brought for an evaluation of sexual assault, a standardized approach to the evaluation, similar to that used for prepubertal children, is necessary. This chapter will highlight differences in the approach for adolescents. The physician should have the opportunity to discuss prevention of sexual assault at every well-adolescent office encounter. This chapter will discuss potential opportunities to discuss prevention in the office and emergency department setting.

Anticipatory Guidance

Because adolescence is generally characterized as a period of good health, it is important for the primary care physician to efficiently use the yearly well appointments for addressing preventable morbidity, mortality, and poor health habits. Abuse issues tend to be a continuation of issues that are related to the home environment.

An important aspect of anticipatory guidance is understanding that the adolescent's development of independence and need for acceptance by peers may influence risk-taking behaviors. Many factors are often interrelated, such as poor self-esteem and depression leading to illicit drug use and further spiraling to other self-destructive activities.

Even the most careful teenagers can find themselves in situations that put them at risk for sexual assault. Common judgment errors are often related to trusting of acquaintances or errors in judgment regarding something as simple as accepting transportation from newly acquired friends. Adolescents should feel comfortable enough to call a parent or a friend at any time of the day or night to provide transportation from a situation where there may be a safety concern or even if there is perceived discomfort at a party or other setting.

Sexuality education guidelines provided by the American Academy of Pediatrics define the role of the pediatrician in identification and prevention of exploitive and risky sexual behavior.[6] A discussion about sexuality during the confidential health care visit should also include education about rape prevention, club drugs, acquaintance rape, Internet safety, intimate partner violence, and the role of alcohol and substance abuse in adolescent sexual assault.

Club Drugs and Acquaintance Rape

To help guide young adults and adolescents regarding potential for assault, the physician must understand and discuss prevention strategies regarding drug-facilitated sexual assault and club drugs. *Club drugs* refer to a wide variety of potentially dangerous substances used by young people in social settings, such as at colleges, clubs, and bars.[7] Club drugs can be used to facilitate a date rape by incapacitating a victim that has unwittingly ingested the drug. The drug incapacitates the victim by causing muscle relaxation and retrograde amnesia. Victims of date rape may present after being found partially clothed or without clothes in unfamiliar surroundings with no recollection of the event. Prevention strategies include being aware of the color, texture, and taste of drinks and refusing prepurchased, open drinks of any kind from strangers and casual acquaintances. Physicians and parents should counsel teens to never leave drinks unattended, even in familiar surroundings.

Other than alcohol, which can also be used for its sedative properties, there are 2 main types of club drugs. Rohypnol (Hoffman-LaRoche, Nutley, NJ), the trade name for flunitrazepam, is a member of the benzodiazepine family. Some street names for these pills are *roofies, roachies,* and *the forget pill.* Manufactured in tablet form, it can be easily crushed and dissolved in liquid. Because it is tasteless and odorless, it can be covertly slipped into a drink. A single dose as small as 1 mg can produce effects for 8 to 12 hours after ingestion.[8,9] When used in combination with alcohol and other depressants, Rohypnol can be fatal.

Gamma-hydroxybutyric acid is also known as GHB. It is a central nervous system depressant and is used in the medical field for sedation. The street names include *grievous bodily harm, G, liquid ecstasy,* and *Georgia home boy.* Gamma-hydroxybutyric acid is usually abused either for its intoxicating, sedative, or euphoric properties or for its growth hormone–releasing effects. Gamma-hydroxybutyric acid can be produced in clear liquid, white powder, tablet, and capsule forms. It can be manufactured in homes with ingredients found and purchased on the Internet. Often used in combination with alcohol, it has been increasingly involved in poisonings, overdoses, date rapes, and fatalities. At higher doses it can slow breathing and heart rate to dangerous levels. Overdose of GHB can occur quickly, and the signs are similar to those of other sedatives: drowsiness, nausea, vomiting, headache, loss of consciousness, loss of reflexes, impaired breathing, and ultimately death.[7–10]

Rohypnol can usually be detected in urine for up to 3 days after ingestion. However, it cannot be detected by routine benzodiazepine screening, and specific testing should be obtained. Gamma-hydroxybutyric acid is cleared more quickly from the body, so it is often more difficult to detect. Because these drugs are not usually part of the routine toxicology screens, the tests must be specifically ordered.

Alcohol and Substance Abuse

Intimate partner violence and other types of sexual assault are associated with alcohol and substance abuse.[11] Use of drugs or alcohol immediately preceding a sexual assault has been reported in cohorts of adolescent victims to be as high as 41% to 68%.[12-14] In addition, alcohol is a major factor in unprotected sex among teens, increasing their risk of becoming pregnant or contracting STIs.[15]

Anticipatory guidance regarding alcohol use should include information regarding the increased risk for sexual assault. Physicians should consider screening pregnant and postpartum adolescents for alcohol abuse, substance abuse, and depression, as well as intimate partner violence.[16-18]

Depending on the history, urine or serum testing for alcohol use should be part of the evaluation of the suspected adolescent sexual assault victim.

Internet Risks

Internet and cell phone communication have created a new realm of exposure to dangers for children and teenagers. Despite parents' best efforts, these methods of communication cannot be well monitored. In addition to posing a hazard for exposure to pornography, the Internet can be a gateway to sex crimes. Most victims of Internet sex crimes are between the ages of 13 and 17.[19,20] Certain youths may be more susceptible to online relationships, particularly those who are depressed, lonely, or having relationship problems with their parents or other adolescents.

Most pedophiles and adult offenders of teenagers do not lie to their victims and do inform them of their age and intentions for sex. In most cases, the offenders have communicated with their victims many times. As a result, the teens feel that they know them well and do not consider them to be strangers. The teens often willingly and knowingly meet with the person. Because the victims do not feel coerced, and in fact consider the offenders their paramours, these types of sex crimes are less similar to date rape and are more often characterized similarly to consensual statutory rape cases.

Prevention strategies that emphasize the "don't take candy from a stranger" rules will not work to prevent these situations. More helpful discussions for teen anticipatory guidance involve information about why these relationships do not work.[19] This includes how the adult may manipulate and use them to gain sexual favors, that the adult does not necessarily care about their well-being, and that the relationship will most likely end quickly with the adult moving on to someone else. The discussion should also include the fact that because most states have laws against computer-facilitated luring or solicitation, these relationships are illegal and the relationship may be exposed publicly.[19]

Intimate Partner Violence

The exact prevalence of intimate partner violence in adolescents is unknown. Among all age groups, it is believed to affect more than 32 million Americans.[21] Intimate partner violence includes physical, sexual, or psychological harm caused by a current or former partner or spouse and can occur among either heterosexual or same-sex couples. Stalking is also often classified as a type of intimate partner violence.

Interpersonal violence in dating situations deserves discussion at every well-adolescent visit for both males and females. Adolescents may witness domestic violence at home or may be victims of violence perpetrated by their boyfriend or girlfriend. Exposure to violence in the home is associated with future community and dating violence as well as substance abuse, suicidal behavior, depression, and other problems.[22,23] Physical assault by a partner is often a continuing problem that may start early in the first relationships of a teenager.[24,25] Dating violence is associated with sexual assault, unsafe sexual acts, substance abuse, eating disorders, and suicide. Studies have shown that there is an increased risk of contracting an STI or human immunodeficiency virus (HIV) among girls who have experienced both physical and sexual dating violence.[24] Violence during a relationship is also associated with an increased risk of pregnancy.[25] Prevention of these relationships may require community efforts to influence both partners through education. Recognition of the problem by recognizing signs of physical abuse and/or screening questions with further referral and assistance to the adolescent is essential.[26]

Runaways

The estimated number of runaway youths is between 500,000 and 1.5 million each year.[27] Runaway adolescents often come from homes where they were subjected to abuse and neglect and are at high risk for physical and sexual abuse while living on the streets.[28,29]

Adolescents With Disabilities

Adolescents with disabilities are at increased risk of sexual abuse and assault. The risks are similar to those of younger children as well as older adults with disabilities. Risk factors are related to increased vulnerability due to communication disorders and inability to seek help or report abuse, increased dependence on others resulting in high exposure, inappropriate social skills, poor judgment, and poor ability to defend themselves physically.[30] Parents of children with any disability may need assistance with finding trustworthy caregivers, recognition of subtle signs of abuse, and education of their children to protect themselves.

See Box 7.1 for a reference for providing anticipatory guidance to adolescents.

Consent Issues and Mature Minor Definitions

When providing care to the teenager who may have been the victim of sexual abuse, 2 main consent issues need to be considered. These issues include the adolescent's ability to consent to sexual activity and to provide consent for confidential health care. While weighing the teen's ability to consent

BOX 7.1
Adolescent Anticipatory Guidance

- Offer resources for sexuality education.
- Promote learning techniques to say "no" to unwanted sexual activity.
- Discuss physical, emotional, and sexual abuse.
- Discuss how to prevent substance abuse.
- Discuss Internet safety and sexual predator behaviors.
- Discuss club drugs.
- Discuss prevention strategies to reduce risk of sexual assault.
- Promote seeking help if there is a fear of any type of danger.
- Promote responsibility and school achievement.
- Promote developing skills in conflict resolution, negotiation, and constructively dealing with anger.
- Advise not to carry a weapon.
- Promote setting up a "code" system where a parent or other caregiver will respond and provide transportation or other need in an emergency.

is based on state and federal consent and confidentiality laws, the physician must also encourage communication by the adolescent to a parent, guardian, or trusted adult.[31]

Each state has specific laws defining the age of consent for sexual activity. The age of consent is set by individual states in the United States and varies between states from ages 16 to 18 years of age. The penalties for the crimes vary based on differences in age as well as specific ages.[32] Internationally, the age of consent varies from 12 to 18 years. A developmentally delayed teenager who is by law of legal age to consent to sexual activity may need the physician to assist in determining ability to consent.

State laws govern the rights of teens to give consent for specific types of medical care and evidence collection. Reproductive rights laws refer to those state laws that ensure access to medical care for teenagers who may have concerns regarding pregnancy, pregnancy prevention, STIs, and related mental health.

Laws regarding consent for health care as well as laws regarding confidentiality of the health information of an adolescent are more clearly defined in some states than in others. In some situations the decision regarding the ability to consent to health care is left to the discretion of the medical provider. In all cases, it is critical for the physician to clearly document the reasons that the teenager was or was not able to give consent. Consent for health care in cases of sexual assault usually involves consent for various steps in the evaluation process. For example, there is a need for consent for physical examination and treatment including STIs, HIV, and pregnancy prevention. Generally, a separate consent is needed for forensic evidence and drug-facilitated sexual assault evidence collection and release as well as con-sent for communication with police, the district attorney's office, etc. In all cases, assent for photographs should be obtained, and in most cases consent is also needed.

Informed consent is obtained when the teenager is capable of understanding the health care condition, the nature and purpose of proposed alternative treatments, and the predictable risks and benefits of the treatments, including no treatment. Factors to consider regarding provision of confidential health care are listed in Box 7.2, adapted from the guidelines of the Society of Adolescent Medicine.[31]

Consent of a parent is required in most cases, and care must be taken to understand individual laws allowing minors to consent to their own health care. In cases of emergency, consent for health care is not necessary, and providers can provide care under implied consent laws.[33] However, even in these situations, consent for forensic evidence collection and release must be obtained.

Mandated Reporting of Statutory Rape

Mandated reporting laws requiring physician reporting of statutory rape crimes to law enforcement agencies are not uniform from state to state. Some states require reporting to law enforcement based on the age of the victim and others do not mandate reporting to law enforcement. Suspected sexual abuse, as variously defined by social services laws in each state and involving an act of abuse

BOX 7.2
Provision of Confidential Health Care Factors to Consider

- Chronological age
- Cognitive development
- Capability of understanding implications of treatment or no treatment
- Health-related and risk-taking behaviors
- Independent status of the teen (financial or other)
- Minor consent state statutes
- Implications of the Health Insurance Portability and Accountability Act
- Pregnancy
- Limits of confidentiality
  - Suspicions of sexual abuse and need for reporting to authorities
  - Risks of homicide or suicide or other danger
  - Sexually transmitted infection reporting health laws
  - Billing and reimbursement procedures
- Prior family communication
- Strategies for involving parents

or neglect by a parent, caregiver, or family member is a mandated report in all states. Although there may be rare exceptions, these laws supersede confidentiality requirements.

The physician's decision of whether to report to law enforcement situations where consensual underage sexual activity matches the definition of statutory rape will depend on the legal requirements of the state in which the act occurred. Many times either reporting or not reporting will raise ethical concerns for the physician. For example, not reporting assumes that the teenager engaged in the sexual activity voluntarily and understood the consequences of sexual activity. Yet most teen pregnancies are the result of such relationships.[34,35] On the other hand, mandatory reporting of consensual sexual acts as a crime and mandatory notification of parents has been shown to limit access to reproductive health care for teenagers.[36–39]

History and Rapport Building

Adolescents generally do not volunteer information regarding sexual activity. Obtaining information about potentially unlawful sexual activity, intimate partner violence, substance abuse, and other risk factors for maltreatment and abuse can be challenging. In general, it is important to include some time in the well-adolescent visit during which the physician can speak alone with the patient regarding these issues.

Gaining trust and building rapport with the adolescent patient is essential for providing good health care. It is particularly important in order to help the teen to truly accept preventive counseling as well as for discussions regarding possible sexual victimization. Important factors that will assist in building trust include scheduling enough time for the discussion and establishing the rules of confidentiality. Confidentiality should be ensured but needs to be qualified regarding breeches due to life-threatening situations and legal requirements. When the teen presents for a sexual assault evaluation, obtaining as much information as possible from alternative sources such as parents, law enforcement, or other investigating agencies will assist the provider in formulating appropriate questions and enable a more focused subsequent discussion while alone with the teen.

Keys to good communication, such as showing respect for the teen, sitting at eye level, and maintaining eye contact and attention are expected to enhance rapport. The provider should assess the teen's emotional and intellectual development and current emotional state and use this to help determine the appropriate vocabulary and pace for the conversation. A standard written tool to assess risk factors has been shown to be helpful in addressing sensitive topics.[40,41] Often the use of a hypothetical situation, such as presenting a sexual assault situation regarding a "friend," can open the door to communication. Beginning the conversation with less sensitive topics and nonthreatening questions may put the teen at ease and can lead into discussions regarding sexuality

BOX 7.3
Suspicious Signs or Symptoms of Sexual Abuse

- Depression or other psychological problems
- Aggression, withdrawal, self-mutilation, fire setting, or other behavioral change
- Possessing unexplained gifts or money
- Unexplained pregnancy or sexually transmitted infection
- Teen was abducted and returned to safety with or without a disclosure of sexual abuse
- Fear of going home with parents, runaway behavior
- Sexual victimization of other children
- Sexually suggestive, inappropriate, or promiscuous behavior or verbalizations
- Requesting oral contraceptive pills despite denial of sexual activity

and possible sexual offenses. Care should be taken to ask non-leading questions and to avoid being judgmental or overly emotional. The provider should be supportive without making promises that cannot be kept. One of the most important factors in putting the adolescent patient at ease may be to explain the next steps in the examination process.[42]

Information regarding the recent menstrual history is important for assessing health as well as pregnancy risks. Physicians should ask about the use of contraception before, during, or after the assault or sexual activity. Because over-the-counter emergency contraception is available in some areas, it is important to ask about the use of these medications. Specific areas of the body involved in the sexual act (vagina, anus, and mouth) must be ascertained.

Box 7.3 lists suspicious signs or symptoms of abuse that can be used as a guide to further evaluate for child abuse and maltreatment in teenagers.

Teens who have been sexually abused may at first be uncomfortable with the examination process and particularly with photography of their genital area. A clear explanation of all steps of the examination as well as obtaining consent for photographs is necessary. Adolescents have been shown to display a reduction in anxiety post-examination even with the use of video colposcopy, suggesting that the examination itself can be therapeutic.[43]

Physical Examination

In general, the physical examination of the suspected adolescent victim of physical or sexual abuse is similar to that performed during the examination for sexual assault on the prepubertal child. Although the physical examination to look for evidence of abuse is frequently normal even in legally proven sexual abuse cases, adolescents should be encouraged to be examined.[13,44,45] The examination and assessment for STIs, pregnancy, and other possibly untreated health issues, particularly in high-risk teens who may infrequently visit the doctor's office, is an opportunity for better health care. When the examination of the suspected abused adolescent demonstrates normal findings, the provider can use the opportunity for reassurance regarding health and well-being and to offer support.

As few people as possible should be present during the physical examination and evidence collection process. The adolescent should be given a choice regarding the presence of parents or other support person(s). Ideally, the parent or guardian should be supportive of the child/adolescent and help decrease anxiety. Law enforcement or child protective agency representatives or others involved in the investigation should not be in attendance. Under no circumstances should the examination be held in the presence of a parent or guardian suspected of perpetrating the abuse. Preparation of the teen for the examination should include an explanation of the equipment, education regarding the steps of the examination, attention to personal physical boundaries and emotional needs, and use of relaxation techniques.[46]

The adolescent sexual assault evaluation should include a complete examination of the entire body to look for injuries in other areas in addition to genital injuries.[13,47–50] This may include the palate, bruises or rope marks to the arms from being held, and breast or chest bruises and/or lacerations. Weapons and physical assault have been reported to be used less frequently in adolescent victims compared with adult sexual assault victims, and nongenital areas have been reported to be injured in only 3% of adolescent victims of suspected sexual assault compared with 9% in adults.[13] Others have documented nongenital injuries in as high as 57% of a cohort of assaulted women aged 11 to 84 years.[51] Factors that may influence whether there are nongenital findings include relationship to the perpetrator and time since the assault. Nongenital trauma findings are increased in situations where there is a history of anal penetration and suggests that more violent perpetrators use this act.[51] Other findings suspicious for sexual abuse, such as cutting, may be apparent on a routine well-adolescent examination.[52]

Whether a teen should be evaluated using a speculum for better visualization of the cervix in the time frame immediately following a sexual assault is not clearly supported nor refuted in the literature. A complete bimanual examination is recommended if there are any signs or symptoms of pelvic inflammatory disease.[53] If it is the first internal examination of the teen, it may be prudent to provide only an external examination with good photodocumentation and later schedule a complete assessment using a speculum and bimanual examination after the teen has recovered and is in less pain. However, if follow-up cannot be ensured; if there is evidence of bleeding from inside the vagina or rectum; if there are signs of abdominal pain, vomiting, or fever; if there are signs of discharge; or if the teen requests a pelvic examination, a complete examination is recommended. In cases where a speculum is not used, it is likely that internal injuries to the vagina or cervix will not be well documented. These might include bruises to the surface of the cervix, cervicitis, human papillomavirus (HPV) lesions, other STI lesions, or tears to the cervix. However, further traumatizing an injured patient solely for the sake of collection of photographic or forensic evidence should be a consideration in determining the need for a speculum examination. Under no circumstances should a speculum examination be forced.

If a speculum examination is performed, water should be used as a lubricant so that evidence collected will not be contaminated. The use of photodocumentation, either through a colposcope fitted with a camera or with a good camera, is recommended for legal purposes.[54]

The positioning of the adolescent for the examination depends on the comfort of the patient. In some cases, the use of the frog-leg position as is used in prepubertal children instead of the stirrups may be appropriate. Use of the knee-chest position in adolescents for visualization of the anal area may be difficult in teens due to discomfort and/or the size of the adolescent. Use of positions that allow the maximum visualization and relaxation of the teen are recommended. Experts have advocated the use of a saline moistened swab, saline "floating" of the hymen, or a Foley catheter or other technique to help visualize the hymen edge.[55,56]

In boys, the physical examination of the genitalia will include the penis, scrotum, and rectum. If there is foreskin, it should be retracted to look for tears of adhesions or other lesions. In boys, physical findings of sexual abuse are not well studied but do occur.[57] In general, it is rare to observe penile injuries, and rectal tears and lacerations heal quickly, leaving little or no scar.

Interpretation of the physical examination findings in female adolescents can be challenging due to the normal fimbriated configuration of the hymen and the rapid regrowth of injured mucosal tissue in this area.[44,47,48] Guidelines are available and were developed by a consensus of experts regarding the interpretation of findings in suspected sexual abuse.[48]

An absence of genital findings commonly observed following sexual intercourse often requires an explanation to the patient, parent, and legal authorities. The elasticity of the tissues and lack of visible injury, rapid healing of mucosal tissue, and the delay in time between the injury and the examination all contribute to the fact that the post-assault examination is often normal.[44] Even when teens report consensual intercourse, the examination is also often normal. Historically, a survey of women indicated that most did not have bleeding or pain after first intercourse.[58] In a study of 36 pregnant adolescents, only 2 had findings consistent with healed penetrating injury.[59] However, a report of expert reviewed photographic documentation of adolescent genital examinations demonstrated that posterior notches and clefts of the hymen were more common among girls, average age of 16 years, admitting to past intercourse (48%) than among girls who denied previous intercourse (3%).[56] An earlier study that did not use photos or magnification reported 81% of 100 sexually active females, average age of 19 years, had complete clefts in the lower part of the hymen between the 2 and 10 o'clock positions.[60] This increased number of findings compared with the later study has been hypothesized to be due to a difference in average ages of teens, with the older teens potentially having had more sexual activity.[56] Even with these higher numbers, a clinically significant number of adolescents who have had sexual intercourse will have normal examination findings.

It is important for the provider to recognize that normal hymenal examinations should not be described and documented as being *intact* because this terminology is often misinterpreted to signify that penetration did not occur. Instead, it is suggested that descriptive terms, such as *pale symmetrical and fimbriated hymen* or other similar wording be used in the medical record documentation. Likewise, the words *perforated hymen* can be misunderstood to denote an abnormal examination and descriptions of the abnormality are more appropriate.

When the examination is abnormal, the provider may question whether the findings are due to abuse or consensual intercourse. In all cases, the history will provide important information. Observation of localized injury is more consistent with consensual activity and injury to multiple sites more consistent with assault.[51] Common sites of anogenital injury in assaulted adolescents have been reported to be generally posterior and include the fossa navicularis, hymen, posterior fourchette, and labia minora, whereas adults tend to have fewer hymen and more perianal injuries.[61] Even without a history of vaginal penetration, as many as 20% of suspected sexually abused adolescents have been reported to have abnormal findings.[51] This further supports the need for an examination even when the history may not refer to an act of penile penetration.

Tampon use and the impact of this on possible changes in the hymen have not been well studied. However, findings thought to be consistent with healed hymenal trauma have been identified in adolescents that used tampons and denied sexual abuse and sexual activity.[56,60]

Laboratory Assessment
Neisseria gonorrhea and *Chlamydia trachomatis* identification can be performed using the usual culture techniques of swabbing, urine specimens, or vaginal or cervical swabs used in nucleic acid amplification tests.[62,63] These are the pathogens that are most commonly reported among adolescents and they can be found in asymptomatic patients.[63] Tests for herpes and HPV are indicated when there are suspicious lesions in the cervical and/or genital area. Identifying a preexisting infection

with an STI may influence the legal case by suggesting that the teen has been involved in consensual sexual activity, and this may affect his or her credibility as a witness. However, not identifying the condition, even if treatment is provided, is not considered to be appropriate medical care.

Tests that are normally considered during a routine pelvic examination may or may not be performed post–sexual assault. For example, a test for cervical cytology (Pap smear) may be indicated if the physician feels that it is unlikely that the patient will return for follow-up and is an important test to evaluate for carcinoma of the cervix.[64] However, this Pap smear may be falsely abnormal due to detection error when inflammation of the cervical os occurs after trauma and the abnormal cells may be misintrepreted.[65] Use of polymerase chain reaction for HPV testing can accurately identify infection and cervical cancer risk, but may also potentially be deferred to a later examination.[66]

Serology for hepatitis B and C and for syphilis should be considered during the evaluation and tested as necessary depending on immunization status and exposure risks. Similarly, testing for HIV should be obtained at baseline, with repeat testing at 4 to 6 weeks and 3 and 6 months.[67]

Testing for possible pregnancy due to sexual abuse or assault can be performed at any time post-assault, but serum beta human chorionic gonadotrophin (ß hCG) is not is not detectable until approximately 10 days post-

fertilization. The American Academy of Pediatrics policy state-ment on emergency contraception recommends prevention of pregnancy in sexual assault situations.[68]

If the history or symptoms indicate the possibility that drugs were used to facilitate the assault, and it is within 96 hours of the possible ingestion, collect evidence for drug-facilitated sexual assault using a standardized kit or using methods recommended through local laboratory policy. History or symptoms may include memory loss or lapse, disheveled or missing clothing, dizziness, or intoxication that is disproportionate to the amount of alcohol reportedly ingested.

Treatment

Adolescent sexual assault victims should be provided with antibiotic prophylactic treatment for chlamydia and gonorrhea infections. Results of STI infections and/or symptoms should guide treatment decisions.[67]

When the nature of the sexual activity has been determined to be a risk for HIV infection, postexposure prophylaxis should be offered as soon as possible and is generally not considered to be effective after 72 hours.[69] Consent for testing and treatment for HIV infection can usually be obtained directly from the adolescent. However, parental support may be an important factor for compliance with the medications as well as for understanding the risks of side effects and toxicities from the drugs.[70-72]

Hepatitis B vaccination is recommended for those who have not received the complete series or those who have negative surface antibodies despite completion of the vaccine series. Similar consideration should be given for hepatitis A vaccination based on exposure risk. In addition, all adolescents should be given the opportunity to be vaccinated for HPV.[73,74]

Adolescent females with a history of exposure to semen are at risk for pregnancy and should be counseled regarding emergency contraception. Optimally, prophylaxis is most effective within 12 hours and is approved by the US Food and Drug Administration up to 72 hours; however, treatment up to 120 hours has been shown to be effective.[68] Treatment with Plan B, a progestin-only contraceptive pill (0.75 mg of levonorgestrel) has decreased side effects of nausea and vomiting and requires only 2 doses of one pill 12 hours apart or both pills at once. A βHCG should be obtained prior to treatment and at a follow-up visit 1 to 2 weeks after treatment.

Mental Health Issues

The victim of sexual abuse or assault should be referred to an appropriate resource for mental health and emotional needs. Identified risk factors for sexual abuse or assault, such as drug and alcohol use or abuse, also need to be addressed. The adolescent may be resistant to a mental health referral, and the physician may need to consider ways to make this referral more successful. For example, care

should be taken to provide follow-up that meets transportation requirements. Confidential health care for the adolescent includes confidential referral to mental health resources, and reproductive rights laws in most states protect the right of the adolescent to receive this without parental or law enforcement notification.

Summary and Physician Role

Prevention of abuse and assault can be addressed at the primary care office visit, and risk factors can be identified with intervention provided at every health care visit. Issues regarding adolescents and sexual assault include more than just a protocol to describe the steps to performing an examination of the adolescent rape victim. However, physicians also need to know and understand the steps in the evaluation as summarized below.

Physician's Role in the Care of the Adolescent Rape Victim[49,75]

- Recognize and stabilize any emergency conditions.
- Obtain information from available sources (police, parent, etc).
- Develop rapport with the adolescent.
- Consider need for parental notification or communication.
- Obtain consent for the examination, photographs, evidence collection, and release.
- Obtain and document the medical history.
- Evaluate, treat, and document all physical injuries.
- Take photographs.

- Obtain cultures, collect forensic evidence, and assess for drug-facilitated sexual assault evidence collection.
- Assess risk for and offer STI prophylaxis including HIV when appropriate and offer vaccinations for HPV and hepatitis.
- Offer emergency contraception.
- Provide counseling as needed for crisis intervention.
- Refer for mental health support or other medical needs and arrange for follow-up.
- Report as required by state law and notify authorities as required.

Acknowledgments

Appreciation for editorial review and assistance with obtaining references is given to Alicia Pekarsky, MD; Amy DiFabio, MD; and Trish Booth, MA.

References

1. Kilpatrick DG, Saunders BE, Smith DW. Youth victimization: prevalence and implications. *Research in Brief.* Washington, DC: National Institute of Justice; 2003. NCJ 194972. http://www.ncjrs.gov/pdffiles1/nij/194972.pdf. Accessed October 5, 2007
2. Davis NS, Twombly J. *State Legislators' Handbook for Statutory Rape Issues.* American Bar Association Center on Children and Law, US Department of Justice August 2005, Volume 8, Number 3. http://www.ojp.gov/ovc/publications/infores/statutoryrape/handbook/welcome.html. Accessed October 5, 2007
3. American Academy of Pediatrics Committee on Adolescence. Care of the adolescent sexual assault victim. *Pediatrics.* 2001;107(6):1476–1479. http://aappolicy.aappublications.org/cgi/reprint/pediatrics;107/6/1476.pdf. Accessed December 27, 2007
4. Davis TC, Peck GQ, Storment JM. Acquaintance rape and the high school student. *J Adolesc Health.* 1993;14:220–224
5. Troup-Leasure K, Snyder HN. Statutory rape known to law enforcement. Juvenile Justice Bulletin, Office of Juvenile Justice and Delinquency Prevention August 2005
6. American Academy of Pediatrics Committee on Psychosocial Aspects of Child and Family Health. Sexuality education for children and adolescents. *Pediatrics.* 2001;108(2):498–502. http://aappolicy.aappublications.org/cgi/reprint/pediatrics;108/2/498.pdf. Accessed December 27, 2007
7. El Sohly MA, Salamone SJ. Prevalence of drugs used in cases of alleged sexual assault. *J Anal Toxicol.* 1999;23:141–146
8. Schwartz RH, Weaver AB. Rohypnol, the date rape drug. *Clin Pediatr (Phila).* 1998;37:321
9. Fitzgerald N, Riley KJ. Drug-facilitated rape: looking for the missing pieces. *Natl Inst Justice J.* 2000;8–15
10. Schwartz RH, Milteer R, LeBeau MA. Drug-facilitated sexual assault date rape. *South Med J.* 2000;93:558–561
11. Horvath MA, Brown J. The role of drugs and alcohol in rape. *Med Sci Law.* 2006;46(3):219–228
12. Seifert SA. Substance use and sexual assault. *Subst Use Misuse.* 1999;34(6):935–945
13. Muram D, Hostetler BR, Jones CE, et al. Adolescent victims of sexual assault. *J Adolesc Health.* 1995;17:372–375
14. White C, McLean I. Adolescent complainants of sexual assault; injury patterns in virgin and non-virgin groups. *J Clin Forensic Med.* 2006;13(4):172–180

15. Shrier LA, Emans SJ, Woods ER, DuRant RH. The association of sexual risk behaviors and problem drug behaviors in high school students. *J Adolesc Health.* 1997;20(5):377–383

16. Harrykissoon SD, Rickert VI, Wiemann CM. Prevalence and patterns of intimate partner violence among adolescent mothers during the postpartum period. *Arch Pediatr Adoesc Med.* 2002;156(4): 325–330

17. El-Bassel N, Gilbert L, Witte S, et al. Intimate partner violence and substance abuse among minority women receiving care from an inner-city emergency department. *Womens Health Issues.* 2003;13(1):16–22

18. Martin SL, Beaumont JL, Kupper LL. Substance use before and during pregnancy: links to intimate partner violence. *Am J Drug Alcohol Abuse.* 2003;29(3):599–617

19. Wolak J, Finkelhor D, Mitchell K. Internet-initiated sex crimes against minors: implications for prevention based on findings from a national study. *J Adolesc Health.* 2004;35(5):e11–e20

20. Wolak J, Mitchell K, Finkelhor D. Unwanted and wanted exposure to online pornography in a national sample of youth Internet users. *Pediatrics.* 2007;119(2):247–257

21. Tjaden P, Thoennes N. Extent, nature, and consequences of intimate partner violence: findings from the National Violence Against Women Survey. Washington, DC: US Department of Justice; 2000. Publication No. NCJ 181867. http://www.ojp.usdoj.gov/nij/pubs-sum/181867.htm. Accessed October 5, 2007

22. Bensley L, Van Eenwyk J, Wynkoop Simmons K. Childhood family violence history and women's risk for intimate partner violence and poor health. *Am J Prev Med.* 2003;25(1):38–44

23. Roberts TA, Klein JD, Fisher S. Longitudinal effects of intimate partner abuse on high risk behavior among adolescents. *Arch Pediatr Adolesc Med.* 2003;157:875–881

24. Decker MR, Silverman JG, Raj A. Dating violence and sexually transmitted disease/HIV testing and diagnosis among adolescent females. *Pediatrics.* 2005;116(2):e272–e276

25. Silverman JG, Raj A, Clements K. Dating violence and associated sexual risk and pregnancy among adolescent girls in the United States. *Pediatrics.* 2004;114(2): e220–e225

26. Knapp JF, Dowd MD. Family violence: implications for the pediatrician. *Pediatr Rev.* 1998;19:316–321

27. Hammer H, Finkelhor D, Sedlak AJ. *Runaway/Thrownaway Children: National Estimates and Characteristics.* Washington, DC: Office of Juvenile Justice and Delinquency Prevention; 2002

28. Powers J, Eckenrode J, Jaklitsch B. Maltreatment among runaway and homeless youth. *Child Abuse Negl.* 1990;14:87–98

29. Thrane LE, Hoyt DR, Whitbeck LB, Yoder KA. Impact of family abuse on running away, deviance, and street victimization among homeless rural and urban youth. *Child Abuse Negl.* 2006;30(10):1117–1128

30. Murphy NA, Elias ER. Sexuality of children and adolescents with developmental disabilities. *Pediatrics.* 2006;118(1):398–403. http://aappolicy. aappublications.org/cgi/reprint/ pediatrics;118/1/398.pdf. Accessed December 27, 2007

31. Ford C, English A, Sigman G. Confidential health care for adolescents: position paper for the Society for Adolescent Medicine. *J Adolesc Health.* 2004;35(2):160–167

32. Madison AB, Feldman-Winder L, Finkel M, McAbee GN. Commentary: consensual adolescent sexual activity with adult partners—conflict between confidentiality and physician reporting requirements under child abuse laws. *Pediatrics.* 2001;107:e16

33. American Academy of Pediatrics Committee on Pediatric Emergency Medicine. Consent for emergency medical services for children and adolescents. *Pediatrics.* 2003;111:703–706

34. Elders MJ, Albert AE. Adolescent pregnancy and sexual abuse. *JAMA*. 1998;280(70):648–664

35. Donovan P. Can statutory rape laws be effective in parenting adolescent pregnancy? *Fam Plann Perspect*. 1997;29:30–34

36. American Academy of Family Physicians, American Academy of Pediatrics, American College of Obstetricians and Gynecologists, Society for Adolescent Medicine. Protecting adolescents: ensuring access to care and reporting sexual activity and abuse. *J Adolesc Health*. 2004;35:420–423

37. Miller C, Miller HL, Kenney L, Tasheff J. Issues in balancing teenage clients' confidentiality and reporting statutory rape among Kansas Title X clinic staff. *Public Health Nurs*. 1999;16(5):329–336

38. Richardson CT, Dailard C. Politicizing statutory rape reporting requirements: a mounting campaign? *Guttmacher Rep Public Policy*. 2005;8(3):1–3. http://www.guttmacher.org/pubs/tgr/08/3/gr080301.pdf. Accessed December 27, 2007

39. Reddy DM, Fleming R, Swain C. Effect of mandatory parental notification on adolescent girls' use of sexual health care services. *JAMA*. 2002;288(14):710–714

40. Cavanaugh RM. Obtaining a personal and confidential history from adolescents: an opportunity for prevention. *J Adolesc Health Care*. 1986;7:118

41. Cottrell LA, Nield LS, Perkins KC. Effective interviewing and counseling of the adolescent patient. *Pediatr Ann*. 2006;35(3):164–173

42. Botash AS. *Evaluating Child Sexual Abuse: Education Manual for Medical Professionals*. Baltimore, MD: The Johns Hopkins University Press; 2000

43. Mears CJ, Heflin AH, Finkel MA, Deblinger E, Steer RA. Adolescents' responses to sexual abuse evaluation including the use of videocolposcopy. *J Adolesc Health*. 2003;33:18–24

44. Adams JA, Harper K, Knudson S, Revilla J. Examination findings in legally confirmed child sexual abuse: it's normal to be normal. *Pediatrics*. 1994;94(3):310–317

45. De Jong AR, Rose M. Legal proof of child sexual abuse in the absence of physical evidence. *Pediatrics*. 1991;88(3):506–511

46. Botash AS. *Child Abuse Evaluation & Treatment for Medical Providers*. http://www.ChildAbuseMD.com. Accessed December 27, 2007

47. Kellogg N, American Academy of Pediatrics Committee on Child Abuse and Neglect. The evaluation of sexual abuse in children. *Pediatrics*. 2005;116:506–512

48. Adams J, Kaplan R, Starling S, et al. Guidelines for medical care of children who may have been sexually abused. *J Pediatr Adolesc Gynecol*. 2007;20(3):163–172

49. Poirier MP. Care of the female adolescent rape victim. *Pediatr Emerg Care*. 2002;18(1):53–59

50. Danielson CK, Holmes MM. Adolescent sexual assault: an update of the literature. *Curr Opin Obstet Gynecol*. 2004;16:383–388

51. Slaughter L, Brown CR, Crowley S, Peck R. Patterns of genital injury in female sexual assault victims. *Am J Obstet Gynecol*. 1997;176(3):609–616

52. Cavanaugh RM. Self-mutilation as a manifestation of sexual abuse in adolescent girls. *J Pediatr Adolesc Gynecol*. 2002;15(2):97–100

53. Blake DR, Duggan A, Quinn T, et al. Evaluation of vaginal infections in adolescent woman: can it be done without a speculum? *Pediatrics*. 1998;102(3):939–944

54. Adams JA, Girardin B, Faugno D. Adolescent sexual assault: documentation of acute injuries using photo-colposcopy. *J Pediatr Adolesc Gynecol*. 2001;14(4):175–180

55. Starling SP, Jenny C. Forensic examination of adolescent female genitalia: the Foley catheter technique. *Arch Pediatr Adolesc Med*. 1997;151(1):102–103

56. Adams JA, Botash AS, Kellogg N. Differences in hymenal morphology between adolescent girls with and without a history of consensual sexual intercourse. *Arch Pediatr Adolesc Med.* 2004;158(3):280–285

57. Spencer M, Dunklee P. Sexual abuse of boys. *Pediatrics.* 1986;78:133–138

58. Whitely N. The first coital experience of one hundred women. *J Obstet Gynecol Nurs.* 1978;July-August:41–45

59. Kellogg ND, Menard SW, Santos A. Genital anatomy in pregnant adolescents: "normal" does not mean "nothing happened." *Pediatrics.* 2004;113(1 Pt 1):e67–e69

60. Emans SJ, Woods ER, Allred EN, Grace E. Hymenal findings in adolescent women: impact of tampon use and consensual sexual activity. *J Pediatr.* 1994;125:153–160

61. Jones JS, Rossman L, Hartman M, Alexander CC. Anogenital injuries in adolescents after consensual sexual intercourse. *Acad Emerg Med.* 2003;10(12):1378–1383

62. Kellogg ND, Baillargeon J, Lukefahr JL, Lawless K, Menard SW. Comparison of nucleic acid amplification tests and culture techniques in the detection of *Neisseria gonorrhoeae* and *Chlamydia trachomatis* in victims of suspected child sexual abuse. *J Pediatr Adolesc Gynecol.* 2004;17(5):331–339

63. Burstein GR, Murray PJ. Diagnosis and management of sexually transmitted disease pathogens among adolescents. *Pediatr Rev.* 2003;24(3):75–82

64. Kahn JA, Emans SJ. Pap smears in adolescents: to screen or not to screen? *Pediatrics.* 1999;103(3):673–674

65. Nanda K, McCrory DC, Myers ER, et al. Accuracy of the Papanicolaou test in screening for and follow-up of cervical cytologic abnormalities: a systematic review. *Ann Intern Med.* 2000;132(10):810–819

66. Moscicki AB. Impact of HPV infection in adolescent populations. *J Adolesc Health.* 2005;37(6 suppl):S3–S9

67. Centers for Disease Control and Prevention. Sexually transmitted disease treatment guidelines 2002. *MMWR Recomm Rep.* 2002;51(R-6):1–78

68. American Academy of Pediatrics Committee on Adolescence. Emergency contraception. *Pediatrics.* 2005;116(4):1026–1035

69. Smith DK, Grohskopf LA, Black RJ, et al. Antiretroviral postexposure prophylaxis after sexual, injection-drug use, or other non-occupational exposure to HIV in the United States: recommendation from the US Department of Health and Human Services. *MMWR Recomm Rep.* 2005;54(RR-2):1–20

70. Havens PL, American Academy of Pediatrics Committee on Pediatric AIDS. Postexposure prophylaxis in children and adolescents for nonoccupational exposure to human immunodeficiency virus. *Pediatrics.* 2003;111(6):1475–1489

71. Babl FE, Cooper ER, Barbara D, Louie T, Kharasch S, Harris J. HIV postexposure prophylaxis for children and adolescents. *Am J Emerg Med.* 2000;18(3):282–287

72. Merchant RC, Keshavarz R, Low C. HIV post-exposure prophylaxis provided at an urban paediatric emergency department to female adolescents after sexual assault. *Emerg Med J.* 2004;21(4):449–451

73. Friedman LS, Kahn J, Middleman AB, Rosenthal SL, Zimet GD, Society for Adolescent Medicine. Human papillomavirus (HPV) vaccine: a position statement of the Society for Adolescent Medicine. *J Adolesc Health.* 2006;39(4):620

74. American Academy of Pediatrics Committee on Infectious Diseases. Recommended immunization schedules for children and adolescents—United States, 2007. *Pediatrics.* 2007;119:207–208

75. Hampton HL. Care of the woman who has been raped. *N Engl J Med.* 1995;332:234–237

Chapter 8

The Anogenital Examination: Diagnostic Dilemmas, Mimics of Abuse

Lori D. Frasier

The evaluation of a child presenting with an anogenital complaint or lesion can be anxiety-provoking for both the clinician and the patient. The clinician is faced with the real possibility that a diagnosis of a condition caused by sexual abuse will result in significant repercussions to the child, family, and community. A misdiagnosis of sexual abuse or failure to recognize a treatable condition can each have devastating consequences. Confounding the problem is that sexual abuse and unrelated anogenital disease are not mutually exclusive, and some conditions are recognized coincidentally during a careful genital evaluation. Most primary care physicians and other medical providers are not trained to recognize the variety of systemic and dermatologic problems that can affect the anogenital area. Dermatologists and other specialists often do not appreciate the possibility of sexual abuse or are reluctant to consider it. This chapter presents a systematic approach to the child with anogenital complaints as well as systemic illnesses that can have an anogenital focus.

General Approach

When a child presents with a genital complaint, a careful medical history, which includes social and family constellations, must be done. The clinician should not focus exclusively on the presenting problem. The whole child, in the context of the family, remains central to the entire evaluation. The examination must include height and weight measurements, the developmental level of the child, general health and hygiene, and a complete general physical examination. With much preparation and explanation to both the parent and the child, a careful and thorough anogenital examination should be performed. See Chapter 3 for guidelines. Only then can a thoughtful, systematic, and differential diagnosis be formulated.

Infectious Processes Localized to the Anogenital Tract

Viral

Human Papillomavirus

A variety of conditions affect the anogenital tract and may present or be confused with the sequelae of sexual abuse. Infectious processes are among the most common seen in children. This section discusses infections caused by viruses, bacteria, fungi, and parasites.

Human papillomavirus (HPV) is one of the most common sexually transmitted infections (STIs) in adults and children. Its significance as an STI is discussed in Chapter 5. The diagnosis of a lesion caused by HPV in children is often made based on the classic appearance of anogenital warts, also known as *condylomata acuminata*. Typical fleshy, verrucous, often pedunculated lesions appear frequently in the perianal area in both sexes but may be present on the scrotum and penis of prepubertal boys. When appearing on the mucosa

of the vestibule, these lesions can appear as either flattened or elevated areas with a whorled or cobblestone appearance (Figures 8.1 and 8.2). A variety of conditions have a verrucous or nodular appearance and can mimic HPV infections. Atypical lesions may require biopsy confirmations. As more experience is gained in the evaluation of such genital lesions, the differential diagnosis of HPV has expanded to include many papular, verrucous, and nodular conditions found exclusively on the anogenital area. This differential diagnosis is listed in Box 8.1. Specific details and presentation of these conditions are listed in the section of this chapter applicable to the condition.

An HPV-related condition, bowenoid papulosis, requires special attention. Bowenoid papulosis is distinguished from condyloma by its histologic similarity to carcinoma in situ.[1] It is most often caused by HPV 16, but other oncogenic HPV types have been implicated. The classic lesions

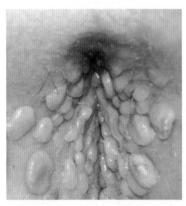

FIGURE 8.1
Typical appearance of perianal condylomata acuminata. Flesh-colored, verrucous lesions.

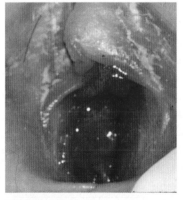

FIGURE 8.2
Less typical appearance on the mucosa of the vestibule, just beneath the clitoris. May have a whorled or cobblestone appearance.

BOX 8.1
Differential Diagnosis of Anogenital Verrucous Lesions

Condyloma acuminatum	Granular cell tumor
Verruca vulgaris	Syringoma
Bowenoid papulosis	Linear epidermal nevus
Condyloma latum	Langerhans cell histiocytosis
Molluscum contagiosum	Skin tags
Lymphangioma circumscriptum	Neurofibromatosis
Cutaneous Crohn disease	Perianal pseudo-verrucous papules and nodules
Darier disease	
Apocrine nevi	

are present in a mirror distribution around mucosal and epidermal skin folds and usually appear as small, flat-topped papules, often with a velvety brown appearance (Figure 8.3). Clinical variants are not uncommon. Hyperpigmented condylomata in children with dark skin are common and may be confused clinically with bowenoid papulosis, necessitating a biopsy. Bowenoid papulosis is generally benign, but progression to invasive carcinoma has been reported. Children

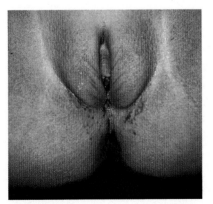

FIGURE 8.3
Velvety, flat-topped lesions typical of bowenoid papulosis, a premalignant condition caused by human papillomavirus.

should be screened for the possibility of sexual abuse. Active nonintervention is an acceptable approach with close follow-up, early gynecologic referral, and Pap smears at regular intervals.[2]

Complicating the diagnosis of HPV is the possibility that it is transmitted sexually, innocently, or vertically. Recent studies suggest that the virus can be transmitted through fomites or other nonsexual mechanisms.[3] Some studies indicate that an infection that is vertically transmitted can persist for several years.[4] Overall, the concern of sexual abuse may be raised by the presence of HPV; however, it does not prove it. A careful medical history, interview, and medical examination, including a directed genital examination, are still essential in the diagnosis of sexual abuse.

Molluscum Contagiosum

Cutaneous infection with *Molluscipoxvirus* is common, affecting up to 10% of children in tropical climates, with an increased incidence in children younger than 5 years.[5] Humans are the only known source of the virus. This infection is easily transmitted by person-to-person contact, autoinoculation, or fomites. Anogenital mollusca are commonly acquired innocently, but sexual transmission is also possible.[6] The incubation period is rapid for immunocompetent patients, at 2 to 8 weeks for individual lesions and 6 to 9 months for an average attack.[6]

Typical lesions are easily recognized as pearly, dome-shaped, 2- to 3-mm papules with a central umbilication. They can occur on any skin site but have a predilection for intertriginous areas, including the inguinal creases and gluteal cleft (Figure 8.4). Clustered in these areas, "agminated" molluscum may be mistaken for condyloma acuminata. A careful search for isolated and extragenital lesions with typical features can confirm the diagnosis clinically. The association of sexual abuse in prepubertal children with genital molluscum is unclear.

Epstein-Barr Virus

Epstein-Barr virus (EBV) has been reported to cause genital ulcers in both sexes that are shallow, painful, and on the mucosa, and they often have a grayish exudate.[7] Such ulcers can be easily confused with the lesions of herpes simplex. Systemic symptoms that suggest infectious mononucleosis are often present, with fever, lymphadenopathy, pharyngitis, and hepatosplenomegaly.[8–11] Such symptoms can also be present in primary herpes simplex infections. A Monospot, EBV titers, or polymerase chain reaction may be helpful in making a diagnosis.

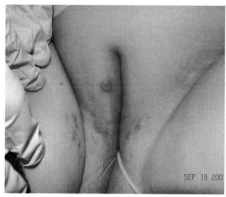

FIGURE 8.4
Genital molluscum in a 10-year-old. A concern of sexual abuse arose because the lesions were thought to be either condyloma or herpes. The central umbilication is typical of molluscum contagiosum.

Herpes Simplex

Herpes simplex viruses (HSVs) cause grouped vesicles on an erythematous base that are easily eroded on mucous membranes (Figures 8.5 and 8.6). Herpes simplex virus types 1 and 2, primary varicella-zoster virus (chickenpox), or shingles in a sacral dermatome can present in a similar fashion. A clinical diagnosis of HSV is not sufficient, and appropriate laboratory testing must be performed to confirm the diagnosis. Sexual abuse should be considered in children with anogenital herpes simplex, although innocent transmission can occur. Herpes simplex virus type 1 is usually found above the waist, but infections can be transmitted to the genital area through autoinoculation from the oral mucosal secretions or innocent heteroinoculation with diapering. A history of a recent episode of herpes gingivostomatitis, recurrent labial herpes, or a herpetic whitlow supports

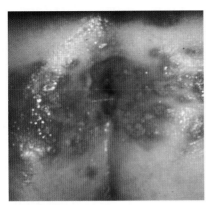

FIGURE 8.5
Herpes simplex virus type 1 in the perianal area of an infant. Note grouped vesicles on an erythematous base.

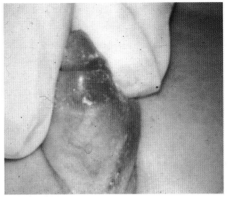

FIGURE 8.6
The same infant with vesicular lesions of herpes simplex virus type 1 on the shaft of the penis.

innocent transmission. Abusive oral/ genital contact can also transmit HSV-1. Either HSV-2 or HSV-1 can be the result of direct sexual contact. However, innocent transmission is possible in the case of HSV-1 or HSV-2.[12] Neither type of anogenital HSV infection can be differentiated by clinical appearance. A variety of blistering and ulcerating conditions have been confused with HSV and those conditions are noted in Box 8.2. Nonspecific viral infections such as influenza, coxsackieviruses, and many respiratory viruses can cause mucosal lesions that may resemble herpes viruses. A general rule is that any virus that results in mucosal ulcerations or vesicles can cause genital lesions.[13]

Other Viruses

In the presence of genital ulcers and clinical signs and symptoms of immunodeficiency, such as infection with human immunodeficiency virus, post–organ transplantation, or other immunosuppressive drug viruses,

such as cytomegalovirus, and human herpesviruses, can cause a variety of mucocutaneous lesions.

Bacterial

Vulvovaginitis

Vulvovaginitis presents in prepubertal girls as genital pain, dysuria, pruritus, erythema, or discharge.[14] Sexual abuse or an STI may have a similar presentation and alone trigger suspicions of sexual abuse. However, the most common etiology of minor

BOX 8.2
**Differential Diagnosis
of Blistering/Ulcerating Diseases**

Herpes simplex virus types 1 and 2
Varicella-zoster virus
Shingles
Crohn disease
Bullous pemphigoid
Pemphigus vulgaris
Behçet disease
Epstein-Barr virus
Contact/allergic dermatitis
Epidermolysis bullosa

vulvovaginitis with scant to moderate discharge is irritation, frequently the result of overzealous or poor hygiene. Resolution of symptoms occurs with the institution of a program of good hygiene and avoidance of irritants or overaggressive cleansing. However, if the discharge is copious, bloody, or foul, vaginal cultures should be obtained.

Many organisms have been reported to cause symptomatic vulvovaginitis in a child, and the differential diagnosis of a vaginal discharge must include STIs and non-venereal pathogens.[15] There are a variety of pathogens now described as causing vulvovaginitis in prepubertal children (Box 8.3). The most commonly reported bacterial pathogens are usually those commonly observed in the respiratory tract such as group A streptococcus, *Haemophilus influenzae,* and *Neisseria meningitides.*[16,17] Group A streptococcus requires particular attention because of the severe irritation, discharge, and vulvitis that it causes.[18] Bleeding can occur due to

mucosal involvement. To an inexperienced examiner, sexual abuse may be the first concern. Group A streptococcus is also the cause of a painful, erythematous, perianal dermatitis (Figure 8.7). The superficially eroded, painful infection has been reported to be confused with anal trauma and may be difficult to distinguish from abrasions. A Gram stain or rapid assay may be done if such a condition is suspected. It is important that routine cultures for non-venereal pathogens are performed even if abuse is suspected and cultures for *Chlamydia trachomatis* or *Neisseria gonorrhoeae* are done.

Vaginal Foreign Bodies

Vaginal foreign bodies may present with a persistent, foul-smelling, serosanguineous discharge. *Staphylococcus aureus* may be the predominant pathogen, or the culture can yield mixed bacteria. The most common vaginal foreign bodies in young girls are small bits of toilet paper that can be gently removed with saline

BOX 8.3
Common Non-Venereal Pathogens in Pediatric Vulvovaginitis

Streptococcus group A	*Corynebacterium*
Streptococcus group B	Gram-negative enteric bacteria
Streptococcus viridans	*Shigella*
Streptococcus pneumoniae	*Salmonella*
Staphylococcus aureus	*Yersinia enterocolitica*
Staphylococcus epidermidis	*Gardnerella vaginalis*
Enterococcus sp.	Anaerobes
Escherichia coli	*Candida albicans*
Haemophilus influenzae	Mycoplasma and other atypicals
Neisseria meningitidis	

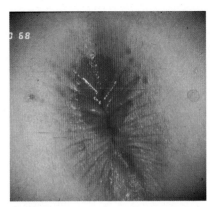

FIGURE 8.7
Perianal group A streptococcal dermatitis
causes erythema and pain and can be
confused with sexual abuse trauma.

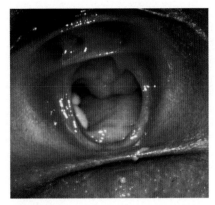

FIGURE 8.8
Foreign body; small bits of toilet paper can
be seen. Discharge is often serosanguineous
and foul smelling.

irrigation (Figure 8.8). Those that cannot be removed with saline irrigation may require anesthesia (Figure 8.9).

Gram-Negative Enteric Bacteria

Due to the proximity of the anus to the vagina and the relatively atrophic nature of the prepubertal vagina, it is not surprising that a variety of gram-negative enteric pathogens can be implicated in symptomatic vulvovaginitis.

Bloody vaginal discharge may also signal the presence of *Shigella, Salmonella,* or *Yersinia* bacteria. Such organisms are rare in developed countries and can accompany enteric and systemic infections. *Shigella* is the most common cause of bloody vaginitis in developing countries.[19] *Shigella flexneri* has been reported to be the cause of chronic vulvovaginitis and may not be accompanied by fever or bloody diarrhea.[20] An index of suspicion is necessary to make the diagnosis.

Fungal/Parasitic

Candida vulvovaginitis deserves a special note because it is often diagnosed clinically in a child with vulvovaginitis. *Candida* is unusual in healthy prepubertal children beyond infancy unless there is a history of recent antibiotic use, diabetes mellitus, immunosuppression, or underlying primary skin disease.[21] There is no link to sexual abuse, but chronic irritation, maceration, and loss of the keratinized epithelial barrier may predispose to candidal overgrowth.

Tinea corporis (ringworm) can affect the anogenital area. When it is isolated to the genital area, it usually appears as an expanding scaly, pruritic macule with central clearing. There is no association with sexual abuse.

Pinworms are a common pediatric condition that typically causes nighttime perianal pruritus when the worms lay their eggs on the perianal skin. Because of close proximity of the

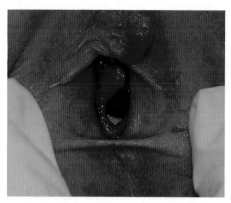

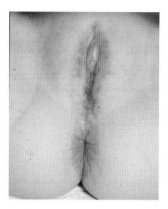

FIGURE 8.9
This child had complained of nearly a year of genital irritation and discharge. Two months before presentation intermittent vaginal bleeding was noted. The examination showed a shiny object in the vaginal vault. Under anesthesia 2 marbles were removed.

FIGURE 8.10
Typical figure eight distribution in lichen sclerosus et atrophicus. The pallor of the affected atrophic skin is not as apparent when the child is also very fair, as in this case.

vestibule in prepubertal girls, pinworms can be present and cause genital itching, secondary excoriation, and redness. This is a diagnosis to consider and treat if pruritus in a child or siblings is a frequent complaint.

Anogenital Conditions Presenting With Primary Anogenital Involvement

This group of conditions is classified as such because of primary involvement of the anogenital area. Although there are occasional systemic manifestations, these are rare. Because of the primary anogenital involvement, sexual abuse concerns are frequently raised.

Lichen Sclerosus et Atrophicus

Lichen sclerosus is a skin condition with features easily misinterpreted as traumatic injury from sexual abuse.[22] The onset of this disorder most commonly occurs in adulthood, but 7%

to 15% of cases occur in children.[23] Girls present with clinical evidence of lichen sclerosus 10 times more often than boys, but histologic evidence of the disease can be detected in at least 10% of boys undergoing circumcision for phimosis.[24] Childhood lichen sclerosus may become apparent at any age, most often between the ages of 3 and 7. Typical lesions appear as shiny, white, well-circumscribed, atrophic patches symmetrically involving the vulva and perianal skin that result in a classic figure eight distribution. Excoriations, purpura, and occasional fissuring and bleeding or bullae may be prominent signs. These features raise suspicions of abusive traumatic injury, but they also help distinguish this condition clinically from vitiligo, which has no skin atrophy (Figures 8.10 and 8.11). Children with long-standing lichen sclerosus may develop phimosis or labial adhesions. Symptoms may

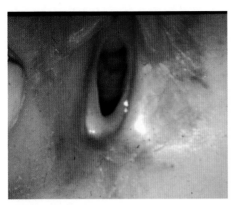

FIGURE 8.11
Shiny, atrophic skin without involvement of
the mucous membranes is the hallmark of
lichen sclerosus.

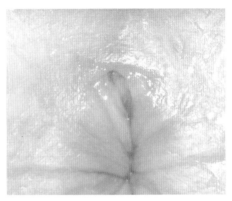

FIGURE 8.12
Perianal lichen sclerosus with fissuring can
lead to stricture, constipation, and possible
encopresis.

be absent, but pruritus and pain are
common. Chronic perianal pain may in
some cases provoke stool withholding
and the development of encopresis
(Figure 8.12).[25] The pathogenesis of
lichen sclerosus is unknown. The rate
of spontaneous remission is high for
children with lichen sclerosus. A single,
uniformly effective treatment has not
been defined.[26,27] High-dose pulsed
topical corticosteroids and topical
nonsteroidal inflammatories have
been used with some success. Current
treatment of perianal lichen sclerosus is
aimed at providing symptomatic relief
and maintaining normal stooling.

Perianal Pseudo-Verrucous Papules and Nodules

Perianal pseudo-verrucous papules and
nodules (PPPN) are an underreported,
benign, cutaneous condition that may
be difficult to distinguish from STIs
such as condyloma acuminatum, condyloma latum, or other conditions
such as cutaneous Crohn disease and
Langerhans cell histiocytosis.[28] They

may appear papular, verrucous, nodular,
or ulcerated. Pseudo-verrucous papules
and nodules occur in the setting of
chronic irritation coupled with skin
contact to stool and urine. A chronic
ulcerative condition with similar pathophysiology occurring in the diaper area
of otherwise healthy infants is referred
to as *Jacquet dermatitis* (Figure 8.13).[29]
This once common condition has
become rare with the widespread use
of superabsorbent disposable diapers.
A similar eruption has been described
in association with urostomies and on
the perineal area of children with
Hirschsprung disease or encopresis
(Figure 8.14).[30] It also may be a component of chronic irritation due to
enuresis.[31] This author observed PPPN
in a child with chronic fecal incontinence secondary to occult spinal dysraphism (Figure 8.15). She was referred
for a sexual abuse evaluation after being
diagnosed with condyloma acuminatum.
Another form of pathophysiologically
related diaper dermatitis classically

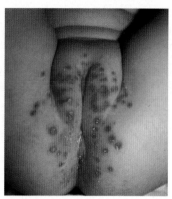

FIGURE 8.13
Erythematous, nodular lesions of Jacquet
diaper dermatitis generally respond to
avoidance of prolonged contact of stool
or urine.

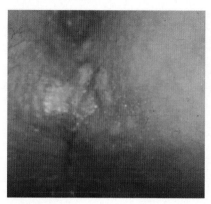

FIGURE 8.14
White papules of pseudo-verrucous papules
and nodules in the genital area of a child
with a history of chronic enuresis. These
cleared when the enuresis was managed.

presents as thick, violaceous papules
and plaques, usually without ulceration.

This condition, called *granuloma
gluteale infantum,* may be due to either
irritation or overuse of potent topical
corticosteroids.[32] Pseudo-verrucous
papules and nodules, granuloma gluteale infantum, and Jacquet erosive
dermatitis are all proposed as variants
of genitocrural dermatitis.[33] Pseudo-
verrucous papules and nodules is a
clinical diagnosis. Skin biopsy is nonspecific. Pseudo-verrucous papules
and nodules will resolve with skin
protection, removal of the precipitating
factors, and recovery of skin barrier
function.

Labial Adhesions

Labia minora adhesions occur in up to
one-third of girls who are not abused.[34]
They are the result of minor chronic
irritation and are most common in
girls younger than 2 years, but they
can be observed at any age. Most

adhesions involve only the posterior
2 to 3 mm of the fourchette, although
they can be anterior or even involve
just the central portion of the labia
minora (Figures 8.16 and 8.17). Most
partial adhesions require no specific
intervention except for emphasis on
good genital hygiene and avoidance of
irritants. More extensive adhesions will
respond to treatment with conjugated
estrogen cream. Adhesions can also be
the result of sexual abuse, but in the
absence of other evidence, the presence
of adhesions is not diagnostic.[35]

Anogenital Conditions That May Have Systemic or Extragenital Involvement

This class of conditions can present in
extragenital locations, but the primary
reason for a referral is often due to the
genital lesion. A careful total body
evaluation may provide clues to the
clinician that lead to proper diagnosis.

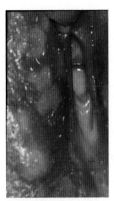

FIGURE 8.15
Nodular, hypopigmented lesions in a
child with occult spinal dysraphism whose
skin was continuously exposed to both
stool and urine.

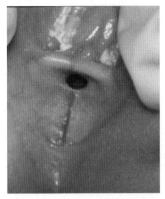

FIGURE 8.16
Nearly complete adhesion of the labia
minor. Note the thin, almost translucent line
of fusion..

Psoriasis

Psoriasis is a chronic condition
that begins in childhood. Typical
skin lesions in children are sharply
demarcated with fine, silvery scales;
a guttate morphology; and truncal
distribution. In infants and toddlers,
psoriasis frequently presents in the
diaper area and skin folds (Figure 8.18).
Inverse psoriasis is another distinct
pattern, involving the anogenital
area, axillae, and ear canals. A linear
distribution has also been described.
Often erythema is the predominant
clinical feature and scaling is minimal,
suggesting other skin diseases such
as candidiasis, contact dermatitis, or
seborrheic dermatitis.[36] The correct
diagnosis is commonly made only after
multiple unsuccessful trials of a variety
of topical medications.

Seborrheic Dermatitis

Infantile seborrheic dermatitis is a
common condition affecting the diaper
area. It presents as greasy yellow scale

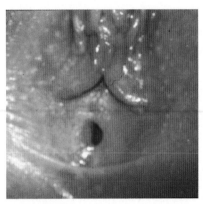

FIGURE 8.17
Partial anterior and partial posterior labia
minora adhesion with central opening.

on an erythematous base and minimal
pruritus[37] Onset is usually within the
first 2 months of life. In addition to the
diaper area, the most common sites of
involvement are the face and scalp. It
may be localized or disseminated.
Flexural areas such as the posterior
auricular sulcus, neck, axillae, and
inguinal folds can also be affected,
but the mucosa is spared. Hypopigmentation is often striking in dark-skinned

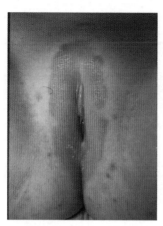

FIGURE 8.18
Genital psoriasis with sharply demarcated areas of hypertrophic epithelium.

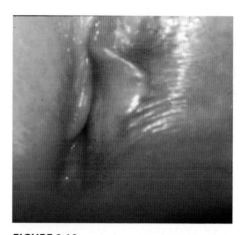

FIGURE 8.19
This small hemangioma had been confused with trauma but was unchanging over time. Note also that the labia minora is fused to the inner surface of the labia majora at the site of the hemangioma.

infants. In severe cases, fissures may develop and become secondarily infected.[38]

Hemangioma of Infancy

Hemangiomas of the anogenital area have been confused with anogenital trauma from sexual abuse.[39] A hemangioma is a benign tumor of vascular endothelium characterized by a proliferative phase and an involutional phase. It is the most common tumor of infancy. The male:female ratio in term infants is 1:3. Ulceration occurs in 5% of hemangiomas. Anogenital lesions, located in an area of friction, and rapidly growing or involuting lesions are at highest risk for ulceration (Figure 8.19.)[40] This has rarely been misinterpreted as sexual abuse. Ulcerated hemangiomas are painful and at risk for secondary infection. Hemangiomas of the anogenital area may also be associated with imperforate

anus, renal anomalies, or abnormalities of the external genitalia.[28,41] In most cases, a hemangioma can be diagnosed by its clinical appearance and pattern of evolution. It may be necessary to perform serial examinations on a child to demonstrate that a lesion is stable and therefore a vascular malformation, not a traumatic injury.

Epidermal nevi are rare lesions that involve the anogenital area along the lines of Blaschko. Blaschko lines were described by Alfred Blaschko in 1901. They are distinct from dermatomes, skin tension lines, and lines of lymphatic drainage. The pattern is linear and whorled, with a midline demarcation. They are usually apparent at birth but may not be recognized until childhood, presenting as smooth, hyperpigmented patches or rough, skin-colored plaques most often on the trunk or extremities[42] (Figure 8.20). Several skin disorders are expressed

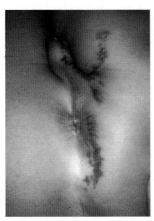

FIGURE 8.20
Verrucous-appearing lesions along the lines of Blaschko can be confused with genital warts. These can also occur on other parts of the body.

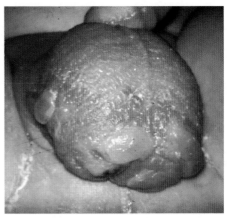

FIGURE 8.21
Bullous impetigo on the scrotum of an infant, which responded to anti-staphylococcal antibiotics.

in this fashion. Epidermal nevi in this area may enlarge and, with time, become verrucous. They can also become inflamed, ulcerated, and painful. Malignant change has rarely been reported. To a clinician unaware of the unique distribution of an anogenital epidermal nevus, condyloma acuminatum may be suspected. This distribution is the only feature that distinguishes this type of nevus clinically from other diagnoses.

Darier disease (also known as *Darier-White disease* or *keratosis follicularis)* is an autosomal-dominant disorder predominantly affecting skin, nails, and mucosa, including vulvar mucosa. Two cases have documented mucosal disease with the histologic features of Darier disease confined to the vulva and groin. In one case, a 5-year-old girl presented with wart-like lesions that initially suggested condyloma acuminatum and sexual abuse.[43]

Fixed drug eruptions may present on the genitalia. These occur in the same location on the body with repeated use of the same medications. Sulfa-containing antibiotics are often implicated. Reintroduction of the suspect drug may be diagnostic.

The anogenital area is a common site for superficial infections with streptococcus or staphylococcus. These lesions generally present as typical erosions with honey-colored crusting, and the diagnosis is not difficult. However, bullous impetigo can be confused with other blistering conditions and abusive burns of the genital area (Figure 8.21).

Lichen planus, lichen nitidus, and lichen striatus are dermatoses that can present with lesions on the anogenital area as well as elsewhere on the body. They are all relatively uncommon, but their presentation on the genital area can be confused with traumatic or

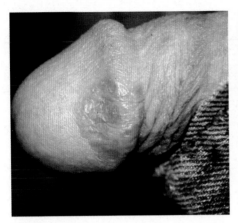

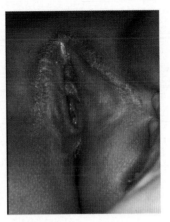

FIGURE 8.22
Typical polygonal plaque on the penis of a child with lichen planus.

FIGURE 8.23
Contact dermatitis. Scaling, hypopigmentation, and thickening of the epidermis help to differentiate this condition from lichen sclerosus.

infectious processes related to sexual abuse. Lichen planus is characterized by pruritic, purple, polygonic papules involving the genitals, but it can also be found on flexor surfaces, mucous membranes, nails, and scalp (Figure 8.22). Wickham striae, or white, lacy, reticulated papules on the buccal mucosa, gingivae, lips, and tongue, are seen in two-thirds of patients. Most cases resolve in 1 to 2 years, but some eruptions persist for 10 to 20 years. Most lesions respond to topical corticosteroids.

Lichen nitidus is characterized by flat-topped, flesh-colored papules in children between 7 and 13 years of age. It has a predilection for the arms, abdomen, and genitals and can be confused with genital warts.

Lichen striatus is characterized by flat-topped papules that arise suddenly in streaks and swirls on the upper back, neck, palms, soles, genitals, and face.

It is usually self-limited, but it can be confused with a linear epidermal nevus.

Contact Dermatitis

Typical irritant contact dermatitis affects the anogenital area in most diapered infants. In children, the condition commonly occurs as a result of erratic cleansing efforts after toileting or overzealous use of potentially irritating products, such as bubble bath. Less often, allergic contact dermatitis can occur in the area. In most cases, the history will support the skin findings, the skin findings are characteristic, and the diagnosis is straightforward. Typical features are erythema and loss of normal skin markings. Scaling, crusting, or even blistering can occur (Figure 8.23). Edema may be marked, especially with contact dermatitis involving the penis, foreskin, or labia. Latex allergies should be considered when marked acute swelling occurs in a setting where exposure to latex can occur (Figure 8.24). When there is a discrepancy, other diagnoses must be considered, including the possibility of abuse. In one reported case, a vesicular allergic contact dermatitis to nickel from a bed-wetting alarm was mistaken for HSV-associated sexual abuse.[44]

Initial treatment is identification and avoidance of the offending contactants, and temporary discontinuation of all but the weakest topical products until skin barrier function is restored (Figure 8.25).

Anogenital Conditions That Have Primary Systemic or Extragenital Involvement

This class of conditions often presents systemically, or else the recognition of anogenital involvement is not common.

Localized Bullous Pemphigoid

Localized vulvar bullous pemphigoid has been reported as being misdiagnosed as sexual abuse, with devastating social consequences.[45–47] This is likely because the earliest clinical manifestations of juvenile bullous pemphigoid are erythema and pruritus. Blisters may be single or grouped, and initial presentation can be limited to one site. Sites of predilection include genitals, face, neck, palms, and soles. It rarely presents in a localized form, limited to the genital mucosa. The diagnosis of localized genital pemphigoid requires a high index of suspicion. The diagnosis was delayed in all 6 reported cases[48] because confirmation depends on skin biopsy of perilesional skin.

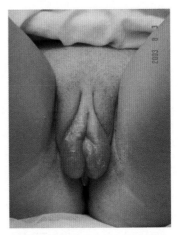

FIGURE 8.24
Severe labial edema was the result of latex allergy. The examiner touched this child wearing latex gloves. (Photo courtesy of Dr. Fred Bruhn.)

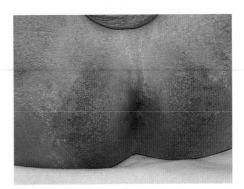

FIGURE 8.25
Perianal contact irritation due to diaper dermatitis. Removal of irritants and protection of the skin with barrier ointments is the key to treatment.

Pemphigus Vulgaris

Pemphigus vulgaris is a rare autoimmune blistering disease with a predilection for mucosal skin.[49] Vulvar erosions may also be an early sign. Although onset is usually in the fifth to sixth decade, a self-limited form of the disease, presenting at birth, can be transmitted via maternal antibodies. Childhood pemphigus is uncommon but has been reported as early as age 3 years. The diagnosis is confirmed by skin biopsy.[50]

Crohn Disease

Crohn disease has been reported to be misdiagnosed as sexual abuse by several authors.[51-55] Crohn disease is a familial inflammatory disorder of the gastrointestinal mucosa that can affect any site from the mouth to the anus. Anal and perianal lesions occur in most patients with Crohn disease and are often unrecognized initial signs, especially in those with active colonic involvement. These include skin tags, fissures, fistulas, ulcers, and abscesses. Similar vulvar lesions may also occur. Marked anal dilation is another ambiguous sign. The correct diagnosis may require a high index of suspicion. Radiologic and endoscopic studies, including bowel biopsy, are confirmatory.

Kawasaki Disease

Kawasaki disease (mucocutaneous lymph node syndrome) is an acute, febrile, vasculitic illness of childhood. Bright red, perineal erythema, evolving into desquamation over 48 hours, is a common and striking feature that can precede development of the diagnostic criteria for the disease.[56] This feature can be confused with sexual abuse in its early stages. This diagnosis should be considered if the child develops other principal clinical signs: persistent fever for 5 days or more, cervical adenopathy,

conjunctival infection, strawberry tongue, palmoplantar involvement, and a polymorphous exanthem. The differential diagnosis suggested by the eruption includes contact dermatitis, seborrheic dermatitis, candidiasis, psoriasis, syphilis, erythema multiforme, staphylococcal scalded skin syndrome, and scarlet fever. Careful examination for other, subtle clinical features of Kawasaki disease as well as typical laboratory findings will support the diagnosis.

Behçet Disease

Described by Behçet in 1937, this syndrome is characterized by recurrent aphthous stomatitis, vulvar ulcers, and ocular inflammation.[57] Behçet disease occurs mostly in those of Far East and Middle Eastern descent. It is rare in children and may be associated with human leukocyte antigen B5 positivity.[58] Almost any organ in the body can be involved, with ocular problems causing the highest morbidity.[59] The vulvar ulcers may be destructive and deep, but they are relatively painless. Scarring and distortion occur with recurrences of the syndrome. The diagnosis is made only after other conditions, such as Crohn disease, granulomatous disorders, and syphilis, are ruled out. Treatment is supportive and nonspecific, and spontaneous resolution can occur.

Purpuric and Petechial Lesions Secondary to Systemic Disease

Purpuric and/or petechial lesions in any location on the child's body have been frequently confused with trauma. Henoch-Schönlein purpura occasionally has been confused with physical abuse because the lesions appear on the buttocks and lower extremities. Sometimes the first presentation of purpura may be on the anogenital area. A careful assessment of the child, as well as hematologic studies, may clarify the diagnosis. Some conditions that can cause purpura and petechiae are listed in Box 8.4. Neoplasms of the anogenital area are fortunately rare in childhood. However, these have been known to cause symptoms and/or lesions that are initially diagnosed as sexual abuse. Langerhans cell histiocytosis is a group of histologically related disorders characterized by cutaneous and visceral infiltration of atypical cells. This author is aware of 2 cases that were initially misdiagnosed as condyloma acuminatum, assumed secondary to sexual abuse. Another report documented similar perianal lesions on a 2½-year-old boy who presented with a lytic skull lesion typical of

BOX 8.4
Disorders That Can Cause Purpuric Lesions

Henoch-Schönlein purpura

Lichen sclerosus

Hemolytic uremic syndrome

Systemic infections (purpura fulminans)

  Neisseria meningitidis

  Streptococcus pneumoniae

  Haemophilus influenzae

Myelodysplastic/myelosuppressive disorders

   Aplastic anemia

   Leukemia

Drugs that interfere with platelet function

eosinophilic granuloma.[60] The classic Letterer-Siwe variant occurs most often in infants and young children with a seborrhea-like rash that typically involves the scalp and anogenital area. Clinical diagnostic clues include atrophy, hemorrhagic lesions, and deep ulcerations.[61] Occasionally skin lesions are nodular[62] (Figures 8.26 and 8.27).

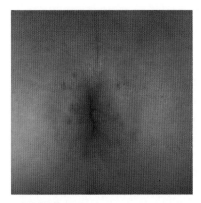

FIGURE 8.26
Nodular lesions of the perianal area shown by biopsy to be Langerhans cell histiocytosis.

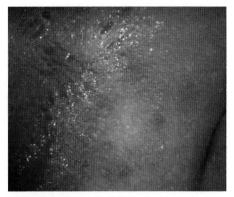

FIGURE 8.27
Hemorrhagic perineal rash of Langerhans cell histiocytosis.

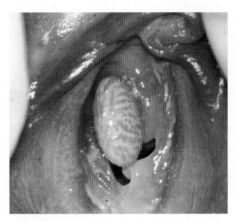

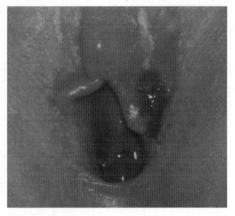

FIGURE 8.28
Urethral prolapse. Unusual appearance of urethral prolapse, which is pale and obscures the urethra. This resolved in less than 3 days with sitz baths.

FIGURE 8.29
A small compression straddle injury occurring between the labia minora and majora. The child fell onto another child's foot on a trampoline.

Rare Neoplasms

Unusual neoplasms serendipitously occurring in the anogenital area have been reported in children. These include apocrine nevi, syringomas, granular cell tumors, and vulvar and scrotal angiokeratomas.[43,63,64] As with other lesions confined to the anogenital area, suspicions of sexual abuse may be raised. This underscores the importance of a biopsy in confirming the diagnosis of any atypical anogenital lesion.

Acquired Structural Abnormalities

Urethral Prolapse

Urethral prolapse is reported to be confused with genital trauma. This condition may present with bleeding and a characteristic doughnut-shaped annular mass visible between the labia minora. It may obscure the hymenal orifice, leaving the appearance of hymenal trauma (Figure 8.28). The peak age of prolapse

is 5 to 8 years, and it seems to appear more often in African American girls.[65] The treatment is conservative topical estrogens and sitz baths; resolution is expected in 1 to 4 weeks.

Non-Abusive Trauma

Straddle injuries are accidental injuries to the genital area that may be difficult to differentiate from those due to sexual trauma. The physician is faced with determining if an accidental etiology is being given to conceal sexual abuse. Understanding the mechanism of trauma may assist in determining if an injury has a plausible explanation. Soft tissues are forcefully compressed between an object and the bones of the pelvis during impact. The result is often a hematoma of the labia majora or labia minora with significant swelling and pain (Figures 8.29 and 8.30). Most straddle injuries are unilateral. Small linear abrasions between the labia majora and upper labia minora, as well

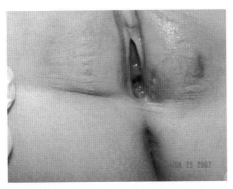

FIGURE 8.30
This 3-year-old child was brought to the
emergency department after falling on the
edge of the bathtub. A small labial bruise
and impact tear raised the concern of
sexual abuse. The hymenal examination
was normal.

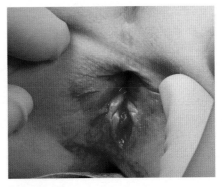

FIGURE 8.31
This anal tear at 5 o'clock in a 3-year-old
occurred when she fell on a toy in the
bathtub.

as small posterior fourchette tears, are
commonly seen in straddle injuries.
Abrasions of the mucous membranes
may occur, but the hymen is rarely
penetrated. Accidental penetrating
injuries generally cause external as well
as internal trauma.[66] A rare exception
is reported to have been caused by a
waterskiing fall.[67] Injuries that crush
the pelvic area can result in "blow outs"
through the vaginal vault, mimicking
penetrating injury.[68] Impalement of the
anus or vagina has also been reported
to have occurred when a child falls
directly on an object.[69] The case in
Figures 8.31 and 8.32 demonstrates this
type of injury. Forced abduction of the
legs has been reported to cause perineal
injury without hymenal injury in 2
cases where girls were rollerblading
and suddenly abducted their legs.[70]

Accidental genital injuries are painful,
and even a young verbal child may
have a clear recollection of the event.
Medical care should be obtained

promptly, particularly if pain and
bleeding are present. If the history
is not consistent with the injury,
then sexual abuse is more likely. In
unclear and unusual cases, a physician
should report to local child protective
authorities. An investigation of the
scene of the accident may provide
evidence that either corroborates the
history of a straddle injury or raises
further suspicion of abuse.

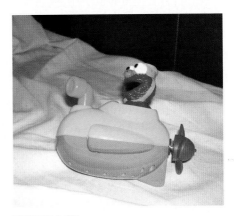

FIGURE 8.32
The father provided the toy that the had
child fallen on in the bathtub.

Masturbation is often questioned as a cause of genital abnormalities, especially hymenal damage in young girls. Most female masturbation is clitoral and not directed toward the vaginal orifice. Insertion of foreign bodies by a child may be associated with a history of sexual abuse, but it certainly occurs in the setting of normal exploration. Self-inserted foreign bodies have not been reported to cause hymenal trauma. Significant injury from masturbation has never been reported and should not be considered in the diagnosis of hymenal trauma that clearly meets the criteria for a vaginal penetrating injury consistent with sexual abuse.

Summary

The evaluation of anogenital conditions in children is a challenging problem. A complete evaluation of the child is essential, as is an understanding of the variety of processes that can present with anogenital involvement. Genital complaints and the appearance of unusual lesions or eruptions on the anogenital area commonly raise the concern of sexual abuse. Many such conditions also have systemic manifestations, and a thorough history and physical examination can provide the clues leading to appropriate diagnoses. Laboratory tests, culture, or biopsy may also be indicated. An accurate assessment with appropriate treatment will ultimately provide the best care possible to the patient.

References

1. Weitzner JM, Fields KW, Robinson MJ. Pediatric bowenoid papulosis: risks and management. *Pediatr Dermatol.* 1989;6(4):303–305
2. Frasier LD. Human papillomavirus infections in children. *Pediatr Ann.* 1994;23(7):354–360
3. Syrjanen S, Puranen M. Human papillomavirus infections in children: the potential role of maternal transmission. *Crit Rev Oral Biol Med.* 2000;11(2):259–274
4. Rice PS, Cason J, Best JM, Banatvala JE. High risk genital papillomavirus infections are spread vertically. *Rev Med Virol.* 1999;9(1):15–21
5. Janniger CK, Schwartz RA. Molluscum contagiosum in children. *Cutis.* 1993;52(4):194–196
6. Bargman H. Is genital molluscum contagiosum a cutaneous manifestation of sexual abuse in children? *J Am Acad Dermatol.* 1986;14(5 Pt 1):847–849
7. Halvorsen JA, Brevig T, Aas T, Skar AG, Slevolden EM, Moi H. Genital ulcers as initial manifestation of Epstein-Barr virus infection: two new cases and a review of the literature. *Acta Derm Venereol.* 2006;86(5):439–442
8. Barnes CJ, Alio AB, Cunningham BB, Friedlander SF. Epstein-Barr virus-associated genital ulcers: an under-recognized disorder. *Pediatr Dermatol.* 2007;24(2):130–134
9. Hudson LB, Perlman SE. Necrotizing genital ulcerations in a premenarcheal female with mononucleosis. *Obstet Gynecol.* 1998;92(4 Pt 2):642–644
10. Lorenzo CV, Robertson WS. Genital ulcerations as presenting symptom of infectious mononucleosis. *J Am Board Fam Pract.* 2005;18(1):67–68
11. Sisson BA, Glick L. Genital ulceration as a presenting manifestation of infectious mononucleosis. *J Pediatr Adolesc Gynecol.* 1998;11(4):185–187

12. Reading R, Ranaan-Eliya Y. Evidence for sexual transmission of genital herpes in children. *Arch Dis Child.* 2007;92(7):608–613

13. Deitch HR, Huppert J, Adams Hillard PJ. Unusual vulvar ulcerations in young adolescent females. *J Pediatr Adolesc Gynecol.* 2004;17(1):13–16

14. Altchek A. Pediatric vulvovaginitis. *J Reprod Med.* 1984;29(6):359–375

15. Gerstner GJ, Grunberger W, Boschitsch E, Rotter M. Vaginal organisms in pre-pubertal children with and without vulvovaginitis. A vaginoscopic study. *Arch Gynecol.* 1982;231(3):247–252

16. Cuadros J, Mazon A, Martinez R, et al. The aetiology of paediatric inflammatory vulvovaginitis. *Eur J Pediatr.* 2004;163(2):105–107

17. Nathanson M, Tisseron B, de Pontual L. Meningococcal vulvovaginitis in a pre-pubertal girl [in French]. *Arch Pediatr.* 2005;12(12):1732–1733

18. Straumanis JP, Bocchini JA Jr. Group A beta-hemolytic streptococcal vulvo-vaginitis in prepubertal girls: a case report and review of the past twenty years. *Pediatr Infect Dis J.* 1990;9(11): 845–848

19. Murphy TV, Nelson JD. Shigella vaginitis: report of 38 patients and review of the literature. *Pediatrics.* 1979;63(4):511–516

20. Baiulescu M, Hannon PR, Marcinak JF, Janda WM, Schreckenberger PC. Chronic vulvovaginitis caused by antibiotic-resistant *Shigella flexneri* in a prepubertal child. *Pediatr Infect Dis J.* 2002;21(2):170–172

21. Banerjee K, Curtis E, de San Lazaro C, Graham JC. Low prevalence of genital candidiasis in children. *Eur J Clin Microbiol Infect Dis.* 2004;23(9):696–698

22. Jenny C, Kirby P, Fuquay D. Genital lichen sclerosus mistaken for child sexual abuse. *Pediatrics.* 1989;83(4):597–599

23. Albers SE, Taylor G, Huyer D, Oliver G, Krafchik BR. Vulvitis circumscripta plasmacellularis mimicking child abuse. *J Am Acad Dermatol.* 2000;42(6):1078–1080

24. Meuli M, Briner J, Hanimann B, Sacher P. Lichen sclerosus et atrophicus causing phimosis in boys: a prospective study with 5-year follow-up after complete circumcision. *J Urol.* 1994;152(3):987–989

25. Loening-Baucke V. Lichen sclerosus et atrophicus in children. *Am J Dis Child.* 1991;145(9):1058–1061

26. Wright JE. The treatment of childhood phimosis with topical steroid. *Aust N Z J Surg.* 1994;64(5):327–328

27. Meffert JJ, Davis BM, Grimwood RE. Lichen sclerosus. *J Am Acad Dermatol.* 1995;32(3):393–416; quiz 417–418

28. Goldberg NS, Hebert AA, Esterly NB. Sacral hemangiomas and multiple congenital abnormalities. *Arch Dermatol.* 1986;122(6):684–687

29. Hara M, Watanabe M, Tagami H. Jacquet erosive diaper dermatitis in a young girl with urinary incontinence. *Pediatr Dermatol.* 1991;8(2):160–161

30. Rodriguez Cano L, Garcia-Patos Briones V, Pedragosa Jové R, Castells Rodellas A. Perianal pseudoverrucous papules and nodules after surgery for Hirschsprung disease. *J Pediatr.* 1994;125(6 Pt 1):914–916

31. Coppo P, Salomone R. Pseudoverrucous papules: an aspect of incontinence in children. *J Eur Acad Dermatol Venereol.* 2002;16(4):409–410

32. Bluestein J, Furner BB, Phillips D. Granuloma gluteale infantum: case report and review of the literature. *Pediatr Dermatol.* 1990;7(3):196–198

33. Robson KJ, Maughan JA, Purcell SD, Petersen MJ, Haefner HK, Lowe L. Erosive papulonodular dermatosis associated with topical benzocaine: a report of two cases and evidence that granuloma gluteale, pseudoverrucous papules, and Jacquet's erosive dermatitis are a disease spectrum. *J Am Acad Dermatol.* 2006;55(5 suppl):S74–S80

34. McCann J, Wells R, Simon M, Voris J. Genital findings in prepubertal girls selected for nonabuse: a descriptive study. *Pediatrics.* 1990;86(3):428–439

35. McCann J, Voris J, Simon M. Labial adhesions and posterior fourchette injuries in childhood sexual abuse. *Am J Dis Child.* 1988;142(6):659–663

36. Farber EM, Mullen RH, Jacobs AH, Nall L. Infantile psoriasis: a follow-up study. *Pediatr Dermatol.* 1986;3(3):237–243

37. Bonifazi E, Meneghini CL. Atopic dermatitis in the first six months of life. *Acta Derm Venereol Suppl (Stockh).* 1989;144:20–22

38. Ruiz-Maldonado R, Lopez-Matinez R, Perez Chavarria EL, Rocio Castanon L, Tamayo L. Pityrosporum ovale in infantile seborrheic dermatitis. *Pediatr Dermatol.* 1989;6(1):16–20

39. Levin AV, Selbst SM. Vulvar hemangioma simulating child abuse. *Clin Pediatr (Phila).* 1988;27(4):213–215

40. Morelli JG. Hemangiomas and vascular malformations. *Pediatr Ann.* 1996;25(2):91, 94–96

41. Girard C, Bigorre M, Guillot B, Bessis D. PELVIS syndrome. *Arch Dermatol.* 2006;142(7):884–888

42. Francis JS. Genetic skin diseases. *Curr Opin Pediatr.* 1994;6(4):447–453

43. Salopek TG, Krol A, Jimbow K. Case report of Darier disease localized to the vulva in a 5-year-old girl. *Pediatr Dermatol.* 1993;10(2):146–148

44. Hanks JW, Venters WJ. Nickel allergy from a bed-wetting alarm confused with herpes genitalis and child abuse. *Pediatrics.* 1992;90(3):458–460

45. Hoque SR, Patel M, Farrell AM. Childhood cicatricial pemphigoid confined to the vulva. *Clin Exp Dermatol.* 2006;31(1):63–64

46. Marren P, Wojnarowska F, Venning V, Wilson C, Nayar M. Vulvar involvement in autoimmune bullous diseases. *J Reprod Med.* 1993;38(2):101–107

47. Levine V, Sanchez M, Nestor M. Localized vulvar pemphigoid in a child misdiagnosed as sexual abuse. *Arch Dermatol.* 1992;128(6):804–806

48. Saad RW, Domloge-Hultsch N, Yancey KB, Benson PM, James WD. Childhood localized vulvar pemphigoid is a true variant of bullous pemphigoid. *Arch Dermatol.* 1992;128(6):807–810

49. Korman N. Pemphigus. *J Am Acad Dermatol.* 1988;18(6):1219–1238

50. Online Mendelian Inheritance in Man, Johns Hopkins University. Benign Chronic Pemphigus; BCPM. Gene map locus 3q21-q24.

51. Stratakis CA, Graham W, DiPalma J, Leibowitz I. Misdiagnosis of perianal manifestations of Crohn's disease. Two cases and a review of the literature. *Clin Pediatr (Phila).* 1994;33(10):631–633

52. Porzionato A, Alaggio R, Aprile A. Perianal and vulvar Crohn's disease presenting as suspected abuse. *Forensic Sci Int.* 2005;155(1):24–27

53. Sellman SP, Hupertz VF, Reece RM. Crohn's disease presenting as suspected abuse. *Pediatrics.* 1996;97(2):272–274

54. Wardinsky TD, Vizcarrondo FE, Cruz BK. The mistaken diagnosis of child abuse: a three-year USAF Medical Center analysis and literature review. *Mil Med.* 1995;160(1):15–20

55. Bourrat E, Faure C, Vignon-Pennamen MD, Rybojad M, Morel P, Navarro J. Anitis, vulvar edema and macrocheilitis disclosing Crohn disease in a child: value of metronidazole [in French]. *Ann Dermatol Venereol.* 1997;124(9):626–628

56. McCuaig CC, Moroz B. Perineal eruption in Kawasaki's syndrome. *Arch Dermatol.* 1987;123(4):430–431

57. Kone-Paut I, Yurdakul S, Bahabri SA, et al. Clinical features of Behçet's disease in children: an international collaborative study of 86 cases. *J Pediatr.* 1998;132(4):721–725

58. Uziel Y, Brik R, Padeh S, et al. Juvenile Behçet's disease in Israel. The Pediatric Rheumatology Study Group of Israel. *Clin Exp Rheumatol.* 1998;16(4):502–505

59. Yesudian PD, Edirisinghe DN, O'Mahony C. Behçet's disease. *Int J STD AIDS.* 2007;18(4):221–227

60. Cavender PA, Bennett RG. Perianal eosinophilic granuloma resembling condyloma latum. *Pediatr Dermatol.* 1988;5(1):50–55

61. Angeli SI, Alcalde J, Hoffman HT, Smith RJ. Langerhans cell histiocytosis of the head and neck in children. *Ann Otol Rhinol Laryngol.* 1995;104(3):173–180

62. Papa CA, Pride HB, Tyler WB, Turkewitz D. Langerhans cell histiocytosis mimicking child abuse. *J Am Acad Dermatol.* 1997;37(6):1002–1004

63. Stephens-Groff SM, Hansen RC, Bangert J. Benign pigmented apocrine vulvar hamartomas. *Pediatr Dermatol.* 1993;10(2):123–124

64. Tay YK, Tham SN, Teo R. Localized vulvar syringomas—an unusual cause of pruritus vulvae. *Dermatology.* 1996;192(1):62–63

65. Emans S, Laufer M, Goldstein D. *Pediatric and Adolescent Gynecology.* 4th ed. Philadelphia, PA: Lippincott Williams & Wilkins; 1998

66. Boos SC. Accidental hymenal injury mimicking sexual trauma. *Pediatrics.* 1999;103(6 Pt 1):1287–1290

67. Perlman SE, Hertweck SP, Wolfe WM. Water-ski douche injury in a premenarcheal female. *Pediatrics.* 1995;96(4 Pt 1):782–783

68. Boos SC, Rosas AJ, Boyle C, McCann J. Anogenital injuries in child pedestrians run over by low-speed motor vehicles: four cases with findings that mimic child sexual abuse. *Pediatrics.* 2003;112(1 Pt 1):e77–e84

69. Rothamel T, Burger D, Debertin AS, Kleemann WJ. Vaginorectal impalement injury in a 2-year-old child—caused by sexual abuse or an accident? *Forensic Sci Int.* 2001;119(3):330–333

70. Herrmann B, Crawford J. Genital injuries in prepubertal girls from inline skating accidents. *Pediatrics.* 2002;110(2 Pt 1):e16

Chapter 9

Nursing Issues Related to Child Sexual Abuse Evaluations

Eileen R. Giardino

Faye A. Blair

The role of the nurse in dealing with child sexual abuse is multifaceted. Nurses evaluate children suspected of experiencing sexual abuse independently and in collaboration with physicians to ensure their optimal treatment. This chapter describes ways in which nurses intervene in areas of sexual abuse and collaborate with other health care and law enforcement professionals to provide care to children who are suspected of experiencing child sexual abuse. Additionally nurses can play an important role in educating professionals about prevention and detection.

Nursing Role in Detection and Reporting of Abuse

Mandated Reporting of Abuse

Nurses are mandated reporters of abuse and therefore need to understand state-specific reporting laws and to whom reports are made.[1] Under every state's statutes, nurses are mandated to report suspected abuse or neglect of a child if they are suspicious or have reason to believe that abuse or neglect exists. Failure to report is a misdemeanor in most states, and the mandated reporter can be held civilly responsible if the failure was either knowing or willful.[2] The scope of nursing practice enables nurses to observe children in all settings from institutional, to school, to home environments. The importance of understanding laws and ethical issues in the area of mandated abuse reporting is essential because nurses encounter questionable situations in all areas of practice that require wisdom in what to do.[3] Nurses who have education and experience in the issues of child sexual abuse are better able to identify signs of abuse in all settings.[4]

Studies of compliance of health care professionals in reporting suspected cases of child abuse show that approximately 40% of subjects were deliberately noncompliant at some point for a variety of reasons.[5] Some reasons for non-reporting include uncertainty of the findings in relation to the consequences to the caretakers and concerns about reprisal or litigation. Greipp[6] studied reasons why nurses do not report child abuse and suggested that nurses and other health care professionals be educated in the reporting process. The issues include the need to understand the problem of abuse, ethical issues related to reporting or non-reporting, intervention protocols, and legal parameters by which reporting should occur. When a nurse is unsure of whether to report an incident, he or she should collaborate with others to decide what is in the best interest of the child.

Public School System— School Nurses

The public school system is the largest reporter of child abuse and neglect.[1] School nurses play a direct role in uncovering abuse among school-children through direct observation and interaction with students. They provide education to classroom teachers about abuse and provide abuse prevention programs to students.[7] It is important that school nurses understand their legal and ethical responsibility as mandated reporters of child abuse. Nurses need to confirm that administrators in their school system also understand the state and professional responsibilities of practice standards of school nurses regarding mandated reporting.[8] Although mandated reporting of abuse to state authorities is required, many state laws prohibit dissemination of confidential

information to school employees after the initial interview of a child to ensure the privacy and protection of children and their families.[9]

Despite a large number of reports filed through school systems, 76% of cases in schools still go unreported.[1] A Nebraska study was conducted to determine if school nurses are in an ideal situation to see potential signs of abuse and maltreatment. Findings showed that school nurses had the ability to identify indicators of emotional abuse in school-aged children.[10] In general, school nurses are instrumental in identifying signs of physical and sexual abuse in the school populations[10] and in developing programs in schools aimed at preventing child abuse by increasing awareness of the problem and attempting to change peoples' attitudes toward the causes of the problem.[8,11]

Nurses in Emergency Departments

Sexually abused children enter the health care system in many ways. Police, child protection workers, and pediatricians often refer parents to the local emergency department (ED) when they suspect sexual abuse. Parents often turn to the ED for immediate help when they are concerned that their child may have been sexually abused. Some communities have child abuse diagnostic and treatment centers that serve to provide medical and mental health services independently, or colocated with law enforcement, and social services to assist in evaluating child sexual abuse. The availability of specialized services varies from community to community, with the ED frequently being the only available place to receive services 24/7. Whenever possible children should be evaluated by professionals who are knolwedgeable about the special needs of child victims and in a child-friendly environment. Parents frequently turn to EDs because of the crisis of a child's disclosure and the belief that they will obtain a definitive diagnosis in a hospital. Although some EDs have skilled professionals available to evaluate child sexual abuse, many do not. Sexual assault nurse examiners (SANE) frequently work in the ED and when available provide evaluation and treatment services.

Triage Nurse in the Emergency Department

Nurses provide care to sexually abused children in the ED from the point of triage through discharge. The triage interview usually consists of questions to elicit the reason the child is visiting the ED for care. Children may disclose abuse to the nurse during the triage interview, but it is common for children to be unwilling to talk about the abuse until they are in a more private setting. Nurses often suspect child sexual and physical abuse in triage because they are the first ones to question the child and caregiver about why they are there.[12]

The triage nurse seeks the underlying reason for the visit, but the interview should not delve into details of the assault. Initial triage assessment for acute injury and safety of the patient is essential. The priority is care of acute injury with preservation of evidence during treatment. Although the triage interview would not be considered an

investigative interview because the health care professional's role is that of diagnosis and treatment, it is important that the nurse ask appropriate questions in the appropriate way for the well-being of the child and for the further interactions that take place regarding the evaluation of suspected abuse.[13]

A child who presents to the ED for sexual assault examination should be triaged as a high-priority patient. Emergency departments that do not routinely take care of child sexual assault victims should transfer the child to a facility that specializes in child abuse. The single most important question to be asked by the triage nurse when a child presents for the concern of sexual abuse is when the last time was that something happened. Most children who present to the ED are presenting long after the last sexual contact and well beyond the time frame in which the SANE would have a role in evidentiary collection.

SANE Training

Nurses play a significant role in the direct evaluation of victims of abuse in the ED setting. It became evident in the late 1970s that this group of patients was receiving suboptimal care in the busy ED. Victims often had long waits to be examined, and physicians and nurses caring for them often lacked the expertise to provide psychological and forensic techniques and training necessary to care for sexual assault victims. The role of the SANE was developed to address the need to give comprehensive care to the sexual assault patient in the ED.[14]

A SANE is a registered nurse who has advanced education and clinical preparation in the forensic examination of sexual assault victims. The SANE offers prompt compassionate care, experience in forensic techniques, psychological support, and comprehensive documentation of relevant findings. The SANE has completed advanced theory and clinical training in the nursing care and treatment of patients who report being victims of violence. Nurses access SANE training through state-sponsored courses, university settings, or private companies. The SANE educational program for adult/adolescent victims comprises at least 40 hours of didactic lessons, usually with additional clinical preceptor hours required. Additional training in pediatric sexual assault is required to treat that age group. Pediatric training includes normal growth and sexual development, special communication techniques, and different findings based on the child's age. The International Association of Forensic Nurses (IAFN) has developed national certification programs for both adult/adolescent and pediatric SANEs.

Training of SANEs and program development began slowly in the 1980s in a few hospitals. Organized national efforts to disseminate these programs started with a group of 31 SANE programs from around the country coming together in Minneapolis in 1992 to form the IAFN (www.iafn.org). This professional organization was founded to develop, promote, and disseminate information about the science of forensic nursing. With the inception of this international organization came a proliferation of SANE programs throughout the United States. The American Nurses Association granted specialty status to this new nursing discipline in 1995. The IAFN has developed standards of practice and education to ensure consistent practice. Today there are SANE programs in every state.

Sexual assault nurse examiners provide many services to the sexual abuse survivor including history taking of the encounter, evaluation, documentation of physical trauma and verbal statements, and collection of forensic evidence. The SANE also maintains a proper chain of evidence and works cooperatively and collaboratively with law enforcement and prosecution.[15] In addition, the SANE works as a case manager and may help survivors navigate the law enforcement system. Along with the forensic examination, the nurse examiner looks for abuse-related injuries and sexually transmitted infections (STIs), and also assesses pregnancy risk. The SANE may intervene with crisis intervention and make arrangements for follow-up counseling.[15]

In an effort to provide comprehensive and competent approaches to the sexual assault evaluation, many EDs employ SANEs as on-call staff. This process ensures that the nurse examiner is skilled in the specifics of the comprehensive examination and that other staff in a busy ED are not pulled away from their responsibilities. Because the staff of many EDs do not perform forensic examinations on a daily basis, it is difficult for them to maintain proficiency. In many hospitals that use nurse examiners, the usual procedure is to page the on-call SANE when the patient arrives to the ED for a sexual abuse evaluation. The SANE completes the interview process and evidentiary examination, provides crisis intervention, evaluates risk for STIs and pregnancy, and coordinates follow-up care.

Sexual assault nurse examiners do not operate in isolation. Physician partners are needed for injury evaluation, ordering medication, and peer review. Some hospital-based programs have protocols for medication administration, while other programs require a physician consultation while in the ED. The use of the colposcope with video or still pictures provides an opportunity for peer review of the examination and ultimate findings. This is especially important in pediatric sexual assault cases, where there are many variations of normal findings.

The goal of the SANE is to document injuries and physical evidence. With meticulous documentation, it is possible that SANE evaluations may help increase prosecution rates in the community, and there is evidence to that desire.[16] One study that included a direct comparison of legal outcomes for SANE cases versus non-SANE cases found strong evidence that prosecution of sexual assault cases was higher in SANE cases.[17]

Nurses are part of community-based programs called Sexual Assault Response Teams (SARTs). A SART is a multidisciplinary team that consists of people and agencies that respond to and work with victims of sexual assault.[18,19] Included on the SART are sexual assault forensic examiners, patient advocates, law enforcement officers, prosecutors, and forensic laboratory personnel. The SART process helps to coordinate all aspects of the sexual assault evaluation and possible law enforcement proceedings. The SANE, in the role of the forensic examiner on the SART, completes the medical/legal examination and maintains the chain of evidence in collecting forensic data.[20]

Role of the SANE in the Emergency Department

The SANE nurse provides comprehensive care to the victim and family. Domains within the role include (a) psychological support for the victim and the victim's family, (b) post-rape medical care, (c) collection and documentation of forensic evidence, and (d) expert testimony at trial.[16]

Sexual assault nurse examiner responsibilities include history taking of the encounter and preparation of the victim and family for the evidentiary examination. Preparation includes explanation at the child's level of understanding of procedures and equipment to be used. The SANE documents physical trauma and verbal statements, collects forensic evidence, and maintains a chain of evidence. Documentation on examination findings would be expected to include patients' demeanor and statements related to the assault not already recorded on the medical forensic history. Such documentation can be admitted as evidence at trial in most states.[19] Depending on the history of the event and the age of the victim, the SANE also assesses need for toxicological evaluation, provides information and treatment for STIs, and judges pregnancy risk. The SANE provides information about further medical care needs, counseling resources, and law enforcement procedures.

Roles of the Nurse in Child Sexual Abuse

The Nurse as Expert Witness

An expert witness in the area of child sexual abuse must be able to render an opinion on which the court can reasonably rely and demonstrate sufficient knowledge of the subject matter through specialized training or practical experience. Relevancy of the witness is determined and the expert's qualifications are properly established. Challenges to the expert's techniques and the basis for his or her opinion will ordinarily focus on how much weight the expert's opinion should be given.[21]

The expert witness renders opinions, testifies to appropriate standards of care in all cases, and explains various medical terms and/or procedures specific to the details of abuse cases.[22] Case law has established SANEs as able to testify as expert witnesses. Although medical providers are generally advocates for patients in their care, the role of expert witness remains objective and factual regarding findings of the examination and evidence obtained.

A professional who possesses the skills, knowledge, training, education, and experience in the content area of abuse may qualify as an expert witness.[23] The nurse who has specialized training and experience in evaluating child sexual and physical abuse qualifies as an expert witness in a court of law. The validity of the nurse to testify in a case stems from experience in working with victims of abuse, specialized training by approved programs, and adhering to chain-of-evidence protocols.[24] A national survey of nonphysician health care providers showed that most nurse practitioners and registered nurses with specialized training in child molestation did qualify as expert witnesses.[25]

Collaboration With Other Health Care Professionals

In all areas of child sexual abuse and assault evaluation, nurses work in partnership with members of the health care team to provide comprehensive and appropriate care and evaluation. In situations where the nurse and other health care professionals work together to complete the sexual assault evaluation, the nurse may play an important role in helping the child to cope as well as possible with the procedures involved in the examination. Thus the nurse may provide information, explain the procedures, and help the child relax as much as possible throughout the process.[26]

Working With Police and Community Resources

Nurses who evaluate children for sexual abuse are an essential part of a team with law enforcement and social service agencies. Community-based team approaches in which the nurse examiner works collaboratively with police and other forensically trained nurses afford a better opportunity to provide consistency in sending reports to law enforcement, as well as more reliable information about details and findings.[15] Nurse examiners play a significant role in helping the victim and family work through the concerns they may have in reporting the assault and dealing with the psychological trauma.[15] Sometimes there are questions about what to expect from the legal system and what the reporting of the incident involves. Also, victims and families may have fears about what to expect and misconceptions about aspects of the process that the nurse can help to clarify or dispel.

Collecting Data: Sexual Assault Tools

Nurses have been instrumental in developing tools that help practitioners collect and document clinical findings of child sexual abuse evaluations. These tools enable nurses and other health care practitioners to uncover abuse, collect data on clinical and forensic evidence, and document evaluation of clients. Thorough evaluations support the potential for successful criminal prosecution through extensive documentation of specific verbal and physical findings. A sexual assault examiner uses the Comprehensive Sexual Assault Assessment Tool (CSAAT) to document investigative subjective data about the victim and the assault pattern, as well as forensic details of the assault.[27] The Sexual

Abuse Comfort Scale is an instrument that can be used in an educational way to determine whether nurses who work with victims of sexual abuse feel comfortable inquiring about or supporting victims of abuse.[28] Because sexual abuse is such an emotionally charged issue, it is important to recognize that there can be vicarious traumatization of health care professionals who care for these children. With this recognition steps can be taken to provide emotional support and training for professionals to learn effective ways of defusing the emotional impact of caring for this population.

Summary

Nurses are directly involved with the care of children suspected of sexual abuse. The implications of a nurse's knowledge of the problem and ability to intervene at all levels of care are tremendous. In every aspect of intervention, the nurse can provide a holistic approach to the many issues involved in the evaluation and treatment of child sexual abuse.

References

1. O'Toole A, O'Toole R, Webster S, Lucal B. Nurses' diagnostic work on possible physical child abuse. *Public Health Nurs.* 1996;13:337–344

2. Freed P, Drake V. Mandatory reporting of abuse: practical, moral, and legal issues for psychiatric home health nurses. *Issues Ment Health Nurs.* 1996b;20:423–436

3. Freed PE, Drake VK. Mandatory reporting of abuse: practical, moral, and legal issues for psychiatric home healthcare nurses. *Issues Ment Health Nurs.* 1999;20:423–436

4.   Flaherty EG, Sege R, Binns HJ, Mattson CL, Christoffel KK. Health care providers' experience reporting child abuse in the primary care setting. Pediatric Practice Research Group. *Arch Pediatr Adolesc Med.* 2000;154:489–493

5.   Zellman GL. Report decision-making patterns among mandated child abuse reporters. *Child Abuse Negl.* 1990;14:325–336

6.   Greipp M. Ethical decision making and mandatory reporting in cases of suspected child abuse. *J Pediatr Health Care.* 1997;11:258–265

7.   Marshall E, Buckner EJ, Perkins J, et al. Effects of a child abuse prevention unit in health classes in four schools. *J Community Health Nurs.* 1996;13:107–122

8.   Oldfield D, Hays BB, Megel ME. Evaluation of the effectiveness of project trust: an elementary school-based victimization prevention strategy. *Child Abuse Negl.* 1996;20:821–832

9.   Administration for Children and Families/Children's Bureau. *Child Abuse Prevention and Treatment Act as Amended by the Keeping Children and Families Safe Act of 2003.* Washington, DC: Department of Health and Human Services; 2003. http://www.acf.hhs.gov/programs/cb/laws_policies/cblaws/capta03/index.htm. Accessed April 21, 2008

10. Pakieser RA, Starr D, Lebaugh D. Nebraska school nurses identify emotional maltreatment of school-age children: a replication of an Ohio study. *J Spec Pediatr Nurs.* 1998;3:137

11. Olds D, Hill P, Mihalic S, O'Brien RA. *Blueprints for Violence Prevention: Prenatal and Infancy Home Visitation by Nurses.* Boulder, CO: Institute of Behavioral Science, Regents of the University of Colorado; 1998

12. McFarlane J, Greenberg L, Weltge A, Watson M. Identification of abuse in emergency departments: effectiveness of a two-question screening tool. *J Emerg Nurs.* 1995;21:391–394

13. Monk M. Interviewing suspected victims of child maltreatment in the emergency department. *J Emerg Nurs.* 1998;24:31–34

14. Ledray LE. *SANE Development and Operation Guide.* Washington, DC: Sexual Assault Resource Serviceand US Department of Justice, Office of Justice Programs, Office for Victims of Crime; 1998

15. Ledray LE, Arndt S. Examining the sexual assault victim: a new model for nursing care. *J Psychoso Nurs.* 1994;32:7–12

16. Campbell R, Patterson D, Lichty LF. The effectiveness of Sexual Assault Nurse Examiner (SANE) programs: a review of psychological, medical, legal, and community outcomes. *Trauma Violence Abuse.* 2005;6:313–329

17. Crandall C, Helitzer D. *Impact Evaluation of a Sexual Assault Nurse Examiner (SANE) Program.* Washington, DC: National Institute of Justice; 2003. NCJ 203276.

18. American College of Emergency Physicians. *Evaluation and Management of the Sexually Assaulted or Sexually Abused Patient.* Dallas, TX: US Department of Health & Human Services; 1999

19. US Department of Justice Office on Violence Against Women. *A National Protocol for Sexual Assault Medical Forensic Examinations: Adults/Adolescents.* 2004. NCJ 206554

20. Smith K, Holmseth J, Macgregor M, Letourneau M. Sexual assault response team: overcoming obstacles to program development. *J Emerg Nurs.* 1998;24:365–367

21. Gillotte SL, Cates SE. The use of expert witnesses in child sexual abuse cases. University of Georgia Center for Continuing Education Web site. http://childabuse.georgiacenter.uga.edu/both/gillote/gillotte_print.phtml. Published 2001. Accessed April 21, 2008

22. Ruiz-Contreras A. Topics in emergency medicine. *SANE.* 2005;27(1):27–35

23. Myers JEB. Expert testimony. In: Myers JEB, ed, *Legal Issues in Child Abuse and Neglect Practice.* Thousand Oaks, CA: Sage Publications; 1998:221–281

24. Ledray LE, Simmelink K. Efficacy of SANE evidence collection: a Minnesota study. *J Emer Nurs.* 1997;23:75–77

25. Kelley SJ, Yorker BC. The role of nonphysician health care providers in the physical assessment and diagnosis of suspected child maltreatment: results of a national survey. *Child Maltreat.* 1997;2:331–340

26. Lawson L. Preparing sexually abused girls for genital evaluation. *Issues Comp Pediatr Nurs.* 1990;13:155–164

27. Burgess AW, Fawcett J. Comprehensive sexual assault assessment tool. *Nurse Pract.* 1996;21:66–78

28. McCay E, Gallop R, Austin W, Bayer M, Peternelj-Taylor C. Sexual abuse comfort scale: a scale to measure nurses' comfort to respond to sexual abuse in psychiatric populations. *J Psych Mental Health Nurs.* 1997;4:361–367

Chapter 10

Psychological Issues

Julie Lippmann

As described in previous chapters, physicians' roles in the identification, reporting, medical evaluation, and treatment of possible sexual abuse are unique and highly specialized. Although responsible physicians must confine their contribution to their own medical "piece of the puzzle," appreciation of relevant psychological issues can inform physician practice by improving comprehension of the dynamics, and sensitivity to the impact, of children's sexual abuse experiences; refining age-appropriate history-taking techniques; and clarifying appropriate referrals for mental health follow-up.

The Case for Mental Health Involvement

The disclosure of possible child sexual abuse inevitably creates an unwelcome crisis in the family—a period of some disorganization, disequilibrium, and distress. However, with it comes the potential for constructive change. Crisis intervention theory recognizes that mental health intervention may be particularly valuable and powerful during this period of flux. Thus the sooner after disclosure the psychologist, psychiatrist, or social worker becomes involved with the family, the more receptive the family members are likely to be.

To convey the nature of mental health intervention in cases of suspected child sexual abuse, this chapter provides an overview, from a psychological point of view, of what the experience of sexual abuse is like for a child and how it may affect the child's current and long-term functioning. The chapter also defines the various roles that mental health professionals may assume in these cases (evaluator, treating therapist, expert witness) and delineates some criteria for determining who needs what. Then, focusing on the evaluation process, the chapter reviews special issues related to forensically defensible and developmentally sensitive interviewing.

The Psychological Impact of Sexual Abuse on Children

Finkelhor and Browne[1] proposed a classic conceptualization that highlighted 4 specific "traumagenic dynamics" inherent in the sexual abuse experience—betrayal, powerlessness, stigmatization, and traumatic sexualization—that contribute to the psychological impact. Yet each child's experience is unique, and one or more of these factors may be more salient than the others in each particular situation. Thus it follows that the resulting psychological impact, in terms of both overt symptomatology and the child's internalized view of himself or herself in relation to the world, differs accordingly.

Although the specific nature of its effects vary widely, most researchers and clinicians concur that sexual abuse poses a significant risk for children both in the short term[2] and throughout the life span.[3–5] Its impact ranges along a continuum, from apparently negligible or neutral effects[6] to very severe and debilitating effects. Whereas a significant proportion of sexually abused children (up to 40%) show no apparent symptomatology,[2,7] comprehensive reviews of the literature find between 46% and 66% of sexually abused children demonstrating significant symptomatology of both an internalizing and an externalizing nature.[3]

The effects of child sexual abuse may be enduring; whether mild or severe, the symptoms evidenced by adult survivors seem to be continuations of childhood problems. Long-term impairment includes depression and anxiety disorders, chronic and/or delayed posttraumatic stress symptoms, revictimization,[8–10] suicidality,[11] and substance abuse, as well as sexual and other behavioral and interpersonal difficulties. Recent research suggests that a history of childhood sexual abuse seems to be related to a constellation of neuropsychological deficiencies as well.[12] The research on adult survivors generally focuses on adults who were not treated for their abuse-related difficulties—many of whom had not, in fact disclosed—as children because such treatment typically was unavailable in the past. Rosenthal et al[13] pointed out that avoidance of associated unpleasant internal experiences may itself be a mediator of long-term abuse-related psychological distress. Current psychotherapeutic intervention is grounded largely in the hope that long-term prognosis for individuals treated in childhood will be better. It is the present generation of child patients that will eventually determine the long-term efficacy of treatment. From the limited data available, it seems that many of the symptoms associated with child sexual abuse can be responsive to treatment and most children's symptoms gradually improve over time, although this improvement may be uneven and may be influenced by other attributional and family factors.[14] However, a smaller but significant proportion of children (particularly those with sexual problems and acting out behaviors)[15] may not improve or may even deteriorate depending on their circumstances.[2,16]

Mediating Factors in Prognosis

The wide variation in psychological impact is likely to reflect diversity in the nature and intensity of different children's abuse experiences.[17] Certain immutable factors, inherent in the abuse itself, as well as ethnic, cultural, and demographic variables seem to affect the nature and severity of the child's distress.[7,18,19] Situations involving violence, penetration, multiple offenders, longer duration, and greater frequency of incidents generally lead to increased problems. Abuse perpetrated by a parent or other person with a very close relationship to the child often tends to take a greater emotional toll. But even abuse by a peer may at times cause adverse outcomes.[20] Both relationship to the perpetrator and child's age at the onset of abuse have been noted as significant mediating factors in some studies, but not in others.[16,21-23] The nature of the problems manifested may be a function of the child's age and sex, with boys typically exhibiting more externalizing behavior problems than girls.[24,25]

Among the factors more amenable to therapeutic intervention are cognitive appraisal and attributional and coping styles. Avoidant coping may be a risk factor for increased psychological distress[13] and specifically for posttraumatic stress disorder (PTSD).[26] In addition to coping strategies, attachment styles and social support have been identified as mediators of the consequences of child sexual abuse.[27,28] Family dysfunction not only creates a risk for sexual abuse but may also exacerbate its negative consequences.[29] Negative abuse-specific internal attributions and shame in particular have been shown to increase depression and PTSD and need therefore be a focus of treatment.[30-33] Age may also be a factor; younger children do not comprehend the implications of their sexual abuse and therefore may be less distressed by it than older, more sophisticated children. But the most significant determinant of eventual prognosis is the belief and support of a non-offending caretaker, usually the mother.[7,34,35] Most mothers do, in fact, believe their children's disclosures and attempt to support and protect them.[36,37] However, children who are victims of incestuous abuse, where maternal support is more likely to be compromised, are most at risk for out-of-home placement, recantation, and an eventually poor outcome.[38-42] Therapeutic and educational intervention with these mothers, often secondary victims themselves, may be key to enhancing their support of their children.[36,43,44]

Nonspecific Symptoms of Distress

As a group, sexually abused children do not self-report clinically significant levels of nonspecific symptomatology, perhaps because of the heterogeneity of the group and their experiences, or the difficulties in identifying abuse-related problems with generic measures. Nevertheless, by clinical observation and parent report, many sexually abused children do manifest any of a wide range of affective and behavioral problems, such as anxiety and fearfulness; depression; low self-esteem; somatic complaints; regressive behavior; problems of attention, concentration, and activity level; and aggressive and self-destructive acting out. All of these are common childhood manifestations of some form of distress, warranting attention and therapeutic intervention, but they are not confined to, nor diagnostic of, sexual abuse. There is no one symptom that characterizes most sexually abused children and no evidence of any single syndrome or profile stemming from exposure to inappropriate sexual experiences.

Posttraumatic Effects

Posttraumatic stress disorder is a psychiatric diagnosis that describes a constellation of anxiety symptoms in direct response to an overwhelming stressor. Symptoms include intrusive phe-nomena such as flashbacks and nightmares, avoidance of stimuli associated with the trauma, and physiological hyper-arousal triggered by trauma-related stimuli. The disorder may present with immediate or delayed onset and may be chronic or episodic in its course. Kaplow and colleagues[26] identified 3 direct paths leading to PTSD symptoms—avoidant coping, anxiety/arousal, and dissociation— all measured during or immediately following disclosure of sexual abuse. Research has documented a high rate of PTSD in sexually abused children, with up to 40% of these children meeting full diagnostic criteria and more than 50% demonstrating at least partial symptoms.[45] However, a diagnosis of PTSD does not prove that a child has been sexually abused; a significant number of physically abused and non-abused psychiatric inpatients,[46] as well as children exposed to other traumatic experiences, have PTSD. A careful examination of the specific qualities of the child's symptoms and the circumstances that trigger them may help the clinician identify the nature of the child's trauma. For example, sexually abused children may be more likely than other children to fear or avoid sexual material, or to demonstrate repetitive reenactments of their trauma in sexualized play with dolls or other children. Although dissociation and self-mutilation—seen as a means to decrease dissociation and other PTSD symptoms—have been shown to be consequences of severe trauma and related to child sexual abuse, they seem not to be unique to that experience.[47–49]

Sexualized Behavior Problems

Only about a third of sexually abused children exhibit significant sexual behavior problems,[50] and certainly sexualized behaviors can also reflect normative processes, family, and other child variables.[51] Nevertheless, the presence of inappropriate sexual behavior serves as a red flag for the possibility of sexual abuse and may be an important psychosocial marker to differentiate sexual abuse victims not only from non-psychiatric but also from other traumatized and psychiatrically disturbed children.[46,52,53] Distinguishing inappropriate from developmentally normal sexual behaviors in children is sometimes difficult. Friedrich et al[54] found that 40% of parents reported that their children touched their own sex parts at home and undressed in front of others. Less common and more problematic is compulsive and/or public masturbatory behavior. Other more explicit behaviors, such as inserting objects in one's vagina or rectum or engaging in oral-genital contact, are reported by less than 1% of the parents of non-abused children. Comparison of parental reports of the observed behavior of sexually abused and non–sexually abused children reveals that those who have been abused demonstrate more sexual behavior in general and engage in more genital sexual activity and sexual behavior that is imitative of adult sexual behavior.[55] Still, although such explicit behaviors are cause for serious concern and investigation, they are not definitive evidence of abuse because they could reflect passive exposure to parental nudity or sexual behavior observed in person or in the media (eg, on videos, television, or computer).

The Multiple Roles of Mental Health Professionals in Cases of Suspected Sexual Abuse

In view of the complexities and legal implications of child sexual abuse cases, the involvement of mental health professionals may be called for at several different phases and for several different purposes. Recognizing the potential conflicts inherent in a blurring of roles, professional guidelines prohibiting dual relationships have prompted clearer definition and separation of the roles of forensic evaluator and therapist.[56–58] Each professional's role must be identified clearly in advance; each must serve in a single capacity. In making a referral for mental health intervention, then, what criteria may the physician use to determine the specific needs in a particular case?

Clinical Versus Forensic Roles

Kuehnle[59] delineates the distinctions between clinical and forensic roles in sexual abuse cases. In a clinical capacity, a mental health professional may serve as psychotherapist for the child and/or child's parents, with the goal of understanding and ameliorating the child's distress. Or, still in the clinical realm, the professional may undertake a clinical evaluation of the child's psychological status, often as a prerequisite for specific treatment planning but not geared toward validating an allegation of abuse. Both of these roles are grounded in the confidential therapeutic relationship and presuppose clients' honest and trustworthy communications.

In contrast, forensic roles involve a service to the judicial system (rather than to the individual child or parent) that is based on obtaining unbiased and uncontaminated data from the various parties, as well as a testing of several possible hypotheses. Operating from a position of investigative neutrality, the forensic professional must use forensically defensible methods to answer specific questions relevant to the court. Thus the mental health evaluation of possible child sexual abuse involves a greater emphasis on obtaining corroborating information from a variety of sources, such as medical evaluations, school reports, prior interviews, and collateral interviews.[56] Similarly, the professional engaged as an expert witness must act as an impartial scientist to educate the court and provide unbiased professional opinions based on established data and methods. The limits of that information and any resulting conclusions must be shared clearly with the court.[60]

Indications for Clinical Evaluation/Treatment

Addressing the diversity of the effects of sexual abuse, Saywitz and colleagues[14] identified 4 different groups of children to be considered for therapeutic intervention, ranging from those who showed no apparent signs of abuse impact (but may develop symptoms later) to those who met full criteria for psychiatric disorders when first assessed. These authors suggested that a continuum of intervention strategies are warranted, ranging from psychoeducation, to short-term cognitive-behavioral treatment for child and non-offending parent, to more comprehensive long-term treatment programs for multiproblem cases.

Although it is generally well accepted that most sexually abused children warrant some form of therapeutic intervention, empirical research on the effectiveness of specific approaches is a relatively recent development. Pretreatment and posttreatment studies comparing treatment and no-treatment groups have showed significant effects of treatment in general, but studies comparing alternative treatments have yielded inconsistent findings.[61] Although a variety of treatment strategies (including individual, group, and family therapy and focused, directive, and more nondirective interventions) have been described in the clinical literature,[62] it is only recently that controlled studies

comparing the effectiveness of different treatment modalities have been conducted. Some recent research demonstrates that sexually abused children with PTSD symptoms tend to improve with abuse-specific treatment[63–65] and that those gains are generally sustained[66]; however, Lanktree and Briere[15] suggest that the improvement in symptoms may be a function of time in treatment.

Controlled study of short-term, individual, cognitive-behavioral interventions found that involving both non-offending parents and their children in treatment was key in ameliorating behavioral symptoms.[63] One such investigation demonstrated that an abuse-focused cognitive-behavioral treatment was significantly more effective in treating internalizing symptoms and sexualized behaviors in preschoolers than was a nondirective, supportive counseling approach.[67] Likewise, a more recent study comparing trauma-focused cognitive-behavioral therapy (TF-CBT) with a more supportive child-centered treatment approach found that those children and caregivers who had completed TF-CBT treatment reported fewer symptoms of PTSD and less shame and abuse-specific parental distress at the conclusion of therapy, and that those improvements were sustained in 6- and 12-month follow-up.[68,69] Generally, although the number of well-controlled treatment outcome studies that randomly assigned clients to different treatments has been relatively small, results consistently favor abuse-specific CBT over other treatment modalities to which it has been compared and find that parental involvement and behavioral interventions are needed to decrease aggression or sexualized behavior problems.[14]

In cases of substantiated sexual abuse, then, it is appropriate for the child to be referred for evidence-based, abuse-focused treatment with a therapist who has specific expertise in this area if possible. Some form of clinical pretreatment evaluation is advised to assess the impact of the abuse, establish specific therapeutic needs, and make recommendations regarding treatment goals for this particular child and family. The likelihood of successful treatment is substantially enhanced when the treatment is matched to the specific needs of the particular child and family. In addition to identifying target symptoms, clinical assessment in child abuse cases must attend to the level of continued risk to the child (eg, if the child continues to have contact with the offending party) and the stance of the caregiver vis-a-vis the child's allegations and openness to change.[62] Where there is no potential court involvement and the specifics of the abuse have been well established, such an assessment in the pretreatment phase of therapy may be undertaken by the treating therapist. In keeping with the confidentiality of the therapeutic relationship, it may be helpful for the therapist to establish in advance with the child and parents the limits of his or her role in any legal proceeding that might ensue in the future (regarding visitation, reunification, etc) and

warrant a separate forensic mental health evaluation.

If ambiguity remains regarding the possibility of sexual abuse, a separate forensic evaluation may be requested to clarify the allegations further prior to referral for therapy. A child who has not made any disclosure of suspected sexual abuse may be referred for nondirective therapy or treatment targeting other symptoms or difficulties. However, the child should not be placed in therapy for ongoing observation with the agenda to elicit the "secret" through exposure to potentially contaminating anatomical dolls or stories encouraging disclosure.

Indications for Forensic Evaluation

A forensic mental health evaluation of allegations of sexual abuse is needed when sexual abuse is suspected but has not been substantiated clearly by the formal legal or child protection agencies mandated to investigate and intervene in these cases. It is hoped that a more extensive and comprehensive evaluation will illuminate and help to clarify what did or did not happen to the child, and that the appropriate legal, protective, and therapeutic intervention may follow from such an assessment. The following complex circumstances typically warrant a comprehensive forensic evaluation:

- Very young or developmentally immature children who are unable to provide the clear and cogent disclosure of abuse often required for formal substantiation

- Allegations of sexual abuse that emerge in the context of contentious divorce, custody, and visitation disputes
- Limited, conflicting, and/or ambiguous disclosures
- Allegations that are recanted at some point after original disclosure
- The medical history is limited in detail but of concern and the medical examination is non-diagnostic, warranting further assessment

Likewise, forensic evaluation may be requested in any cases in which there is current or anticipated court involvement, be it criminal prosecution of the alleged offender, a civil suit, or family court litigation either between family members or among family members and other parties (eg, when child protective services seeks guardianship of a child alleged to have been abused). It is prudent for forensic evaluation of the original allegations to take place early in the process, before the child is involved in ongoing therapy or exposed to other influences that can potentially complicate future legal issues.

Professional Guidelines for Conducting Sexual Abuse Evaluations

At this time, no formal credential or definitive standard of practice exists at either state or national levels for professionals conducting sexual abuse evaluations. However, both the American Professional Society on the Abuse of Children[70] and the American Academy of Child and Adolescent Psychiatry[56] have developed comprehensive guidelines emphasizing

qualifications of the evaluator and forensically defensible methods. They concur that mental health professionals conducting such evaluations should have formal graduate-level training in child development, assessment of children, and assessment of child sexual abuse, as well as knowledge of the current literature and research on child sexual abuse, interview techniques, assessment tools, memory and suggestibility, and false allegations. Sharing with all parties the limits of their confidentiality, they must define themselves in this endeavor as neutral and impartial scientists who collect, organize, and integrate data from multiple sources to understand behavior and render a probabilistic opinion regarding the likelihood of various hypotheses.[59] Keuhnle[71] outlines the strengths of using a scientist-practitioner model for these evaluations, based on empirically established relationships between data and the behavior of interest, rather than on subjective opinions. Even within the field, controversy exists regarding the appropriateness of providing an opinion regarding the ultimate legal issue—that a particular party is guilty of sexually abusing the child. Conclusions must be cautious and empirically based for presentation in the legal context. Reviewing the literature on evaluator competency, Herman[72] offered evidence that many mental health professionals lack the requisite levels of training, knowledge, and skills to perform high-quality evaluations or to address the complexity underlying decisions regarding the validity of sexual abuse allegations, and finds that approximately one-fourth of the decisions made by mental health evaluators involve either false-positive or false-negative errors.[73] Given the lack of a reliable empirically based foundation for determining whether sexual abuse actually occurred, recognized authorities in the field opine that it is irresponsible or even unethical for evaluators to offer such expert opinions.[72-74] It is important to recognize that psychologists have no particular expertise in deciphering truthfulness and ought not to provide testimony regarding credibility. (For discussion of appropriate psychological testimony, see Ceci and Hembrooke,[75] Goldstein,[76] and Myers et al.[77])

The Evaluation Process

The physician referring for a comprehensive mental health evaluation may expect a forensic evaluation of the allegations of sexual abuse, an assessment of the impact of any such abuse on the child's overall psychological functioning, and recommendations regarding appropriate intervention for the child and family.

Sources of Information

To enhance the comprehensiveness and objectivity of the evaluation, the mental health professional should gather information from multiple sources using multiple methods. In addition to obtaining information directly from the child and non-offending parent or guardian, the psychologist may speak to a number of other parties, including the "fresh complaint" witness (ie, the person

to whom the child made his or her original disclosure); the child's siblings, if appropriate; the child protection worker; the prosecution investigator or investigating police officer; and others who might be involved with the child, such as the examining physician, teacher, nurse, counselor, and babysitter or other caretaker.

When possible, the alleged offender should be interviewed as well; this is particularly important in cases where he or she is the child's parent and where the allegations emerge in the context of custody and visitation issues. However, unless ordered to participate by the court, alleged offenders may decline to participate in the evaluation, often on the advice of their attorneys; in such cases, their refusals and reasons provided should be documented in the resulting evaluation reports. When an alleged offender is willing to come in, the interview generally should be an individual one. Although some evaluators may see the alleged offender together with the child (particularly when custody is at issue), the risks and benefits of that practice must be weighed carefully. It is possible that a child may be traumatized by such a reunion or feel pressured to recant. Even where a child appears willing and eager to meet with the alleged offender, observations of their interaction in session are not likely to reveal whether sexual abuse has occurred. Children may remain quite close to someone who has been sexually inappropriate with them; likewise, there are many other reasons besides the possibility of abuse that some children may appear to be estranged from, angry with, or fearful of a parent or caretaker. Psychological evaluation of an alleged offender is a particularly difficult process due to a higher level of denial and absence of a typical test profile; most guidelines for such evaluations are geared toward assessing known offenders and focus on risk of recidivism and treatment issues.[78,79] Unless the evaluator in the case has specific expertise in such evaluations, the clinical interview with the alleged offending parent must be limited to obtaining history and his or her perspective on the allegations; any formal assessment of the alleged offender should be deferred to another professional holding that specialized expertise. A team approach may be advisable in such cases.

Methods of Assessment

The evaluator must draw on a variety of sources of data and integrate them with information from the documented case history and collateral contacts. Sources of information include review of official reports, clinical interviews with the child and parents, observations of their behavior and affect, and administration of standardized psychological assessment instruments.

Psychologists use a variety of assessment devices, including standardized observation systems, behavior rating scales, self-report psychological measures, projective techniques, and children's drawings. They should be familiar with the psychometric properties of measures and use only those with adequate reliability and validity; otherwise, any data derived from the measure are questionable. Instruments should be administered only to children within the designated age range and used only for the purposes intended. Self-report behavior measures are face-valid, and respondents can either deny or exaggerate the presence of symptoms. Projective testing and artwork may be useful in understanding the personality functioning of the client, but they do not indicate sexual abuse and their use in forensic settings is generally discouraged.[79-81] Thus, although many of these assessment devices are quite useful in describing the particular behaviors, symptoms, developmental/cognitive abilities, and underlying personality dynamics of the child, there are currently no assessment tools that offer the sensitivity and specificity to reliably differentiate sexually abused from non–sexually abused children.[59,71]

Recently, several standardized instruments have been developed that target symptomatology more specific to the effects of trauma and sexual abuse. Among those that psychologists may find useful in the evaluation process are the following:

- Child Sexual Behavior Inventory—Revised[81]
- Trauma Symptom Checklist for Children[82]
- Trauma Symptom Checklist for Young Children[83]
- Children's Impact of Traumatic Events Scale—Revised[84]

- Child Dissociative Checklist[85] or Adolescent Dissociative Experiences Scale[86]
- Children's Attributions and Perceptions Scale[87]

Although helpful in detecting and assessing trauma-related symptoms and reactions, these measures also must be interpreted cautiously. Sexually abused children are a heterogeneous group; they demonstrate different symptoms, and many children manifest none at all. Thus no single measure can accurately detect a sexually abused child.

Domains of Information

A comprehensive mental health evaluation should include history and current information relating to the following domains:

1. Identifying/referral information, including pending child protection and legal issues
2. History and background of the allegations
3. Characteristics of the alleged abuse and circumstances and context of disclosure
4. Findings of any medical evaluation and prior investigative procedures
5. Medical, developmental, psychosocial, and academic histories of the child
6. Family history and dynamics, including histories of physical and/or sexual abuse, mental illness, substance abuse, domestic violence, other criminal activity or impulse control problems, divorce, custody and visitation issues, and other risk factors

7. History of other childhood traumas, including neglect, physical or emotional abuse, early loss, abandonment, separations, and placements
8. Description of child's support resources and coping skills
9. Description of the child's behavioral and emotional functioning prior to, during, and following the alleged abuse and disclosure, including nonspecific symptoms of distress, specific posttraumatic symptoms, sexualized behavior problems, and other trauma-related problems (ie, quality of attachment/relationships; affect regulation; dissociation; self-image; beliefs, attributions, and distortions related to the alleged abuse experience; shame and self-blame; and risky, destructive behaviors)

Observations of the child during his or her individual evaluation sessions allow for assessment of mental status and developmental/cognitive level, particularly as these relate to the verbal abilities and concept formation required for a standard abuse interview (ie, number, time, size, color, truth vs lie, real vs make believe), as well as of the child's level of activity and emotional and behavioral responses to neutral versus abuse-related discussion. While developing rapport, the clinical interview may also elucidate the child's current (and previous) living situation(s), school and peer relationships, likes and dislikes, worries and problems, and other general information. It is in the individual session(s) with the child that abuse-related investigative interviewing takes place.

Investigative Interviewing of Children

Forensic interviewing of children is a specialized skill, a fact-finding process geared to help children relate their experiences accurately and completely. Children are interviewed about the possibility of sexual abuse when something has occurred to raise suspicion that such abuse might have taken place. Perhaps the child has made a purposeful disclosure or a spontaneous but unintentional comment, or perhaps he or she has engaged in sexualized behavior that raises concern. Suspicion may arise from medical findings or adult observations, which then prompt an adult to question a child directly. Any of these may be indications of sexual abuse, but they might also occur in a child who has not been sexually abused. Therefore, professionals investigating the possibility of sexual abuse must adopt a hypothesis-testing (not a hypothesis-confirming) approach. Rather than assume that the child must have been abused and view the interview as a way of extracting a disclosure, an investigative interviewer must generate and systematically test out each of the feasible explanations for suspicious statements or behavior, both within and outside the interview.

Medical professionals evaluating allegations of sexual abuse do not interview children but rather obtain a medical history from the child or adolescent. The cornerstone of diagnosis and treatment is the medical history. Medical professionals evaluating children for sexual abuse are focused on diagnosing the health-related impact of sexual contact and are required to obtain histories to understand a child's history, not for forensic, but rather for treatment purposes. However, it is important that any professional speaking to children about these issues have a good understanding of the factors influencing children's disclosures and the potential impact of their conversations on the children's statements.

The Process of Disclosure

Rather than resist their abusers and come forward immediately to tell, most children, trapped in an ongoing pattern of escalating abuse by someone they love and trust, find it very difficult to disclose. Force or direct threat of harm occurs in a significant number of cases[38]; in many others, subtle emotional coercion, bribes, covert misuse of authority, and the power of the relationship itself are used to maintain the child's silence. In his seminal article, coining the term *child sexual abuse accommodation syndrome,* Summitt[88] described the dynamics of the experience for children who are sexually abused by someone with whom they have a close and trusting relationship and why they may be more likely to remain silent and find a way to accommodate to this untenable situation. If and when they do reveal their abuse, their disclosures may be delayed, unconvincing, and/or eventually recanted. More recently, controversy regarding the manner by which sexual abuse victims typically disclose their experiences has prompted renewed empirical study of these issues.[89–91]

In fact, research corroborates that most sexual abuse is not immediately disclosed and reported to the authorities. Retrospective studies of adults abused as children indicate that fewer than half of the victims had told anyone at the time of their victimization, few had actually reported their abuse to the authorities, and a large proportion had never revealed their abuse to anyone until asked specifically in the course of the research.[91–94] Much of that index abuse may have occurred prior to the advent of mandated reporting laws in the mid-1970s, and rates of formal reporting have increased dramatically in recent years. Yet, in their comprehensive review of 11 such retrospective research studies of disclosure conducted since 1990, London et al[89] concluded that only about one-third of adults who had suffered sexual abuse as children revealed that abuse to anyone during childhood. Likewise, the results of a number of recent studies of children concurred that delayed disclosures remain common[89] and that abuse is often revealed not by intentional disclosure but by observation of an accidental comment or suspicious behavior, particularly in the cases of young children.[95] Children (like adults) are more likely to report sexual abuse when asked; reported rates of abuse in clinical outpatient settings rose from 6% to 31% when the children were asked specifically about any history of sexual abuse.[64]

Even when questioned directly, however, some children may initially deny their abuse or eventually retract original disclosures. Rates of denial and recantation vary widely across studies and may reflect such factors as the developmental level of the children— with school-aged children more likely to disclose when interviewed professionally than preschoolers— and whether the child has disclosed prior to that formal interview, a strong predictor of subsequent formal disclosure.[89] Selection biases in sampling are also important to consider. For example, when sample cases are selected from cases being criminally prosecuted, fewer denials or recantations are noted; this may well reflect a circular circumstance in which prosecutors are more likely to pursue those cases in which the child's disclosure has been clear and consistent throughout.[90,91] Likewise, in studies of cases in which the sexual abuse remains unclear, it is possible that some instances of children's denial or retraction may occur because the original abuse allegations were false. London et al[89] maintained that those studies demonstrating the highest levels of denial and retraction were those in which the abuse was less clearly substantiated. For example, going back retrospectively to follow the process by which 116 of their cases of sexual abuse had originally come to light, Sorenson and Snow[95] found in their 1991 study that, in almost three-fourths of these cases, the children had not indicated that they had been abused when first questioned; and only gradually did tentative and, at times, inconsistent disclosures emerge, eventually solidifying into more cogent and detailed disclosures. However, although the reported percentages vary, recent summaries of cases in which child sexual abuse was confirmed by external corroboration (sexually transmitted infections [STIs], pornographic pictures, witnesses to or confessions of the abuse) concur that gradual disclosure by children is quite common, suggesting the need at times for subsequent or repeated interviews.[38,96] For example, when first questioned by professional interviewers, fewer than half of a sample of 28 children with known STIs disclosed their sexual abuse.[97] Although 63% of the children with supportive caretakers disclosed, only 17% of those with unsupportive caretakers revealed their abuse during this initial interview. This suggests that parental belief in the allegations may be a key factor in the disclosure process.[97] Likewise, in a study by Dubowitz et al,[98] 25% of the children presenting medical findings indicative of sexual abuse provided no verbal information disclosing that abuse when interviewed even by skilled interviewers. Reviews of research on recantation similarly found significant variation, with rates ranging from 4% to 27%, again depending on methodology, sampling, and substantiation.[89] Most recently Malloy and colleagues[99] examined the prevalence and predictors of recantation among child sexual abuse victims ranging in age from 2 to 17 years whose cases had been substantiated by filings in dependency court. In their study, a recantation rate of 23% was noted, with abuse victims who were more vulnerable to familial adult influences (ie, younger children,

those abused by a parent figure and who lacked the belief and support of a non-offending caretaker) more likely to recant.

The Interviewer's Dilemma in Cases of Suspected Child Sexual Abuse

As described previously, it is difficult for children to disclose sexual abuse. The reasons center on the dynamics of the abuse experience and the pressures on children to keep the secret, protect the abusers they may love and trust, and maintain the integrity of their families. Children are embarrassed, ashamed, fearful, and avoidant of conversations about sexual interactions. Even when their genitals are touched in a socially acceptable context, such as a medical examination, children are quite reluctant to report that their private parts have been touched.[100] Only when questioned in a very direct, leading manner did most of the girls who had experienced a genital examination acknowledge that the doctor had touched their private areas; and even then, several did not. However, when questioned in that unacceptably leading fashion, there were a couple of young children who assented to questions about genital examinations when they had not, in fact, had them.[100]

This study illustrates the dilemma that an interviewer faces when talking to children about possible sexual abuse. Children may not disclose genital contact unless asked specifically and directly—and maybe not even then. Specific, direct questions may increase the chance of accurate disclosure, but they may also pose a small, undefined, but serious risk of obtaining a false report. Thus the interviewer is always balancing the relative risk of false-negatives versus false-positives. Specifically, when sexually abused children are unable to provide a cogent disclosure, their abuse is not substantiated and protective and therapeutic interventions may not be available; these children may remain vulnerable to continued abuse. On the other hand, a person falsely accused of child sexual abuse faces criminal prosecution and, if convicted, possible punishment by incarceration. In the family court arena, false-positive results may separate children unnecessarily from innocent parents or other caretaking figures.

Concerns about the possible confounding effects of repeated, highly leading, and coercive interviews, primarily on young children, were highlighted in the case of *State v Michaels*.[101] This 1994 New Jersey Supreme Court decision provided for pretrial taint hearings to scrutinize the interviews of child victims/witnesses and to ascertain whether the questioning was so flawed as to impeach the reliability of the children's statements. This ruling illustrates the implications of the recent shift in the investigation and prosecution of child sexual abuse cases from a focus on children's credibility to scrutiny of interviewing methods, and it underlines the need for state-of-the-art, forensically defensible interviewing techniques. In view of these concerns, the National Children's Advocacy Center has developed and tested guidelines for extended

forensic evaluations with reticent children, recommending that, should several interviews be needed, they be conducted by a single interviewer, be structured sensitively to build rapport, and avoid repetitive and suggestive questioning.[102]

Child-Centered, Developmentally Sensitive Interviewing

The ability to elicit accurate accounts from young children depends on the interviewer's understanding of developmental capacities and limitations—attention, memory, concept formation, language, and self-representation—because these affect the fundamental skills needed for reporting auto-biographical events.[103]

Language and Concept Formation

It is obvious that young children's language (ie, articulation, vocabulary, rules of syntax, conversational competence) and understanding of concepts develop gradually. Comprehensive reviews of children's language development and implications for forensic interviewing[59,103-105] suggest the following:

- Adults should not use baby talk, use words beyond the scope of the child's knowledge, or guess at what a child is trying to say or express.
- Adults should use short sentences, preferably in a simple subject-verb-object construction, and address only one concept or question at a time.

- Pronouns may be ambiguous and confusing to young children; use proper nouns for greater clarity. Follow-up questions can help to clarify identification of the referent.
- Avoid introducing new words, such as the names of body parts, until the child uses them.
- Avoid using negatives and double negatives, as well as tag questions (those ending in questions like "isn't it?" or "didn't he?"), which imply an answer.
- Use only concepts that the child understands. It is helpful to test out the child's usage of such concepts (eg, who, what, when, where, why, how; on vs in, over vs under) in a neutral context before using them in abuse-related questions. Typically, children learn to answer what, who, and where questions before when, how, and why.
- Until the ages of 8 to 10 years, children's ability to respond accurately to questions about the time of an event is very limited. If it is necessary to try to assess a time frame for the event, use links to special events, television shows, and other external markers.
- With young children, concepts of number, size, and color may not yet be established reliably. Just because a child can count or recite the days of the week does not mean that he or she is able to identify when or how many times an event occurred.

These authors point out that the usual patterns of adult-child conversation do not empower children to provide new information and can be problematic in the forensic interview context. Typically, children assume that the adults know all the answers and that their questions are tests to see if children can get them right. Unless trained otherwise, children are more likely to guess than to say they do not know; if a question is repeated, they assume that their response was wrong and change their answer, trying to respond with what the adults want to hear.

Memory

A robust finding in memory research is that what adults and children describe from their free recall ("Tell me everything you remember….") is most likely to be accurate, if limited. Memory research with young children[106] indicates that although memory generally improves with age, even very young children have the capacity for accurate memory of salient events that they have personally experienced. They remember central facts—such as who did what to whom—more than peripheral detail. Despite impressive evidence of their memory capacities, young children's autobiographical report of events differs in several important ways from the reports of older children and adults.[103] Young children have more difficulty recognizing what event is being discussed, and they are likely to shift focus during the course of the conversation; their repeated accounts of the same events may seem less consistent because they tend to address different aspects of the experience at different times. Preschoolers also have more difficulty with source monitoring—identifying whether they learned something from their own personal experience, from conversation, or from television—a capacity that is relevant when considering the possibility that a child's statements may have been contaminated by conversations with others. Moreover, although their recognition memory is good, young children's free, spontaneous recall for events is further limited by their lack of sophisticated strategies for memory retrieval. As children develop, their narratives become more complete and coherent. But young children are dependent on cues or "scaffolding" to assist in retrieval.[107]

This highlights the special dilemma facing those who interview very young children: Although their memories are accurate, these children's capacity for spontaneous recall is limited by their development; they need specific cues (direct questions, props, etc) to focus their attention and help with memory retrieval. However, these more directive questions have the potential to be leading. And, ironically, it is just these very young children who are the most susceptible to being misled by suggestive questioning.

Suggestibility

Research on children's vulnerability to the influences of suggestion has increased dramatically since the mid-1980s, and this continues to be a major issue in the field. Reviews of the recent research literature[103,107–109] concur that, although most children are quite accurate in their reports of personally experienced events, younger children may be more vulnerable

to suggestion than older children; preschoolers, and especially 3-year-olds, seem to be at greatest risk for succumbing to biased and suggestive interviewing techniques. By the time children are 9 or 10 years of age, they seem to be no more suggestible than adolescents or adults—which is not to say that they, too, cannot be misled. Moreover, although there is evidence that children more often resist suggestions about significant events that involve their bodies than those about other experiences, some children do misreport even inappropriate touches under certain circumstances. Factors that may affect memory—time delay between the event and questioning, ambiguous or less salient events—also affect children's suggestibility. Other factors reflect the interview situation itself. Specific or misleading questions are more likely to elicit misinformation than are open-ended questions. Young children are more likely to be misled by adults of high status or when questioned in a detached and authoritative manner rather than a friendly and generally supportive manner.[110] Likewise, although quite accurate when first interviewed, children are more likely to be misled when questioned repeatedly in an intimidating or coercive way. When asked repeatedly to think about or envision events that had never really occurred (eg, catching their fingers in a mousetrap), some young children eventually came to report, with impressive perceptual detail, that the events had actually happened, and they even came to believe their stories fairly tenaciously. In fact, professionals shown videotapes of these children's statements were unable to distinguish between the true and the fictitious reports.[111]

Although children may be influenced more readily about pleasant rather than unpleasant events, it is possible, when the misleading suggestion is strong and repeated, to induce false reports of negative events as well.[112] Such findings emphasize again the complexity of the interviewer's dilemma, illustrating both the beneficial and the harmful effects of using suggestive techniques with preschoolers. For those children who were initially reluctant to speak about unpleasant but true events, the use of repeated interviews with suggestive components helped them gradually to disclose those events; however, those same techniques prompted some children eventually to assent to events that had never occurred. Whereas most of the studies demonstrating potential suggestibility used repeated and numerous misleading questions, there seems to be little concern over the use of a single abuse-specific question, particularly when posed by neutral interviewers in single interviews of school-aged children.[103]

In discussing the potentially contaminating influences in children's interviews, Bruck et al[113,114] emphasize that interviewer bias (ie, a priori beliefs about the occurrence of certain events) not only may result in misleading or suggestive questions, but also, in a more general way, may guide the interviewer's questions in a way that reveals only confirmatory evidence and neglects exploration of alternative or disconfirming information. They suggest that interviewer bias, more than the number of leading questions per se, determines the risk of eliciting false information. There is also the danger of stereotype inducement, in which questions or comments depict a generally negative view of the alleged perpetrator (eg, that he or she is bad or does bad things), and which, in turn, may influence the child's statements and interpretation of events. It is important to recognize that all of these sources of suggestion are not confined to the interview situation; they may also be of concern when considering the potential effects of children's previous and repeated interactions with parents and others. Children's resistance to leading questions may be affected by the expectations or stereotypes implanted outside of the interview situation, as well as by interviewer bias and interpretation of events.[108,115,116]

Helping Children Relate Their Experiences Accurately and Completely

In view of these concerns, several researchers have explored ways to improve children's resistance to suggestion and maximize the amount of accurate information they are able to provide. Saywitz and colleagues[117,118] demonstrated that children can be trained to answer questions more accurately when they are given specific instructions and practice. Minimizing the authority differential, interviewers can convey to children that, having not been there, they really need the children's input to understand what happened and that it is important to tell truthfully everything that they remember. Children may be taught that it is all right to say "I don't know" when appropriate or to decline to respond. They may be given permission to correct the interviewer and to ask for clarification if something is unclear. Trained in this manner, school-aged children have been shown to be more resistant to misleading or suggestive questioning.[119]

Lamb et al[120,121] developed and tested an interview format that emphasizes the use of open-ended questioning and encouragement of spontaneous narratives during the early, rapport-building phase of the interviews. Rather than asking the typical closed introductory questions that tend to elicit short, often one-word answers, this protocol asks children to "tell all about" themselves and to describe events "from the very beginning to the very end," which trained children to produce narrative responses. They found that the amount of information and detail provided by children in real sexual abuse cases using this experimental protocol was significantly greater than the amount elicited through more typical investigative interview techniques. And because the information was provided primarily through spontaneous recall rather than specific, focused questions, its reliability was considered to be superior. Their empirical research findings have prompted the development of a structured interview protocol by the National Institute of Child Health and Human Development that translates

into a practical interview instrument for use by forensic investigators.[122,123]

In addition to their underlying formal, structured protocols,[124] these research findings have been applied more generally in guidelines for forensically defensible interviewing practice. Although specific interview practices vary widely, there seems to be consensus[59,73,103] about the following basic principles:

- Children should be interviewed as soon as possible after the alleged event.
- Interviewers should begin the interview with alternative hypotheses rather than a predetermined conclusion. They should remain neutral and be open to varying interpretations of the child's statements.
- Interviewers should not be authoritarian or coercive in any way. They should avoid providing information to the child, telling the child what others have said, or denigrating the alleged perpetrator. A relaxed, child-centered demeanor and generally supportive, friendly attitude is helpful, particularly with young children. However, differential reinforcement to specific responses must be avoided.
- Interviews must be conducted at the child's developmental and language levels. Verbal interviews cannot be the primary source of information with toddlers or others without adequate language and conceptual understanding.[107]

- Children learn to participate in interviews. Begin with a period of rapport-building, during which the child becomes comfortable with the interviewer and environment, learns the "rules" for answering questions accurately, and practices being informative.
- Interviews should center on open-ended questions as much as possible. Allow the child's free recall/narrative to proceed uninterrupted. When focused questions are needed to raise additional topics or clarify details, questions that offer the most choice should be used, and they should be followed by open-ended prompts. To avoid providing misleading suggestions, be especially cautious in using directive questions with preschool-aged children, and do not use leading questions.
- Adjunctive aids, props, cueing techniques, and anatomical drawings or dolls are to be used only after the child has made a disclosure, and only where necessary for further clarification. Be aware of the limitations of such techniques and the guidelines for their appropriate use.[124,125] For example, use of dolls has been shown to correlate with the production of more fantastic details and, when used with young children, to produce suggestive play and contradictory details.[126]
- Interviews go through a series of phases, from rapport-building through introductory information—truth and lies, rules, and practice interviewing regarding neutral events—before introduction of the topic at hand. The child is encouraged to provide a free narrative of the event before being questioned more specifically for further clarification and detail. Interviews should end with more neutral topics and closure, and they should afford opportunity for the child to provide additional information later if needed.

Again, it's important to recognize that the physicians' roles in cases of suspected sexual abuse involve medical history taking, not forensic interviewing per se; examining physicians do not therefore typically use the same format and procedures in talking to their child patients as do investigative interviewers or mental health evaluators. However, their medical history taking should follow similar principles, be unbiased, be developmentally sensitive, and be as open-ended as is feasible to avoid confusion or contamination.

Reporting Evaluation Conclusions and Recommendations

At the conclusion of a comprehensive mental health evaluation, the evaluator must finally integrate and interpret the various data collected from all sources—interviews, observations, assessment tools, reports, and collateral information from others—and present the findings in a formal written document.

Integrating the Evidence

In a coherent and detailed manner, the evaluator should delineate the various possible explanations regarding the child sexual abuse allegations and the weight to be accorded to the child's statements and behaviors. In this way, professionals are able to provide information about the complexity and limitations of the state of knowledge regarding sexual abuse while providing a useful perspective on the present concerns to the legal decision-maker.[73] A forensic evaluator seeks out corroborating evidence—medical evaluation reports, eyewitness reports, and fresh complaint witness testimony—when present. Often, however, such external confirmation is unavailable, and the evaluator must rely on the child's history, symptoms, statements, and presentation.

Which aspects of the child's verbal report are relevant to his or her reliability? There is very little empirical evidence to support the efficacy of particular markers or validation criteria; however, the consistent clinical observations of well-respected professionals in the field suggest certain criteria that warrant consideration and may provide some useful direction for the evaluator. Appropriate caution must be exercised in applying any of these criteria; they need to be considered in light of the child's developmental level, interpretation of the sexual abuse experience, and relationship with the perpetrator. Faller[127] synthesized the results of a number of publications that addressed validation criteria and, from that analysis, derived the following 8 criteria that appear to have some consensual validity and that Kuehnle[59] also describes in detail:

1. *Timing and circumstance of disclosure:* spontaneity, absence of influence
2. *Language congruent with developmental level:* child's perspective, vocabulary
3. *Quantity and quality of details:* explicitness; unusual, idiosyncratic, sensorimotor details; increasingly progressive sexual acts
4. *Developmental appropriateness versus precocity of sexual knowledge and/or eroticization*
5. *Repetition over time:* internal and external consistency; consistency of core elements and salient details, but some expected inconsistency over time in details
6. *Description of offender behavior:* coercion, threats, bribes or rewards, secrecy, pressures to comply or recant
7. *Plausibility of abuse:* rich and varied description rather than rote recitation
8. *Emotional reaction of the child during the interview:* congruence with allegations

Myers[128] cites additional statement components that are afforded weight in judicial decisions of reliability, including the child's or adult's motives to fabricate, quantity and quality of previous questioning, the child's correcting the interviewer, and the child's belief that disclosure might lead to punishment. Such information may help to determine if the child may have been confused or "contaminated" by others' questioning or statements.

Diagnostic Formulation

Child sexual abuse is an event, not a psychiatric diagnosis or discrete clinical syndrome. [71] Because sexually abused children respond differently to their experiences, one cannot "diagnose" the occurrence of sexual abuse on the basis of a child's behavior or emotional symptoms. However, a full diagnostic formulation (which may include a 5-axis *Diagnostic and Statistical Manual of Mental Disorders, Fourth Edition* psychiatric diagnosis or more descriptive narrative formulation) contributes to assessing the impact of any abuse experience on the child—as well as the child's vulnerability and risk of further victimization or other dangerous, destructive, or self-destructive behavior—and determining appropriate and specific recommendations for treatment.

Conclusions and Recommendations

The forensic evaluation report informs the court, the child protective agency, and/or the parents of the findings of the evaluation in a clear and scientific manner; conclusions must be supported by the data. Alternative hypotheses, and the data to confirm/support or negate these competing hypotheses, are presented and weighed, and the strengths and limitations of the evidence must be provided.

Recommendations should follow directly from the evaluation findings and address, as specifically as possible, the questions posed at referral, such as those regarding appropriate placement and the advisability and circumstances of contact, visitation, and/or reunification with the alleged perpetrator. However, the evaluators should not offer conclusions or recommendations regarding individuals whom they have not evaluated. Therapeutic recommendations should stipulate the appropriate modality, orientation, goals, and approximate duration of treatment.

Mindful of the implications and potential consequences of evaluation conclusions in these often complicated and ambiguous cases, it is critical for the responsible evaluator to be aware of not only what can be concluded with a reasonable degree of certainty but also, and perhaps more important, what cannot be ascertained from the data.

References

1. Finkelhor D, Browne A. The traumatic impact of child sexual abuse: a conceptualization. *Am J Orthopsychiatry.* 1985;55:530–541
2. Kendall-Tackett KA, Williams LM, Finkelhor D. Impact of sexual abuse on children: a review and synthesis of recent empirical studies. *Psychol Bull.* 1993;113:164–180
3. Browne A, Finkelhor D. Impact of child sexual abuse: a review of the research. *Psychol Bull.* 1986;99:66–77
4. Finkelhor D. Early and long-term effects of child sexual abuse: an update. *Prof Psychol.* 1990;21:325–330
5. Friedrich WN, Fiher JL, Dittner CA, et al. Child sexual behavior inventory: normative, psychiatric, and sexual abuse comparisons. *Child Maltreat.* 2001;6:37–49
6. Rind B, Tromovitch P, Bauserman R. A meta-analytic examination of assumed properties of child sexual abuse using college sample. *Psychol Bull.* 1998;124:22–53

7.   Conte JR, Schuerman JR. Factors
     associated with an increased impact of
     child sexual abuse. *Child Abuse Negl.*
     1987;11:201–211
8.   Arata CM. Child sexual abuse and sexual
     revictimization. *Clin Psychol Sci Pract.*
     2002;9:135–164
9.   Classen CC, Plaesh OG, Aggarwal R.
     Sexual revictimization: a review of the
     empirical literature. *Trauma Violence
     Abuse.* 2005;6:103–129
10. Haskell L. Revictimization in women's
     lives: an empirical and theoretical account
     of the links between child sexual abuse
     and repeated sexual violence. *Diss Abstr
     Int section A: Human and Social Sciences.*
     2000;60:2813
11. Briere J, Runtz M. Suicidal thoughts and
     behaviours in former sexual abuse
     victims. *Can J Behav Sci.* 1986;18:413–423
12. Navalta CP, Polcari A, Webster DM,
     Boghossian A, Teicher MH. Effects
     of childhood sexual abuse on neuro-
     psychological and cognitive function
     in college women. *J Neuropsychol Clin
     Neurosci.* 2006;18:45–53
13. Rosenthal MZ, Hall MLR, Palm KM,
     Batten SV, Follette VM. Chronic
     avoidance helps explain the relationship
     between severity of childhood sexual
     abuse and psychological distress
     in adulthood. *J Child Sex Abuse.*
     2005;14:25–41
14. Saywitz KJ, Mannarino AP, Berliner L,
     Cohen JA. Treatment for sexually abused
     children and adolescents. *Am Psychol.*
     2000;55:1040–1049
15. Lanktree C, Briere J. Outcome of therapy
     for sexually abused children: a repeated
     measures study. *Child Abuse Negl.*
     1995;19:1145–1155
16. Briere J, Elliott DM. Prevalence and
     symptomatic sequelae of self-reported
     childhood physical and sexual abuse
     in a general population sample of men
     and women. *Child Abuse Negl Int J.*
     2003;27:1205–1222
17. Berliner L, Elliott DM. Sexual abuse of
     children. In: Briere J, Berliner L, Bulkley
     JA, Jenny C, Reid T, eds. *The APSAC
     Handbook on Child Maltreatment.*
     Thousand Oaks, CA: Sage; 1996
18. Clear PJ, Vinent J, Harris GE. Ethnic
     differences in symptom presentation of
     sexually abused girls. *J Child Sex Abuse.*
     2006;15:79–98
19. Ruggiero K, McLeer S, Dixon J. Sexual
     abuse characteristics associated with
     survivor psychopathology. *Child Abuse
     Negl.* 2000;24:951–961
20. Sperry DM, Gilbert BO. Child peer sexual
     abuse: preliminary data on outcomes and
     disclosure experiences. *Child Abuse Negl.*
     2005;29:889–914
21. Beitchman J, Zucker K, Hood J, daCosta
     G, Akmen D, Cassavia E. A review of the
     long-term effects of child sexual abuse.
     Child Abuse Negl. 1992;16:101–118
22. Kaplow JB, Widom CS. Age of onset of
     child maltreatment predicts long-term
     mental health outcomes. *J Abnorm
     Psychol.* 2007;116:176–187
23. Ullman SE. Relationship to perpetrator,
     disclosure, social reactions and PTSD
     symptoms in child sexual abuse survivors.
     J Child Sex Abuse. 2007;16(1):19–36
24. Friedrich WN, Beilke RL, Urquiza AJ.
     Behavior problems in young sexually
     abused boys: a comparison study. *J
     Interpers Violence.* 1988;3:21–28
25. Holmes WC, Slap GB. Sexual abuse of
     boys: definition, prevalence correlates,
     sequelae, and management. *J Am Med
     Assoc.* 1998;280:1855–1862
26. Kaplow JB, Dodge KA, Amaya-Jackson L,
     Saxe GN. Pathways to PTSD, Part II:
     sexually abused children. *Am J Psychiatry.*
     2005;162:1305–1310
27. Shapiro DL, Levendovsky AA. Adolescent
     survivors of childhood sexual abuse: the
     mediating role of attachment style and
     coping in psychological and interpersonal
     functioning. *Child Abuse Negl.*
     1999;23:1175–1191

28. Tremblay C, Hebert M, Piche C. Coping strategies and social support as mediators of consequences in child sexual abuse victims. *Child Abuse Negl.* 1999;23:929–945

29. Alexander PC. Application of attachment theory to the study of sexual abuse. *J Clin Consult Psychol.* 1992;60:185–195

30. Cohen JA, Mannarino AP. Addressing attributions in treating abused children. *Child Maltreat.* 2002;7(1):82–86

31. Fiering C, Taska L, Chen K. Trying to understand why horrible things happen: attribution, shame, and symptom development following sexual abuse. *Child Maltreat.* 2002;7:26–41

32. Fiering C, Taska L. The persistence of shame following sexual abuse: a longitudinal look at risk and recovery. *Child Maltreat.* 2005;10:337–349

33. Fontes LA. Sin verguenza: addressing shame with Latino victims of child sexual abuse and their families. *J Child Sex Abuse.* 2007;16(1):61–83

34. Everson MD, Hunter WM, Runyan DK, Edelson GA, Coulter ML. Maternal support following disclosure of incest. *Am J Orthopsychiatry,* 1989;59(2):198–207

35. Gomes-Schwartz B, Horowitz J, Cardarelli A. *Child Sexual Abuse: The Initial Effects.* Newbury Park, CA: Sage; 1990

36. Deblinger E, Hathaway CR, Lippmann J, Steer R. Psychosocial characteristics and correlates of symptom distress in nonoffending mothers of sexually abused children. *J Interpers Violence.* 1993;8:155–168

37. Sirles E, Franke PJ. Factors influencing mothers' reactions to intrafamilial sexual abuse. *Child Abuse Negl.* 1989;13:131–139

38. Elliott DM, Briere J. Forensic sexual abuse evaluations: disclosures and symptomatology. *Behav Sci Law.* 1994;12:261–277

39. Coohey C. How child protective service investigators decide to substantiate mothers for failure-to-protect in sexual abuse cases. *J Child Sex Abuse.* 2006;15(4):61–81

40. Hunter WM, Coulter ML, Runyan DK, Everson MD. Determinents of placement for sexually abused children. *Child Abuse Negl.* 1990;14:407–418

41. Malloy LC, Lyon TD. Caregiver support and child sexual abuse: why does it matter? *J Child Sex Abuse.* 2006;15:97–103

42. Pintello D, Zuravin S. Intrafamilial child sexual abuse: predictors of postdisclosure maternal belief and protective action. *Child Maltreat.* 2001;6:344–352

43. Deblinger E, Steer R, Lippmann J. Maternal factors associated with sexually abused children's psychosocial adjustments. *Child Maltreat.* 1999a;6:13–20

44. Koverola C. Perpetuating mother-blaming rhetoric: a commentary. *J Child Sex Abuse.* 2007;16:137–143

45. McLeer S, Deblinger E, Henry D, Orvashel H. Sexually abused children at high risk for post-traumatic stress disorder. *J Am Acad Child Adolesc Psychiatry.* 1992;31(5):875–879

46. Deblinger E, McLeer SV, Atkins MS, Ralphe DL, Foa E. Post-traumatic stress in sexually abused, physically abused, and nonabused children. *Child Abuse Negl.* 1989;13:403–408

47. Briere J, Gil E. Self-mutilation in clinical and general population samples: prevalence, correlates, and functions. *Am J Orthosychiatry.* 1998;68:609–620

48. Friedrich WN, Jaworski TM, Huxsahl JE, Bengston BS. Assessment of dissociative and sexual behaviors in children and adolescents with sexual abuse. *J Interpers Violence.* 1997;12:155–171

49. Putnam FW. Dissociative phenomena. In: Tasman A, ed. *Annual Review of Psychiatry.* Washington, DC: American Psychiatric Press; 1991:159–174

50. Friedrich WN. Sexual victimization and sexual behavior in children: a review of recent literature. *Child Abuse Negl.* 1993;17:59–66

51. Drach KM, Wientzen J, Ricci LR. The diagnostic utility of sexual behavior problems in diagnosing sexual abuse in a forensic child sexual abuse evaluation clinic. *Child Abuse Negl.* 2001;25:489–503

52. Friedrich WN, Trane ST, Gully KJ. Re: It is a mistake to conclude that sexual abuse and sexualized behavior are not related: a reply to Drach, Wientzen, and Ricci (2001). *Child Abuse Negl.* 2005;29:297–302

53. Kolko DJ, Moser JT, Weldy SR. Behavioral/emotional indicators of sexual abuse in psychiatric inpatients: a controlled comparison with physical abuse. *Child Abuse Negl.* 1988;12:529–541

54. Friedrich WN, Grambsch P, Broughton D, Kuiper J, Beilke RL. Normative sexual behavior in children. *Pediatrics.* 1991;88:456–464

55. Friedrich WN, Grambsch P, Damon L, et al. Child sexual abuse inventory: normative and clinical comparisons. *Psychol Assess.* 1992;4:303–311

56. American Academy of Child and Adolescent Psychiatry. Practice parameters for the forensic evaluation of children and adolescents who may have been physically or sexually abused. *J Am Acad Child Adolesc Psychiatry.* 1997;36:423–442

57. American Psychological Association. Ethical principles of psychologists and code of conduct. *Am Psychol.* 1992;47:1597–1611

58. Committee on Ethical Guidelines. Ethical principles of psychologists and code of conduct. *Am Psychol.* 2002;57:1060–1073

59. Kuehnle K. *Assessing Allegations of Child Sexual Abuse.* Sarasota, FL: Professional Resource Press; 1996

60. Committee on Ethical Guidelines for Forensic Psychologists. Specialty guidelines for forensic psychologists. *Law Hum Behav.* 1991;15:655–665

61. Finkelhor D, Berliner L. Research on the treatment of sexually abused children: a review and recommendations. *J Am Acad Child Adolesc Psychiatry.* 1995;34:1408–1423

62. Saunders B, Berliner L, Hanson R, eds. *Child Physical and Sexual Abuse: Guidelines for Treatment (Final Report: January 15, 2003).* Charleston, SC: National Crime Victims Research and Treatment Center; 2003

63. Deblinger E, Lippmann J, Steer R. Sexually abused children suffering posttraumatic stress symptoms: initial treatment outcome findings. *Child Maltreat.* 1996;1:310–321

64. Lanktree C, Briere J, Zaidi L. Incidence and impact of sexual abuse in a child outpatient sample: the role of direct inquiry. *Child Abuse Negl.* 1991;15:447–453

65. Stauffer LB, Deblinger E. Cognitive behavioral groups for nonoffending mothers and their young sexually abused children: a preliminary treatment outcome study. *Child Maltreat.* 1996;1:65–76

66. Deblinger E, Steer R, Lippmann J. Two-year follow-up study of cognitive behavioral therapy for sexually abused children suffering post-traumatic stress symptoms. *Child Abuse Negl.* 1999;23:1371–1378

67. Cohen JA, Mannarino AP. A treatment outcome study for sexually abused preschool children: initial findings. *J Am Acad Child Adolesc Psychiatry.* 1996;35:42–50

68. Deblinger E, Mannarino AP, Cohen JA, Steer RA. A follow-up study of a multisite, randomized, controlled trial for children with sexual abuse-related PTSD symptoms. *J Am Acad Child Adolesc Psychiatry.* 2006;45:1474–1484

69. Cohen JA, Deblinger E, Mannarino AP, Steer R. A multisite, randomized controlled trial for children with sexual abuse-related PTSD symptoms. *J Am Acad Child Adolesc Psychiatry.* 2004;43:393–402

70. American Professional Society on the Abuse of Children. *Guidelines for Psychosocial Evaluation of Suspected Sexual Abuse in Young Children.* Chicago, IL: American Professional Society on the Abuse of Children; 1990

71. Kuehnle K. Child sexual abuse evaluations: the scientist-practitioner model. *Behav Sci Law.* 1998;16:5–20

72. Herman S. Improving decision making in forensic child sexual abuse victims following disclosure. *Law Hum Behav.* 2005;29:87–120

73. Kuehnle K, Kirkpatrick H. Evaluating allegations of child sexual abuse with complex child custody cases. *J Child Custody.* 2005;2:3–39

74. Melton GB, Limber S. Psychologists' involvement in cases of child maltreatment: limits of role and expertise. *Am Psychol.* 1989;44:1225–1233

75. Ceci SJ, Hembrooke H, eds. *Expert Witnesses in Child Abuse Cases.* Washington, DC: American Psychological Association; 1998

76. Goldstein AM, ed. *Forensic Psychology: Emerging Topics and Expanding Roles.* Hoboken, NJ: John Wiley & Sons; 2006

77. Myers JEB, Bays M, Becker J, Berliner L, Corwin D, Saywitz K. Expert testimony in child sexual abuse litigation. *Neb Law Rev.* 1989;68:1–145

78. Becker JV, Murphy WD. What we know and do not know about assessing and treating sexual offenders. *Psychol Public Policy Law.* 1998;4:116–137

79. Bow JN, Quinnell FA, Zaroff M, Assemany A. Assessment of sexual abuse allegations in child custody cases. *Prof Psychol Res Pract.* 2002;33:566–575

80. Lilienfeld S, Wood JJ, Garb HN. The scientific status of projective techniques. *Psychol Sci Public Interest.* 1999;1:27–66

81. Garb HN, Wood JM, Nezworski MT. Projective techniques and the detection of child sexual abuse. *Child Maltreat.* 2000;5:161–168

82. Briere J. *Trauma Symptom Checklist—Children for Children.* Odessa, FL: Psychological Assessment Resources; 1996

83. Briere J. *Trauma Symptom Checklist for Young Children (TSCYC) Professional Manual.* Odessa, FL: Psychological Assessment Resources; 2005

84. Wolfe VV, Gentile C, Michienzi T, Sas L, Wolfe DA. The Children's Impact of Traumatic Events Scale: a measure of post-sexual abuse PTSD symptoms. *Behav Assess.* 1991;13:159–383

85. Putnam FW. *Child Dissociative Checklist (Version 3.0–2/90).* Bethesda, MD: Laboratory of Developmental Psychology, National Institute of Mental Health; 1990

86. Armstrong J, Putnam FW, Carlson EB, Libero DZ, Smith SR. Development and validation of a measure of adolescent dissociation: the Adolescent Dissociative Experiences Scale (A-DES). *J Nerv Ment Dis.* 1997;185:491–497

87. Mannarino AP, Cohen JA, Berman SR. The Children's Attributions and Perceptions Scale: a new measure of sexual abuse-related factors. *J Clin Child Psychol.* 1994;23:204–211

88. Summit RC. The child sexual abuse accommodation syndrome. *Child Abuse Negl.* 1983;7:177–193

89. London K, Bruck M, Ceci SJ, Shuman DW. Disclosure of child sexual abuse: what does the research tell us about the way that children tell? *Psychol Public Policy Law.* 2005;11:194–226

90. Lyon TD. Scientific support for expert testimony on child sexual abuse accommodation. In: Conte JR, ed. *Critical Issues in Child Sexual Abuse* Newbury Park, CA: Sage Publications; 2002:107–138

91. Olafson E, Lederman CS. The state of the debate about children's disclosure patterns in child sexual abuse cases. *Juv Fam Court J.* 2006;57:27–40

92. Finkelhor D, Hotaling G, Lewis IA, Smith C. Sexual abuse in a national survey of adult men and women: prevalence, characteristics, and risk factors. *Child Abuse Negl.* 1990;14:19–28

93. Russell DEH. *Sexual Exploitation: Rape, Child Sexual Abuse, and Workplace Harassment.* Beverly Hills, CA: Sage; 1984

94. Smith D, Letourneau EJ, Saunders BE, Kilpatrick DG, Resnick HS, Best CL. Delay in disclosure of childhood rape: results from a national survey. *Child Abuse Negl.* 2000;24:273–287

95. Sorenson T, Snow B. How children tell: the process of disclosure in child sexual abuse. *Child Welfare.* 1991;70:3–15

96. Lyon TD. False denials: overcoming biases in abuse disclosure research. In: Pipe M, Lamb M, Orbach Y, Cederborg A, eds. *Disclosing Abuse: Delays, Denials, Retractions and Incomplete Accounts.* Mahwah, NJ: Erlbaum; 2007

97. Lawson L, Chaffin M. False negatives in sexual abuse disclosure interviews. *J Interpers Violence.* 1992;7:532–542

98. Dubowitz H, Black M, Harrington D. The diagnosis of child sexual abuse. *Am J Dis Child.* 1992;146:688–693

99. Malloy LC, Lyon TD, Quas JA. Filial dependency and recantation of child sexual abuse allegations. *J Am Acad Child Adolesc Psychiatry.* 2007;46:162–170

100. Saywitz KJ, Goodman GS, Nicholas G, Moan S. Children's memories of physical examinations that involve genital touch: implications for reports of child sexual abuse. *J Consult Clinical Psychology.* 1991;59:682–691

101. *State v Michaels,* 642 A2d 1372 (NJ 1994)

102. Carnes CN, Nelson-Gardell D, Wilson C, Orgassa UC. Extended forensic evaluation when sexual abuse is suspected: a multi-site field study. *Child Maltreat.* 2001;6:230–242

103. Poole DA, Lamb ME. *Investigative Interviews of Children.* Washington, DC: American Psychological Association; 1998

104. Saywitz KJ. Improving children's testimony: the question, the answer, and the environment. In: Zaragoza M, Graham J, Hall G, Hirschman R, Ben-Porath Y, eds. *Memory and Testimony in the Child Witness.* Thousand Oaks, CA: Sage; 1995:113–140

105. Walker AG. *Handbook on Questioning Children: A Linguistic Perspective.* Washington, DC: American Bar Association Center on Children and the Law; 1994

106. Fivush R. Developmental perspectives on autobiographical recall. In: Goodman GS, Bottoms BL, eds. *Child Victims, Child Witnesses.* New York, NY: Guilford; 1993:1–24

107. Hewett SK. *Assessing Allegations of Sexual Abuse in Preschool Children: Understanding Small Voices.* Thousand Oaks, CA: Sage; 1999

108. Bruck M, Ceci S J. Amicus brief for the case of State of New Jersey v Michaels presented by the Committee of Concerned Social Scientists. *Psychol Public Policy Law.* 1995;1:272–322

109. Ceci SJ, Bruck M. The suggestibility of the child witness: a historical review and synthesis. *Psychol Bull.* 1993;113:403–439

110. Goodman GS, Bottoms BL, Schwartz-Kenny BM, Rudy L. Children's testimony about a stressful life event: improving children's reports. *J Narrat Life Hist.* 1991;1:69–99

111. Ceci SJ, Crotteau-Huffman M, Smith E, Loftus EW. Repeatedly thinking about non-events. *Conscious Cogn.* 1994;3:388–407

112. Bruck M, Ceci SJ, Hembrooke H. Children's reports of pleasant and unpleasant events. In: Read D, Lindsay S, eds. *Recollections of Trauma: Scientific Research and Clinical Practice.* New York, NY: Plenum Press; 1997:199–219

113. Bruck M, Ceci SJ, Hembrooke H. Reliability and credibility of young children's reports: from research to policy and practice. *Am Psychol.* 1998;53:136–151

114. Bruck M, Ceci SJ, Hembrooke H. The nature of children's true and false narratives. *Dev Rev.* 2002;22:520–554

115. Clarke-Stewart A, Thompson W, Lepore S. Manipulating children's interpretations through interrogation. Paper presented at: Biennial Meeting of the Society for Research on Child Development; May 1989; Kansas City, MO

116. Leichtman MD, Ceci SJ. The effects of stereotypes and suggestions on preschoolers' reports. *Dev Psychol.* 1995;31:568–578

117. Saywitz KJ, Moan S, Lamphear V. The effect of preparation on children's resistance to misleading questions. Paper presented at: Meeting of the American Psychological Association; 1991; San Francisco, CA

118. Saywitz KJ, Snyder L. Improving children's testimony with preparation. In: Goodman GS, Bottoms BL, eds. *Child Victims, Child Witnesses: Understanding and Improving Testimony.* New York, NY: Guilford Press; 1991:117–146

119. Saywitz KJ, Goodman GS. Interviewing children in and out of court: current research and practice implications. In: Briere J, Berliner L, Bulkley JA, Jenny C, Reid T, eds. *The APSAC Handbook on Child Maltreatment.* Thousand Oaks, CA: Sage; 1996

120. Lamb ME, Sternberg KJ, Esplin PW. Making children into competent witnesses: reactions to the amicus brief in re *Michaels. Psychol Public Policy Law.* 1995;1:438–449

121. Lamb ME, Sternberg KJ, Esplin PW. Conducting investigative interviews of alleged sexual abuse victims. *Child Abuse Negl.* 1998;22:813–823

122. Sternberg K, Lamb M, Esplin P, Orbach Y, Hershkowitz I. Using a structured interview protocol to improve the quality of investigative interviews. In: Eisen M, ed. *Memory and Suggestivity in the Forensic Interview.* Mahway, NJ: Erlbaum; 2002:409–436

123. Yuille JC, Hunter R, Joffe R, Zapurniuk J. Interviewing children in sexual abuse cases. In: Goodman GS, Bottoms BL, eds. *Child Victims, Child Witnesses: Understanding and Improving Testimony.* New York, NY: Guilford Press; 1993:95–115

124. Boat BW, Everson MD, American Professional Society the Abuse of Children. *Practice Guidelines—Use of Anatomical Dolls in Child Sexual Abuse Assessment.* Chicago, IL: APSAC; 1995

125. Faller K. Anatomical dolls: their use in assessment of children who may have been sexually abused. *J Child Sex Abuse.* 2005;14:1–21

126. Thierry K, Lamb M, Orbach Y, Pipe M. Developmental differences in the function and use of anatomical dolls during interviews with alleged sexual abuse victims. *J Consult Clin Psychol.* 2005;73:1125–1134

127. Faller KC. Evaluating young children for possible sexual abuse. Paper presented at: San Diego Conference on Responding to Child Maltreatment; 1993; San Diego, CA

128. Myers JEB. *Legal Issues in Child Abuse and Neglect.* Newbury Park, CA: Sage; 1992

Chapter 11

Prevention and Treatment of Child Sexual Abuse

Melissa K. Runyon

Esther Deblinger

Child sexual abuse is a public health problem of epidemic proportions that affects children and families from all ethnic, social, cultural, socioeconomic, and gender groups. Although the overall rates of child sexual abuse may be declining in the United States, this worldwide problem remains highly prevalent, with 1 in 12 (82 per 1,000) having experienced some form of sexual victimization.[1] Moreover, emotional and behavioral reactions to child sexual abuse are quite variable, ranging from mild to severe. Some children may present with mild, short-lived immediate aftereffects, while others may suffer significant difficulties that may persist throughout their lives.

Despite the alarming rates of child sexual abuse, little attention has been given to prevention work aimed at reducing the risk of sexual abuse. There are 3 levels of prevention when approaching any public health problem: primary, secondary, and tertiary. According to the definitions set forth by the UK Department of Health,[2]

primary prevention would involve providing education and intervening with children before the sexual abuse occurs. The next level, secondary prevention, involves early detection and treatment of child sexual abuse to promote health, while tertiary prevention focuses on reducing the impact of the child sexual abuse and promoting well-being through active treatment, such as mental health counseling. Obviously, pediatricians can play an important role in all levels of prevention work given their ongoing and trusted relationships with families. Unfortunately, it seems that many pediatricians receive very limited training and have insufficient knowledge of the dynamics and presenting symptoms of child maltreatment.[3] According to the American Academy of Pediatrics (AAP),[4] pediatricians are important supports to guide children and families when sexual abuse occurs. Thus it is important for all pediatricians to have an understanding of the basic facts and myths about child sexual abuse and some familiarity with community experts who evaluate and treat children who may have experienced sexual abuse. American Academy of Pediatrics guidelines indicate that pediatricians may obtain disclosures during routine physical examinations; when sexual abuse is suspected by a parent, social service worker, or law enforcement professional; and/or when a child is brought to a pediatric office or emergency department for an acute illness or injury, or a suspected assault. It is critical, therefore, for pediatricians to be familiar with the clinical and legal definitions of child sexual abuse and the state statutes that require professionals to report when they have reason to suspect such abuse. The goal of this chapter is to provide pediatricians with some practical guidance to address the issue of child sexual abuse, healthy sexual development, and body safety skills with children and their caregivers.

Primary Prevention

Research has indicated that children lack knowledge about sexual abuse and body safety and may not perceive inappropriate sexual touches as sexual or "not OK."[5] High-quality, evidence-based programs that teach children abuse-response skills[6,7] may result in improvements in children's awareness, knowledge, and comfort level with disclosing inappropriate sexual touches, which may, in turn, decrease the reoccurrence of abuse.

While child sexual abuse is a serious public health problem, research has indicated that most parents do not discuss these issues with their children.[8,9] Some studies have indicated that about half of parents discuss child sexual abuse with their preschool children, with those parents who report greater levels of personal involvement with child sexual abuse either by having a relationship with someone who had been abused or a personal history of child sexual abuse being more likely to initiate those discussions (Deblinger E, Thakkar-Kolar RR, Berry EJ, Schroeder CM. Caregivers' efforts to educate their children about child sexual abuse: a replication study. UMDNJ-SOM CARES Institute. Unpublished paper.) According to Kenny et al,[10] education about healthy sexuality and sexual development should include discussions of child sexual abuse, begin by the age of 3, and be initiated by parents and other important figures in the child's life. These authors also suggest that it is equally important to discuss body safety with children as it is to discuss traffic, bicycle, and fire safety, which are safety issues that are commonly addressed by parents, pediatricians, and other professionals with children at a very young age.

Research has indicated that parents generally support the ideas that body safety skills should be taught at home and be included as a part of the curriculum in preschools and child care centers.[9] Despite these beliefs, studies demonstrate that children lack knowledge about child sexual abuse, body safety, and the correct medical terms for their genitalia.[5,10–12] In fact, one study reported that half of the children in their sample, regardless of their abuse history, were unable to correctly identify an inappropriate sexual touch or advance.[13]

Indeed, pediatricians have the potential to provide general education about child sexual abuse and body safety to children with no history of sexual abuse during annual physical examinations. In fact, a recent survey of 605 parents demonstrated that 98% of the parents thought pediatricians should discuss normal sexual development and 96% welcomed sexual abuse education. While parents welcomed such discussions, they reported that only 44% of their pediatricians discussed normal sexual development and only 29% reported that discussions of sexual abuse and/or body safety were initiated by their children's pediatrician.[14] Recent authors have suggested that physicians take a role in the primary prevention of child sexual abuse by assisting parents through incorporating discussions of sexual development, body safety, and child sexual abuse into routine anticipatory guidance.[15]

Research has consistently indicated that after their participation in self-protection programs, children demonstrate significant increases in knowledge about sexual abuse and body safety skills.[5,16] While studies including school-aged children have shown even greater gains,[17] children of all ages (preschool, school-aged, adolescence) have demonstrated gains in their ability to identify potentially abusive situations and differentiate between OK and not OK touches.[18,19] There are a number of strategies that can optimize children's learning when introducing self-protection skills. For example, children retained significantly more information if these concepts were introduced in schools or other settings outside the home, if the parent was actively involved.[7,9,18] As cited by Kenny and her colleagues,[10] the positive benefit of including the parent is most likely related to the parent providing the child with repeated exposure to the safety education in their home environment, encouraging the use of the skills, and providing positive feedback to children for their behavioral rehearsal of these skills.[20] Encouraging children and parents to routinely discuss these issues may open communication lines and increase the ease by which children and families communicate about potentially anxiety-provoking topics.[21,22] Kenny et al[10] provide a comprehensive literature review of self-protection/prevention programs and summarize those elements that enhance children's learning: "To achieve the best results, self-protection programs should incorporate parental involvement, opportunities for practice, repeated exposure, and concepts such as identification of potentially abusive situations, age-appropriate sex education, and body safety skills. Self-protection skills should be introduced when children are developmentally capable of learning the medical names of their genitalia, or as early as age 3. Therefore, teaching self-protection skills begins in the home with the parent and progresses from preschool to high school." Another recent review of the empirical and conceptual prevention/education literature refuted common concerns about these programs (eg, increasing children's anxiety), while highlighting the benefits.[23] Based on his review, Finkelhor reported that these programs do not seem to produce increased anxious or noncompliant behavior among children; nor do they seem to be associated with increased tendencies for children to misinterpret appropriate physical contact. Rather Finkelhor[23] suggests that primary prevention programs may have enhanced the sensitivity of adults called on to respond to children's disclosures and may have contributed to the declines in child sexual abuse rates found since 1993.

Pediatricians may have the potential to play an important role in primary prevention through their interactions with children and families in cases where there are no known or suspected child sexual abuse allegations. It is recommended that pediatricians address issues of child sexual abuse and body safety, in conjunction with other safety issues (ie, traffic, bicycle, and fire safety), during routinehealth maintenance assessments after completing a head-to-toe examination of the child (M. Finkel, personal communication, 2007). According to Finkel, this presents an opportunity to begin a dialogue about personal safety with the parent and child as described in Box 11.1. In general, pediatricians can begin by emphasizing 3 primary topics related to body safety and safety skills with parents: (1) children should be given as much independence with genital care at as early an age as possible, (2) children should be taught the names of body parts as early as the age of 3, and (3) parents can model their own personal need for privacy and appropriate boundaries to teach children appropriate boundaries.

The physician should rely on his or her clinical judgment in terms of the parents' comfort and participation in providing anticipatory guidance regarding body safety. Pediatricians can begin by encouraging parents to give children, at a very early age, as much independence as possible with the care of their genitals. Parents can begin by demonstrating (modeling) for children how to adequately clean their genitals while bathing and while going to the bathroom. After demonstrating for children, parents can begin to observe children and provide guidance, praise, and performance feedback to facilitate children learning to adequately clean their genitals. For example, just as parents repeatedly remind their children to buckle their seat belt when they are riding in a car and wear their helmets while riding a bicycle, they should remind their children to wash their private parts while bathing and wipe their private parts when using the bathroom.

Given the prevalence of child sexual abuse in very young children, it seems important for pediatricians and parents to work collaboratively to introduce body safety concepts to children as young as 3 years of age. With very young children, however, pediatricians are encouraged to discuss the issues with parents in advance and use words and phrases that are both developmentally and culturally sensitive. For example, some parents prefer not to teach their young children the doctors' names for the private parts (ie, penis, vagina, breast, and butt) due to their own discomfort

BOX 11.1
Sample Dialogue About Body Safety and OK and Not OK Touches

Pediatrician:	There are lots of rules of body safety and I want to ask you some questions. What do you do when you get in the car to keep safe? or What do mommy and/or daddy do when they get in the car to keep them safe?
Child:	Strap me in.
Pediatrician:	That's right! They put your seat belt on to keep your body safe!
Pediatrician:	Do you ride a bike?
Child:	Yes.
Pediatrician:	What do you do when you ride a bike to keep your body safe?
Child:	Wear a helmet.
Pediatrician:	That's great! You wear a helmet to keep your head safe.
Pediatrician:	Do you like to swim?
Child:	Yes.
Pediatrician:	What do you need to do to be safe in the water?
Child:	Wear a thing that makes me float.
Pediatrician:	We have another important rule that has to do with the parts of your body covered by your bathing suit. Do you know the names of those parts?
Child:	Children may not respond, may appear embarrassed, or may respond with a myriad of names for their private parts. *Note to Pediatrician:* If the name the child provides is not the anatomically correct term, then say, "A lot of kids call it what you told me but you're a big girl/boy and I want you to learn the grown-up words." Proceed to teach the child appropriate terms and have them say the terms aloud and positively reinforce their response. Then explain, "We also call the parts covered by your bathing suit your private parts. Do you know why they are called that?"
Child:	No.
Pediatrician:	They are called that because they belong to you. Do you know who's allowed to touch your private parts?"
Child:	Nobody.

BOX 11.1, continued
Sample Dialogue About Body Safety and OK and Not OK Touches

Pediatrician:	They are called private parts because they belong to you and you can touch your private parts, Mommy, Daddy or anyone Mommy or Daddy says can when you need help or a doctor when Mommy or Daddy are in the room. Has anyone ever touched your private parts when it was not OK?
Child:	No. (If yes ask who and proceed accordingly.)
Pediatrician:	(If no.) That's great! It is important to know about OK and not OK touching. If anyone ever touches your private parts or makes you touch theirs, do you know what to do?
Child:	Tell.
Pediatrician:	That's right! Tell at least 2 adults, and if they say don't tell or they say keep it a secret you always tell because secrets are never OK and you won't get into any trouble. Do you have any questions for me?
Child:	No.
Pediatrician:	Now I am going to take a look at your private parts and nothing is going to hurt.

or familial habits/preferences. This should be respected, although after a brief explanation of how the use of the medical terms for private parts may demonstrate greater parental comfort and may increase the child's ability to effectively communicate about their bodies, especially if they need to disclose possible sexual abuse, most parents agree to teach their children these words.[18] When children are young and parents still assist them with bathing, parents can review the doctors' names of the genitals each time until the child is able to independently label their genitals. In some instances, pediatricians may choose to discuss sexual abuse, practicing safe sex, and issues of sexual development, as well as other potentially problematic issues (eg, drug use, depression, etc) with

adolescents in private. While this may increase some teenagers' willingness to share, it is important to remind teens of a pediatrician's mandated obligation to report abuse and/or other problems that may place the adolescent at risk for being a danger to themselves or others. To encourage open lines of communication, it may be important to provide the teen with a choice to share this information with his or her parent(s) or have the pediatrician share the information with the teen present. The pediatrician may want to prepare the parent first to increase the likelihood that the interaction between the parent and teen is positive, which may increase the likelihood that the teen approaches the parent in the future to discuss difficult topics (ie, substance abuse, teen sexuality).

According to the AAP,[4] pediatricians may also want to introduce, in collaboration with parents, body safety skills or the "no-go-tell" concept[6,7,21,24] to children between the ages of 3 and 5. It is important to emphasize that we do not expect children to be able to stop abuse, and we do not want to convey this message to them. Rather, it is important to give children a vocabulary and teach them skills to increase their abilities to actively disclose any age-inappropriate sexual contacts. This is crucial given the pressures, threats, and other factors that lead children to remain silent about sexual abuse for days, weeks, months, and/or years. Initially, it is important to introduce the concepts of *OK, not OK,* and confusing touches. We recommend the use of the terms *OK* and *not OK* instead of good and bad touches, because a sexual touch between a child and an adult or older child is inappropriate; however, the same touch between consenting adults is acceptable.[6,7,11,24] In assisting children in developing healthy sexuality, we want to avoid insinuating that any sexual behavior is bad. Not OK touches "are touches that are against the rules"[24,25] and may include hugs from strangers, kicking and hitting, and inappropriate sexual touches. OK touches may include hugs, kisses, and pats on the back from people with whom we are familiar. Confusing touches are those where, "you aren't sure if a touch is OK or not OK."[24,26] In these instances, children are encouraged to talk to a trusted adult to help them determine if a confusing touch is not OK. Stauffer and Deblinger[24,25] developed workbooks for children that assist parents and/or professionals in teaching these concepts, as well as body safety skills, to children. After teaching children to differentiate between OK and not OK touches, it is important to teach them how to respond if someone attempts to give them a not OK touch. Pediatricians and parents can begin discussions by presenting children with "what if" scenarios depicting a number of potentially dangerous situations and asking the child how they would respond. Parents can repeatedly review these scenarios and ask children related questions, such as "Who can you tell if someone tries to give you a not OK touch?" It is equally important, based on the research described previously, to have children practice saying no, running away, and telling a grown-up in response to a variety of potentially dangerous situations. Parents should be encouraged to rehearse responding in a supportive and positive manner when their children disclose the situations before they practice the role-play with their children.

Parents can also be educated about modeling appropriate personal boundaries for their children. Caution should be taken to avoid exposing children to sexual relations between parents, pornographic materials in the home, and/or sexually explicit television programs. Parents can begin teaching personal boundaries by closing the bathroom or bedroom doors and saying, "I need my privacy." They can encourage children to close their doors when bathing and changing clothes. Depending on the family's cultural and religious beliefs, parents may want to communicate to their children that if they masturbate this should be done in private as well. First, it may be necessary for parents to repeatedly remind children of these personal boundary rules. As children begin to implement these personal boundary rules, parents can offer praise and positive reinforcement to facilitate children learning these rules.

Box 11.1 demonstrates an example of how to communicate with a school-aged child and their parent(s) about personal safety and child sexual abuse. The conversation is being conducted with a school-aged child with no known or suspected history of child sexual abuse that incorporates many of the elements that research has identified as important in teaching children body safety skills.

Secondary and Tertiary Prevention

When pediatricians and/or other professionals provide information about healthy sexual development, child sexual abuse, and body safety, it is possible that children may disclose child sexual abuse.[27] In fact, there appears to be some evidence that high-quality school-based body safety education programs may lead to increased disclosures of sexual victimization.[23] As such, when pediatricians provide body safety information, it is important for them to be prepared to respond when a child discloses child sexual abuse. If a child discloses child sexual abuse, it is important to be supportive, clarify the

child's terms, and ask non-leading questions, such as, "Tell me more about that." When asking questions, use the child's words as much as possible. For example, "Tell me more about Pop Pop touching you on your kitty cat." However, the child should be asked to clarify what he or she means by "kitty cat." If it is clinically indicated, the pediatrician may talk to both the child and/or caretaker together or independently to inform them of the clinician's legal responsibility to report the concerns about possible sexual abuse to authorities who help to protect children from harm. If the non-offending parent is accompanying the child, the parent may be involved in making the report again depending on the pediatrician's clinical judgment and circumstances of the case. The primary goal here is to obtain sufficient information to make a report to the child abuse hotline to initiate the investigatory process. Please refer to Chapter 2 in this edition for more details on how to conduct a developmentally sensitive, medically sound history.

As noted previously, general pediatricians may play a critical secondary prevention role by detecting sexual abuse earlier than might otherwise occur. Verbal disclosures are, in fact, the most common way sexual abuse is discovered. In addition, with patients who have known histories of child sexual abuse, pediatricians may also be instrumental in providing some additional body safety education and/or encouraging family participation in educational programs offered in the schools and/or specialized therapy offered in the community. This may be very important given child sexual abuse victims' increased rate of re-victimization and the evidence documenting the benefits of providing secondary body safety education and structured, educational mental health therapy to this population.[24,28]

Although general pediatricians play a critical role in identifying and reporting suspected sexual abuse, a pediatric and/or mental health child abuse specialist may be in a better position to comprehensively assess the child's overall physical and/or emotional well-being, the level of parental distress and support available to the child, and the need for treatment in the aftermath of allegations of child sexual abuse.[4] Given their possible role in referring and/or encouraging families to obtain the needed medical and mental health services, it is important for pediatricians to have an understanding of the potential benefits and value of specialized medical and mental health services. (See Chapter 3 for benefits of the medical examination.) Thus it is helpful for pediatricians to have an understanding of effective mental health treatments and how they may mediate the emotional impact of child sexual abuse. A brief review of the treatment literature is offered here to provide information about effective treatments in general, as well as treatment components that are critical for children presenting with specific problems.

Available Treatments for Child Sexual Abuse

In a review of the literature, Ramchandani and Jones[29] identified 12 studies involving randomized clinical comparisons. Most examined the effectiveness of cognitive-behavioral therapy (CBT) for assisting children and their non-offending caregivers to overcome the impact of child sexual abuse. One involved individual therapy for preschool children and their caregivers.[30,31] The results of this investigation demonstrated that the children and parents participating in CBT, when compared with non-directive supportive therapy (NST), had greater improvements on children's behavioral problems and sexualized behaviors. These gains were maintained at 1 year with only 14% and 7% in the clinical range on the Children's Sexual Behavior Inventory and Children's Behavior Checklist for CBT compared with 40% and 33% for NST. Deblinger et al[7] compared the utility of NST and CBT group therapies for young children who have been sexually abused and their non-offending mothers. They found that mothers in the cognitive-behavioral groups showed significantly greater reductions in their intrusive thoughts and their negative parental emotional reactions about the sexual abuse compared with those participating in the parent NST groups. While there were no differences in children's abuse-related distress across the parallel child NST and CBT treatment groups, children assigned to CBT demonstrated greater improvement with respect to the knowledge regarding body safety skills.

Results of the effectiveness of CBT for older children also have varied depending on the study design and treatment modalities being studied. For example, Berliner and Saunders[32] found no additional benefit to including stress inoculation training and gradual exposure component and processing to a structured group program. In another study, Celano et al[33] compared abuse-focused individual psychotherapy to NST for African American females and found no differences between groups for children. Cohen and Mannarino[31] compared individual CBT and NST for youth aged 7 to 14 and found significantly greater improvements in children's depression levels for children assigned to CBT. However, there were no significant differences between the 2 treatment groups in children's behavior problems or sexualized behaviors. Deblinger et al[34] compared 3 individual CBT treatments (parent only, child only, and parent and child) with a community comparison. The findings of this investigation suggested that children's post-traumatic stress disorder (PTSD) symptoms seemed to improve most significantly when the child was directly involved in the CBT treatment (ie, child only or parent and child conditions). On the other hand, the parents' direct involvement in CBT treatment led to greater reductions in children's levels of depression, externalizing behaviors, and greater improvements in effective parenting skills compared with the treatment conditions that didn't directly involve the parents in CBT treatment (ie, child only and community). Significant gains

on the above outcome measures held across the 2-year follow-up period.[35] In another investigation examining the efficacy of individual CBT treatment with this population, King et al[36] found greater improvements in PTSD for children involved in both CBT conditions compared with a wait list control. However, they found no differences between CBT conditions involving the child only or both the parent and child until the 3-month follow-up when they found that children in the parent and child condition were reporting less fear.

In the largest and only multisite treatment outcome study involving children 8 to 14 years old who have experienced sexual abuse, children and their non-offending parents were randomly assigned to trauma-focused cognitive behavior therapy (TF-CBT) or client-centered therapy.[28] The results of this investigation, of alternative individual therapy approaches, demonstrated that children assigned to TF-CBT showed significantly greater improvements with respect to PTSD, depression, behavior problems, shame, and abuse-related attributions. Parents also assigned to TF-CBT showed similar outcomes with greater improvements on their own levels of depression, abuse-specific distress, support of the child, and effective parenting practices. At 6- and 12-month follow-ups, children and caregivers assigned to TF-CBT continued to report fewer symptoms of PTSD, feelings of shame, and abuse-specific parental distress.

There are only a few studies that have examined treatments other than CBT (psychodynamic[37,38]); however, no conclusions about the effectiveness of these treatments compared with other treatments can be made given that no comparison was made to alternate treatments. Alternate modalities (ie, group vs individual) of treatment were compared. For example, Trowell et al[37] found that those receiving individual therapy demonstrated greater reductions in PTSD symptoms than those receiving group therapy; however, there were no differences between the therapy conditions in overall global functioning. Baker[38] found group participation compared with individual therapy to be associated with improvements in self-esteem but not with any of the other outcome measures.

Although the empirical literature concerning the treatment of child sexual abuse remains limited, some conclusions can be drawn from the above studies. Cohen and Mannarino,[31] for example, identified parental support as the strongest predictor of positive outcomes for children. Given these and other findings, it seems critical to include the parent in the child's treatment to produce optimal outcomes for children.[34] Moreover, by assisting the parents in coping with their child's sexual abuse, we are assisting them with their personal distress, while also helping them be more supportive and effective therapeutic resources for their children. It also should be noted that most treatment outcome investigations seem to demonstrate the value of

relatively short-term, time-limited (12–18 sessions) therapy, which may be both comforting to parents and cost-effective in terms of the ability to reach more children.

While most children who have suffered sexual abuse do not necessarily exhibit sexual acting out behaviors, when they do it is very important to address these behaviors immediately Age-inappropriate sexual behaviors may be conceptualized as behaviors that are learned, similar to any other behaviors. As such, consistent behavioral interventions on behalf of the parent and child are important and have been found to be effective with regard to reducing these behaviors in young children.[37] In a follow-up of children with sexual behavior problems who participated in short-term group programs with their parents, 2% of the CBT participants, compared with 10% of the play therapy group participants, had documented sexually acting out problems 10 years after their group experiences.[39] In fact, children in the CBT group were no more likely to exhibit sexual acting out behaviors than youngsters in the general population (3%) during this 10-year period.[39] Given this perspective, it seems to be important to use behavioral strategies and involve children and parents in the treatment process to optimize outcomes in reducing sexualized behaviors or other behavior problems in general.

It should also be noted that the findings of several research investigations suggest that children's involvement in trauma-focused CBT treatment programs provide effective opportunities for children to learn, write, and talk about their child sexual abuse experiences while also processing their related thoughts and feelings. These structured programs seem to be particularly valuable in helping children overcome PTSD and distorted cognitions, as well as feelings of shame.

In general, it seems likely that children and adolescents may benefit from some education and/or therapy in the aftermath of child sexual abuse regardless of whether they are exhibiting a full-blown psychiatric disorder. Most controlled treatment comparisons have not required children to meet criteria for PTSD[28,30,34] because many traumatized children's symptom presentations differ developmentally and do not necessarily mirror that of adult traumatic stress presentations.[40,41] While only a minority of children with a history of sexual abuse present with symptoms sufficient to meet full *Diagnostic and Statistical Manual of Mental Disorders* diagnostic criteria for PTSD and/or other psychiatric disorders, most children referred for treatment present at least some symptoms of PTSD.[42] Moreover, many of these youngsters may feel confused and have distorted perceptions of personal boundaries, sexuality, and/or interpersonal relationships. In addition, children who have suffered sexual abuse may be at increased risk for future victimization.[43,44] These issues may generally be addressed through a structured course of trauma-focused therapy that includes sexual abuse education and body safety skills training as well as other affective, cognitive, and parenting skill-building components. It should be noted, however, that education and support can begin with the pediatrician providing basic information to children who have disclosed sexual abuse in the context of their comprehensive medical evaluation prior to sending them to a mental health clinician for further evaluation and treatment.

In sum, child sexual abuse is a widespread public health problem that breeds in silence and affects both girls and boys from preschoolers to teenagers. As noted earlier, it seems that most parents would welcome pediatric guidance and support in addressing this issue with their youngsters. Ultimately, however, it is important to emphasize that despite body safety education, children themselves are unlikely to stop sexual abuse from occurring. Rather, prevention efforts may be most successful when the goals include (1) increasing child sexual abuse public awareness and educational programs in schools or other community settings; (2) incorporating child sexual abuse information in medical and graduate school training programs; (3) developing and using effective multidisciplinary investigatory procedures; and (4) developing, implementing, and disseminating empirically validated treatment approaches for adult and juvenile sex offenders as well as adult and child survivors of sexual abuse. These objectives are most likely to be achieved through the combined efforts and input of health care, mental health, law enforcement, and education professionals as well as parents and youth.

When prevention fails and the pediatrician suspects sexual abuse, it is important that the pediatrician not only ensure that the child receives a skilled medical assessment to substantiate the concerns but also recognize that in substantiated cases the primary impact of sexual abuse on the child is psychological. With this in mind it behooves the pediatrician to identify and refer all children who have been sexually abused for an evaluation of the psychological impact of the abuse and to receive abuse-focused therapy.

Suggested Resources for Parents and Children

Aboff M. *Uncle Willy's Tickles: A Child's Right to Say No.* 2nd ed. Washington, DC: Magination Press; 2003

Bell R. *Changing Bodies, Changing Lives: A Book for Teens on Sex and Relationships.* 3rd ed. New York, NY: Three Rivers Press; 1998

Chaiet D, Russell F. *The Safe Zone: A Kid's Guide to Personal Safety.* New York, NY: Harper Trophy; 1998

Freeman L. *It's My Body: A Book to Teach Young Children How to Resist Uncomfortable Touch.* Seattle, WA: Parenting Press; 1984

Girard LW. *My Body Is Private.* Morton Grove, IL: Albert Whitman; 1984

Hader E, Brown S. *Play it Safe with SASA: A Board Game for Children Ages 4–14.* 1985

Hindman J. *A Very Touching Book…for Little People and for Big People.* Baker City, OR: Alexandria; 1983

Kirberger K. *No Body's Perfect: Stories by Teens About Body Image, Self-Acceptance, and the Search for Identity.* New York, NY: Scholastic, Inc.; 2003

Madaras L, Madaras A. *My Body, My Self for Girls.* 2nd ed. New York, NY: Newmarket Press; 2000

Madaras L, Madaras A. *My Body, My Self for Boys.* 2nd ed. New York, NY: Newmarket Press; 2000

Mayle P. *Where Did I Come From?: The Facts of Life Without Any Nonsense and With Illustrations.* New York, NY: Kensington; 1975

Mayle P. *What's Happening to Me? A Guide to Puberty.* New York, NY: Kensington; 2000

Ottenweller J. *Please Tell!: A Child's Story About Sexual Abuse (Early Steps)* Center City, MN: Hazelden Publishing; 1991

Spelman C. *Your Body Belongs to You.* Morton Grove, IL: Albert Whitman; 1997

Stauffer L, Deblinger E. *Let's Talk About Taking Care of You!: An Educational Book About Body Safety.* Hatsfield, PA: Hope for Families, Inc.; 2003

References

1. Finkelhor D, Ormond R, Tyrner H, Hamby SL. The victimization of children and youth: a comprehensive, national survey. *Child Maltreat.* 2005;10:5–25
2. UK Department of Health. Definitions of primary, secondary, and tertiary prevention. 2007. http://www.dh.gov.uk/en/publicationsandstatistics. Accessed January 7, 2008

3. Vandeven AM, Newton AW. Update on child physical abuse, sexual abuse, and prevention. *Curr Opin Pediatr.* 2006;19(2):201–205

4. American Academy of Pediatrics Committee on Child Abuse and Neglect. Guidelines for the evaluation of sexual abuse of children: subject review. *Pediatrics.* 1999;103(1):186–191

5. Wurtele S, Owens J. Teaching personal safety skills to young children: an investigation of age and gender across five studies. *Child Abuse Negl.* 1997;21:805–814

6. Deblinger E, Runyon MK. Reducing the children's risk of sexual revictimization. Seminar presented at: 2000 American Professional Society on Abused Children; 2000; Chicago, IL

7. Deblinger E, Stauffer L, Steer R. Comparative efficacies of supportive and cognitive behavioral group therapies for children who were sexually abused and their non-offending mothers. *Child Maltreat.* 2001;6(4):332–343

8. Tutty LM. Child sexual abuse prevention programs: evaluating Who Do You Tell. *Child Abuse Negl.* 1997;21:869–881

9. Wurtele S, Kvaternick M, Franklin C. Sexual abuse prevention for preschoolers: a survey of parents' behaviors, attitudes, and beliefs. *J Child Sex Abuse.* 1992;1:113–128

10. Kenny MC, Thakkar-Kolar Ryan EE, Runyon MK, Capri V. Child sexual abuse: from prevention to self-protection. *Child Abuse Review.* 2008;17:36–54

11. Wurtele SK. Enhancing children's sexual development through child sexual abuse prevention programs. *J Sex Educ Ther.* 1993;19:37–46

12. Wurtele S, Kast L, Melzer A. Sexual abuse: prevention education for young children: a comparison of teachers and parents as instructors. *Child Abuse Negl.* 1992;16:865–876

13. Miller-Perrin C, Wurtele S, Kondrick P. Sexually abused and non-abused children's conceptions of personal body safety. *Child Abuse Negl.* 1990;14:99–112

14. Thomas D, Flaherty E, Binns H. Parent expectations and comfort with discussion of normal childhood sexuality and sexual abuse prevention during office visits. *Ambul Pediatr.* 2004;4(3):232–236

15. Sapp MK, Vandeven AM. Update on childhood sexual abuse. *Postgrad Obstet Gynecol.* 2005;25(22):1–7

16. Hébert M, Lavoie Piché C, Poitras M. Proximate effects of child sexual abuse prevention program in elementary school children. *Child Abuse Negl.* 2001;25:505–522

17. Berrick JD, Barth RP. Child sexual abuse prevention: research review and recommendations. *Soc Work Res Abstr.* 1992;28(4):6–15

18. Boyle C, Lutzker J. Teaching young children to discriminate abuse from nonabusive situations using multiple exemplars in a modified discrete trial teaching format. *J Fam Violence.* 2005;20(2):55–69

19. Wurtele SK. School-based child sexual abuse prevention: questions, answers, and more preventing violence in relationships: interventions across the life span questions. In: Lutzker JR, ed. *Handbook of Child Abuse Research and Treatment.* New York, NY: Plenum Press; 1998:501–513

20. Roberts JA, Miltenberger RG. Emerging issues in the research on child sexual abuse prevention. *Educ Treat Child.* 1999;22:84–102

21. Deblinger E, Heflin AH. *Treating Sexually Abused Children and Their Nonoffending Parents: A Cognitive Behavioral Approach.* Newbury Park, CA: Sage Publications; 1996

22. Deblinger E, Runyon MK. Understanding and treating feelings of shame in children who have experienced maltreatment. *Child Maltreat.* 2005;10(4):364–376

23. Finkelhor D. Prevention of sexual abuse through educational programs directed toward children. *Pediatrics.* 2007;120(3):640–645

24. Stauffer LB, Deblinger E. Cognitive behavioral groups for nonoffending mother and their young sexually abused children: a preliminary treatment outcome study. *Child Maltreat.* 1999;1:65–76

25. Stauffer LB, Deblinger E. *Let's Talk About Taking Care of You: An Educational Book About Body Safety for Preschool Children.* Hatfield, PA: Hope for Families, Inc.; 2003

26. Stauffer LB, Deblinger E. *Let's Talk About Taking Care of You: An Educational Book About Body Safety for Young Children.* Hatfield, PA: Hope for Families, Inc.; 2004

27. Currier L, Wurtele S. A pilot study of previously abused and non-sexually abused children's responses to a personal safety program. *J Child Sex Abuse.* 1996;5:71–87

28. Cohen J, Deblinger E, Mannarino A, Steer R. A multisite, randomized controlled trial for children with sexual abuse-related PTSD symptoms. *J Am Acad Child Adolesc Psychiatry.* 2004;43(4):393–402

29. Ramchandani P, Jones DPH. Treating psychological symptoms in sexually abused children: from research findings to service provision. *Br J Psychiatry.* 2003;183:484–490

30. Cohen JA, Mannarino AP. A treatment outcome study for sexually abused preschool children: initial findings. *J Am Acad Child Adolesc Psychiatry.* 1996;35(1):42–50

31. Cohen JA, Mannarino AP. Interventions for sexually abused children: initial treatment findings. *Child Maltreat.* 1998;3(1):17–26

32. Berliner L, Saunders BE. Treating fear and anxiety in sexually abused children: results of a controlled 2-year follow-up study. *Child Maltreat.* 1996;1:194–309

33. Celano M, Hazzard A, Webb C, et al. Treatment of traumagenic beliefs among sexually abused girls and their mothers: an evaluation study. *J Abnorm Child Psychol.* 1996;24:1–17

34. Deblinger E, Lippmann J, Steer R. Sexually abused children suffering posttraumatic stress symptoms: initial treatment outcome findings. *Child Maltreat.* 1996;1:310–321

35. Deblinger E, Steer R, Lippmann J. Maternal factors associated with sexually abused children's psychosocial adjustment. *Child Maltreat.* 1999;4:13–20

36. King NJ, Tonge BJ, Mullen P, et al. Cognitive-behavioural treatment of sexually abused children: a review of research. *Behav Cogn Psychother.* 1999;27:295–309

37. Trowell J, Kolvin I, Weeramanthri T, et al. Psychotherapy for sexually abused girls: psychopathological outcome findings and patterns of change. *Br J Psychiatry.* 2002;180:234–247

38. Baker CR. A comparison of individual and group therapy as treatment of sexually abused adolescent females (PhD, University of Maryland). *Diss Abstr Int.* 1987;47:4319B

39. Carpentier MY, Silovsky JF, Chaffin M. Randomized trial of treatment for children with sexual behavior problems: ten-year follow-up. *J Consult Clin Psychology.* 2006;74(3):482–488

40. Runyon MK, Faust J, Orvaschel H. Differential symptom pattern of post-traumatic stress disorder (PTSD) in maltreated children with and without concurrent depression. *Child Abuse Negl.* 2002;26:39–53

41. Scheeringa MS, Peevles CD, Cook CA, Zeanah CH. Toward establishing procedural, criterion, and discrminant validity for PTSD in early childhood. *J Am Acad Child Adolesc Psychiatry.* 2001;40:52–60

42. McLeer S, Deblinger E, Henry D, Orvaschel H. Sexually abused children at high risk for post-traumatic stress disorder. *J Am Acad Child Adolesc Psychiatry.* 1992;31(5):875–879

43. Arata CM. From child victim to adult victim: a model for predicting sexual revictimization. *Child Maltreat.* 2000;5(1):28–38

44. Boney-McCoy S, Finkelhor D. Is youth victimization related to trauma symptoms and depression after controlling for prior symptoms and family relationships? A longitudinal, prospective study. *J Consult Clin Psychol.* 1996;64(6):1406–1416

Interdisciplinary Approaches to Child Maltreatment: Accessing Community Resources

Philip V. Scribano

Angelo P. Giardino

Child maltreatment is a multifaceted problem that is addressed ideally in an interdisciplinary fashion in which various disciplines participate jointly in a clinical process that is team-oriented, collaborative, and focused on providing the child and family with the best care possible.[1,2] At a direct service, face-to-face clinical level, the interdisciplinary team shares the responsibility to carefully collect and process the components of a sensitive and thorough evaluation.[3,4] Ideally, at a community level, a variety of agencies and service providers come together to fashion a comprehensive network of services directed at assisting children and families as they progress from crisis to health.[5,6]

This chapter focuses on the direct clinical teamwork needed to work with children and families who are dealing with sexual abuse, given this type of maltreatment most commonly uses a multidisciplinary approach; it also describes the broader teamwork

required among the various agencies and community resources on which health care professionals may need to call to best serve the children and families.

Interdisciplinary Approaches

Interdisciplinary approaches in the health care setting, although effective, are notorious for being difficult to organize, labor intensive, and costly.[7] With the rapid changes that have occurred in health care economics, the human and financial resources required for interdisciplinary direct service and community activity are at risk. Medical insurers have often selected the short-sighted option of cutting interdisciplinary services as a way to reduce short-term costs. Similar efficiency and cost issues have become prominent in traditional social service agencies, including those providing child protective services (CPS).[8] Responding to this general trend, the Pew Health Professions Commission[9] called for an almost complete reorientation of clinical training to highlight the necessity of interdependence and cooperation that takes a long-term view on the cost-benefit ratio of teamwork. In the Commission's words:

> *Interdisciplinary strategies are increasingly the only viable pathway to address complex problems. These strategies lead to a more effective sharing of resources and more creative responses to problems. Initially, this will take more time as effective teamwork strategies are developed across the health care disciplines. However, over time the investment will produce new approaches to teaching, learning, and clinical practice.[9]*

Team Approach to Work in Child Maltreatment

Teamwork in the health care setting is not new, and its clinical value has been recognized and advocated for almost 4 decades.[9-13] The benefits of teamwork are well-known and include improved information sharing among clinicians, joint decision-making and joint planning among team members, a variety of collaborative educational approaches, and the chance to provide mutual support for team members.[2,4,7] This chapter will specifically address teams that focus on assessment/ investigation in contrast to treatment teams, which focus primarily on the psychotherapeutic treatment of child maltreatment survivors.

The idea of applying collaborative, interdisciplinary concepts to child maltreatment occurred in the late 1960s and has remained a central tenet to such work.[1,5,13-15] The interdisciplinary approach was initially described as a series of individuals with different backgrounds coming from different disciplines and traditions who contribute to the solution of the same problem.[16] This remains the central framework used in today's team approach. The benefits to such teamwork in addressing child maltreatment are many and are detailed below. Prominent national organizations and governmental agencies have called for an interdisciplinary model to address child maltreatment at both the individual child and the community levels.[1,5,6,13,14,17] In the early 1990s, a national effort through the US Department of Justice Office of Juvenile Justice and Delinquency Prevention and the US Department of Health and Human Services National Center for Child Abuse and Neglect provided recommendations to promote joint investigations focused on fostering interdisciplinary work in child maltreatment investigations and treatment planning.[17] The stated rationale for a coordinated response to child maltreatment listed the following reasons based on professional experiences:

- Reduction in the number of interviews that the child must endure
- Minimization of the number of people involved in the cases
- Enhanced evidence quality that is discovered for both criminal prosecution and civil litigation

- Provision of information essential for medical diagnosis and treatment, and to CPS and other family service organizations
- Decreased likelihood of conflicts between and among various involved agencies[17]

The concept of an organized and formal grouping of professionals to work with child maltreatment led to the development of the concept of the multidisciplinary team (MDT).[2,18] An MDT is a group of professionals that agrees to work in a coordinated and collaborative way to address the problem of child abuse and neglect.[2] A child abuse MDT is best described[13] as "A group of professionals who work together in a coordinated and collaborative manner to ensure an effective response to reports of child abuse and neglect. Members of the team represent the government agencies and private practitioners responsible for investigating crimes against children and protecting and treating children in a particular community. An MDT may focus on investigations; policy issues; treatment of victims, their families, and perpetrators; or a combination of these functions."

The composition and organization of an MDT is quite variable. An MDT may be established by an interested and motivated primary care provider or a group of institutionally based clinicians or at the direction of a government office or agency.[6,13] From the first publications that describe MDTs, regardless of how it is established or by whom, the goal of the MDT has been to ensure that the multidimensional needs of the child and family are attended to during the child maltreatment investigation and treatment interventions.[2,19,20] Out of the premise that uncoordinated efforts to address child maltreatment may cause additional harm to victims due to subjecting these children to potentially insensitive procedures, MDTs have become the standard care approach to child maltreatment. In addition, those MDTs that emphasize community-wide goals rather than individual agency concerns will have greater success in collaboration.[15] As of 1999, 36 states had legislation requiring MDTs on cases of child abuse,[21,22] and by 2002, all 50 states had legislation that mandated cross-referral of these cases among professional agencies.[21,23]

Various MDT models exist and vary based on need, locality, and setting. Examples of team types include treatment teams, case management teams, case consultation teams, multidisciplinary teaching teams, resource development teams, and mixed model teams,[4,15] with the mixed model being the most common type and exercising multiple functions. Teaching hospitals at academic health sciences centers are often central in the establishment and staffing of MDTs and have been using such teams for more than 40 years.[13] Additionally, a number of MDTs have emerged in community settings where social services agency staff and primary care practitioners agree to come together and collaborate on evaluation, treatment, and prevention.[6,14,24] As such, several of the more common MDT structures are listed below.

Multidisciplinary interview centers.
Focusing on the management of
child sexual abuse and the forensic
interview only, these MDTs include
law enforcement, CPS, and prosecuting
attorneys to interview child victims
and develop strategies based on the
disclosure of sexual abuse.[25]

*Traditional hospital-based and
community-based child abuse teams.*
In the hospital or community setting,
these MDTs review all types of child
maltreatment in their locale and
develop strategies to address the various
issues pertaining to the case findings.[14]

Child advocacy centers. These are
community-based, child-focused,
facility-based programs that support
MDTs to work together in the investigation, treatment, management, and prosecution of child sexual abuse.[26] This
MDT structure has been well-received
in a wide range of communities (rural
vs urban), and the model adapts to the
community it serves. As such, it has
become the most common MDT that
addresses child sexual abuse in the
United States, and will be described in
more detail in this chapter.

The benefits of an effective MDT
include the following:

- Less system-inflicted trauma to
  children and families
- Increased agency performance,
  including enhanced accuracy of
  investigations and more appropriate
  interventions
- Efficient use of limited community
  resources

- More capable professionals as they
  develop collaborative skills
- Recognition of the difficulty inherent
  in maltreatment-related work
  and the opportunity to develop a
  professional network that decreases
  the sense of isolation and risk of
  professional burnout[13]
- Increased effectiveness as defined by
  greater ability to charge a crime and
  to obtain confessions by perpetrators
  of sexual abuse[27]

Dinsmore[17] reported that a coordinated
system for the investigation of child
maltreatment requires 4 essential
components.

- Education of all participating
  disciplines in the dynamics of
  victimization, child development,
  and the criminal justice process as
  it relates to children and families
- Establishment and maintenance of
  consistent reporting practices
- Commitment to high-quality
  investigations and the elimination
  of duplication between and among
  agencies
- Sensitive treatment of child victims
  and their families throughout the
  investigation and judicial process

The MDT concept found its niche with
the establishment of a variety of inter-
agency/provider organizations that
work to make the evaluation of suspected sexual abuse as responsive as
possible to the child and family who
have been subjected to such victimization. The best example of this type of
MDT is the approximately 400 child

advocacy centers (CACs) throughout the country. The concept of a "one-stop" systems approach whereby services can be made more accessible and efficient through colocation and coordination of services normally provided by more than one agency is the hallmark of CAC infrastructures.[28] The nonprofit membership organization for CACs is the National Children's Alliance (NCA), which assists the development and maintenance for accreditation as associate or full members based on NCA credential standards for CACs (Table 12.1). The NCA works with the federal government through the Victims of Child Abuse Act (enacted into law in 1990), which required the US Department of Justice Office of Juvenile Justice and Delinquency Prevention to coordinate with CACs to provide technical assistance to the 4 designated regions (Northeast, Southern, Midwest, and Western).[29] In addition, as of 2005, 36 states have enacted legislation that mandates the use of MDTs, and many specify the CAC model as the preferred MDT in jurisdictions where a CAC exists. Many states have also included funding streams to support this model as well (NCA, personal communication, 2007).

By virtue of the priorities in coordination, CACs have traditionally strived to decrease the need for the child to repeatedly recount the history of his or her maltreatment by using interviewers trained in child development and forensic interview skills to conduct these interviews while the other MDT members observe the interview by one-way mirror or video-monitoring

technology.[13,30,31] Given the evidence that suggests repeated interviews may increase the likelihood that the child perceives the investigation experience as harmful,[32,33] may increase the child's trauma symptoms,[34] and increase the likelihood of inaccurate or false details,[35] it would seem appropriate to continue to pursue the goal of coordinated, multidisciplinary care using the child advocacy center model.

Additional features of CACs include specific guidelines for the interviewing of children, the role and responsibilities of the multidisciplinary team, interagency agreements, medical forensic medical examination standards, access to treatment services, affiliation with a victim advocate, and procedures for case tracking and reviews.[26] The middle ground between a therapeutic versus judicial model of child protection is a key feature and strength of CACs, which allows for a thorough investigation while offering extensive therapeutic services to the child and other family members as they navigate the realities of a child abuse system response.[28] Child advocacy centers may have diverse structures, with some being hospital-based and others not, and this is often based on the resources and the needs of the community. While there remains little empiric evidence to demonstrate the effectiveness of the CAC model, there has been some work conducted in a rural county with a CAC that demonstrated increased law enforcement investigations,greater substantiation of sexual abuse, and more children receiving medical examinations and

TABLE 12.1
National Children's Alliance (NCA) Standards for Accredited Members[a]

NCA Standard	Definition
1. Child-appropriate/child-friendly facility	A comfortable, private, child-friendly setting that is both physically and psychologically safe for clients.
2. Multidisciplinary team	A multidisciplinary team for response to child abuse allegations includes representation from law enforcement, child protective services, prosecution, mental health, medical, victim advocacy.
3. Organizational capacity	A designated legal entity responsible for program and fiscal operations has been established and implements basic sound administrative practices.
4. Cultural competency and diversity	Promotes policies, practices, and procedures that are culturally competent. Cultural competency is defined as the capacity to function in more than one culture, requiring the ability to appreciate, understand, and interact with members of diverse populations within the local community.
5. Forensic interviews	Conducted in a manner that is of a neutral, fact-finding nature, and coordinated to avoid duplicative interviewing.
6. Medical evaluation	Specialized medical evaluation and treatment are to be made available to child advocacy center (CAC) clients as part of the team response, either at the CAC or through coordination and referral with other specialized medical providers.
7. Therapeutic intervention	Specialized mental health services are to be made available as part of the team response, either at the CAC or through coordination and referral with other appropriate treatment providers.
8. Victim support/advocacy	Victim support and advocacy are to be made available as part of the team response, either at the CAC or through coordination with other providers, throughout the investigation and subsequent legal proceedings.
9. Case review	Team discussion and information sharing regarding the investigation, case status, and services needed by the child and family are to occur on a routine basis.
10. Case tracking	CACs must develop and implement a system for monitoring case progress and tracking case outcomes for team components.

[a]National Children's Alliance Standards for Accredited Members (http://www.nca-online.org/pages/page.asp?page_id=4032).

being referred for treatment compared with the standard CPS investigation.[30] In addition, MDTs are thought to improve the investigation by virtue of greater interagency communication and reduction in evidence collection gaps when information is shared across agency investigators.[36] Studies that evaluated the impact of CACs on children, families, systems, and communities are currently being completed, with preliminary results demonstrating a greater prevalence of coordinated investigations, greater number of children receiving forensic medical examinations, significant increase in mental health referrals, and greater satisfaction of parents and caregivers with the investigation.[37]

An MDT is functional and healthy when there are common goals, a mutual understanding of professional roles and responsibilities, and an atmosphere characterized by open communication.[18] While it would seem intuitive that healthy MDTs should translate into improved outcomes for the children and families they serve, this causal relationship remains unclear because there has been so little outcomes research on the MDT.[15] Ideally, practice on such teams should be guided by formal protocols that minimize the chance for failure to adhere to agreed-on standards and to assess relevant outcomes.[1,5,17,18] Specifically, such formal or written protocols may be most helpful when they address (a) the roles and responsibilities of the

different professionals and agencies involved; (b) the steps that must be accomplished at each stage of the process or intervention, time frames for completion of each step, and responsibility for who carries out the protocol; and (c) practical advice for handling both routine and special issues that may arise.[5] Conflict is inevitable in teamwork, and the success of the team is not measured in the amount of conflict but, rather, in the effectiveness with which it is resolved.[13,38] Members need not agree on every point, but resolution must occur in a manner in which the mission of the team and the goal and focus of serving children and families are not compromised. Consensus is a goal but not a requirement in an MDT. Conflicts related to core issues need constructive attention that takes adequate time to build consensus. The team should quickly address peripheral issues that are not central to effective work with children and families and move on to more important primary issues that need discussion and resolution of any ambiguities of the case.[15,39,40] In interdisciplinary work related to child maltreatment, conflict frequently revolves around tension associated with decision-making, interpersonal relationships, competition, territorialism, and perceived lack of cooperation.[5] See Box 12.1 for points to remember when facing conflicts.

BOX 12.1
Points to Remember When Faced With Conflict[a]

- Do not lose sight of the team purpose outlined in the mission statement.
- Look forward to opportunity, not backward to blame.
- Be respectful. Consider each person's point of view. Listen to one another.
- Be sure each position is understood. Restate the other position in your own words.
- Clarify the opposing point of view. Find something positive in each view. Avoid defending your point of view until you understand the other.
- Voice the opposing point of view.
- State your position clearly and firmly, but without excessive emotion.
- Once you have been heard, do not continue to restate your position.
- Avoid personalizing your position, and stay focused on the issue.
- Offer suggestions rather than mere criticism of other points of view.
- Remember that conflict with a team is natural, and work toward a mutually agreeable resolution.
- Base resolutions on consensus, not abdication of responsibility or integrity.
- Keep focused on the team's agreed-on purpose, and refer to your protocol for guidance.

[a]Adapted from Ells M. *Forming a Multidisciplinary Team to Investigate Child Abuse.* Rockville, MD: Office of Juvenile Justice and Delinquency Prevention; 2000. http://www.ncjrs.org/html/ojjdp/portable_guides/forming/contents.html. Accessed March 29, 2007.

The Health Care Setting: Roles and Responsibilities of Clinicians

A variety of clinicians from various disciplines may become involved with the child and family at the direct, face-to-face level. Types of professionals working in the health care setting include physicians, nurses, health care social workers, and mental health professionals.

Regarding the evaluation and treatment of child sexual abuse, physicians are trained to perform the medical evaluation, which includes a medical history, a physical examination, and laboratory/diagnostic testing.[41] The physician is responsible for careful documentation and interpretation of the evaluation's findings. In addition

to the direct work with the child and family, the physician on the team is often asked to provide testimony in court proceedings and to render expert opinions about the medical findings. Legal outcomes such as perpetrator guilt have been associated with the quality and outcomes of medical assessments.[42] The outcomes of those assessments further support the importance of medical providers' participation in the MDT.

The roles for nurses in the evaluation and treatment of child sexual abuse have been evolving over the years, spanning the traditional roles of providing direct patient care and assisting the child and family in dealing with their responses to maltreatment as well as to their involvement with the health care system. Advanced practice nurses, such as pediatric nurse practitioners, have enhanced clinical training and can perform the actual clinical child maltreatment evaluations after advanced training and experience in the field. In addition, sexual assault nurse examiners (SANE) programs have developed in the last 2 decades and provide support in the collection of evidence for acute sexual assault examinations in the emergency department, and can provide a significant contribution to the MDT in this setting. See Chapter 9 for further discussion of the role of nurses in caring for children suspected of having been sexually maltreated.

The health care social worker provides a wide range of support services throughout the evaluation process, including assessing the child's and family's strengths and challenges, interfacing with external agencies such as law enforcement and CPS, and assisting the family in understanding the implications of a report being made and the options available to them. Health care social workers who have received additional, intensive training in interviewing techniques have also conducted the interviews of children as the designated team member of an MDT. The health care social worker on many teams serves as a natural liaison with both CPS and law enforcement personnel.

Mental health service providers, including psychiatrists, psychologists, licensed clinical social workers, and other mental health professionals,

assist in the initial evaluation and provide treatment after the assessment. Mental health professionals are a vital component of the interdisciplinary approach directed at the evaluation and treatment of child sexual abuse owing to their roles in ameliorating the short- and long-term impact of such maltreatment. In addition, there is a growing body of literature that would indicate that a crucial component of mental health services for child maltreatment should include improvements in non-offending caregiver support,[43–46] which has been shown to be predictive of greater resiliency, less distress, greater likelihood for disclosures, and less chance for recantation with greater parental support.[47–50]

The health care team often interfaces with other potential team members external to the health care setting. These external team members may include professionals from CPS, law enforcement, the prosecutor's office and the courts, school personnel, and a variety of child advocates. Table 12.2 lists the various disciplines that may be involved in the evaluation and investigation of child sexual abuse and outlines the role/contribution that can be expected from each.

Roles and Responsibilities of Agencies and Services

When evaluating suspected child sexual abuse, the child, family, and health care team typically become involved with a large number and variety of community and governmental

TABLE 12.2
Roles and Responsibilities of Professional Team Members

Discipline	Main Role	Comments
Pediatrician/pediatric nurse practitioner[a–c]	• Identifies and reports suspected child abuse • Completes accurate medical evaluation, including history, physical examination, and collection of laboratory specimens • Completes accurate forensic evaluation including photo-documentation and/or collection of evidence (for acute sexual assault) • Provides medical treatment and mental health referral for child and family • Ensures follow-up for high-risk clinical concerns that may not rise to the reporting threshold • Interprets and provides expert testimony regarding examination (general and anogenital) and forensic evidence • Participates in community efforts to prevent child sexual abuse • Trains medical/nonmedical professionals on the medical aspects of child sexual abuse	Training, knowledge, and experience essential to adequately manage the medical and forensic aspects of child maltreatment
Nurse[d,e]	• Identifies patient needs • Provides appropriate services • Assists practitioner in the collection of evidence (sexual assault nurse examiner)	• Four factors affect the nurse's role: nursing skills, perception of role, nursing knowledge and practice guidelines, and expectations of others on team
Health care social worker[a,f]	• Role is variable but often includes some level of team coordination • Carefully assesses family strengths and risks • Facilitates access to community services and supports • Serves as liaison to child protective services (CPS) and law enforcement personnel • Supports other team members	• Knowledge of child development, abuse dynamics, and legal process essential • Skills at interviewing, gathering information, and working with all disciplines necessary

TABLE 12.2, continued
Roles and Responsibilities of Professional Team Members

CPS worker[a,g]	• Gathers reports of suspected abuse • Provides initial assessment • Acts as liaison to other disciplines in investigation (ie, law enforcement) • Develops individualized service plan • Delivers and/or coordinates services being provided • Provides updates to court, if involved • Conducts community activities around awareness and prevention	• Knowledge of regulatory and legal issues essential • Collaboration skills necessary
Law enforcement personnel[a,h]	• Conducts initial assessment • Engages in possible immediate intervention and protection of child • Leads criminal investigation and evidence collection • Prepares case findings to present to prosecutor • Awareness of other disciplines' contributions to overall investigation necessary	• Professional training in child sexual abuse investigations essential • Awareness of other disciplines' contributions to overall investigation necessary
Prosecutor[a]	• Manages court proceedings if case goes to trial • Prepares child for court • Facilitates victim advocacy services • Collaborates with other disciplines around community-based efforts dealing with child sexual abuse	• Experience with criminal and juvenile court proceedings essential • Decision to file charges and proceed to court often rests on severity of abuse and perceived ability to prove the case
Child advocate[a,c]	• Protects needs and interests of child in court proceedings • Conducts independent investigation • Determines child's treatment needs depending on jurisdiction	• May or may not be an attorney

TABLE 12.2, continued
Roles and Responsibilities of Professional Team Members

Mental health service providers[a,c,i,j]	• Identifies and reports suspected child maltreatment • Provides mental health assessment • Provides treatment • Interprets findings and provides expert testimony on them • Assesses caregivers' baseline psychosocial risk factors, treatment needs	• May include principals, teachers, school counselors, and other school personnel

a DePanfilis D, Salus MK. *A Coordinated Response to Child Abuse and Neglect: A Basic Manual*. Washington, DC: US Department of Health and Human Services, National Center on Child Abuse and Neglect; 1992b.
b Schmitt BD, ed. *The Child Protection Team Handbook*. New York, NY: Garland; 1978
c Sgroi SM, ed. *Handbook of Clinical Intervention in Child Sexual Abuse*. Lexington, MA: Lexington Books; 1982.
d Bridges CI. The nurse's evaluation. In: Schmitt BD, ed. *The Child Protection Team Handbook*. New York, NY: Garland; 1978:65–81.
e Ledray LE. *Sexual Assault Nurse Examiner Development and Operation Guide*. Washington, DC: US Department of Justice Office of Justice Programs; 1999. NJC170609. http://www.ojp.usdoj.gov/ovc/publications/infores/sane/saneguide.pdf.
f Carroll CA. The social worker's evaluation. In: Schmitt BD, ed. *The Child Protection Team Handbook*. New York, NY: Garland; 1978:83–108.
g DePanfilis D, Salus MK. *Child Protective Services: A Guide for Caseworkers*. Washington, DC: US Department of Health and Human Services, National Center on Child Abuse and Neglect; 1992a.
h Bockman HR, Carroll, CA. The law enforcement's role in evaluation. In: Schmitt BD, ed. *The Child Protection Team Handbook*. New York, NY: Garland; 1978:149–152.
i Bond JR. The psychologist's evaluation. In: Schmitt BD, ed. *The Child Protection Team Handbook*. New York, NY: Garland; 1978:121–133.
j Stern HC. The psychiatrist's evaluation of the parents. In: Schmitt BD, ed. *The Child Protection Team Handbook*. New York, NY: Garland; 1978:109–120.

agencies. Child protective services is legally mandated to provide protection and safety and is responsible for the reporting, investigation, and treatment aspects related to alleged child sexual abuse. Law enforcement personnel often become involved to address safety and to establish whether a crime has been committed. If the law enforcement investigation establishes enough evidence to charge a crime (through investigative interviews and collection of evidence), the prosecutor in that jurisdiction becomes involved for criminal court proceedings. The prosecutor may also become involved when the CPS investigation identifies concerns regarding the parent's ability to protect the child from maltreatment, and this legal proceeding will occur in the juvenile court system. The benefits for coordinated, collaborative team approaches to the investigation and treatment have already been described.

Joint Investigation Concept

The Police Foundation and the American Public Welfare Association collaborated to identify models that best characterized the kinds of joint investigation models that have evolved between law enforcement and CPS agencies.[25] The models vary in the amount of formal collaboration that occurs between law enforcement and CPS agencies, with the most

comprehensive model identified by
these organizations representing the
investigative agencies, being the CAC.[25]

CAC Model

As described previously, a CAC is a
specifically designed physical space
in which law enforcement and CPS
investigators are all located and
in which children are interviewed
in a comfortable, child-friendly
environment. Not all CACs have
an ideal physical setup that includes
colocation of CPS and police. However, the CAC approach is inherently
collaborative and multidisciplinary/
interdisciplinary in practice. The
minimum requirements of a CAC
include the following[25]:

- Preinterview and post-interview
  MDT discussions
- Scheduled case reviews
- Involvement of the prosecutor's
  office
- Joint training programs
- A system of case tracking and
  follow-up

Because the interview is so central
to the CAC mission, some CACs may
have interview specialists on staff
who conduct the forensic interview on
behalf of the rest of the MDT members.
Regardless of which team member
conducts the forensic interview, specific
training is required to conduct these
types of interviews, and ongoing
peer review has become a mainstay
activity to ensure quality of this effort
in the MDT.[51,52]

Multidisciplinary Interview Center Model

To reduce repeated interviewing in this
model, law enforcement and CPS agree
to meet and conduct joint investigative
interviews, but the collaboration and
agency support is neither as formal
nor as comprehensive as in a CAC
model. A steering committee, rather
than an independent board, advises on
procedures and policies, limited staffing
is available, and the model is dependent
on agency budget contributions. Like
the CAC, the multidisciplinary interview center should include similar
minimum requirements to function
as an interdisciplinary team. Where
feasible, the multidisciplinary interview
center may lay the groundwork for the
formation of a full-scale CAC in which
more staff time and independent funding can enable further programmatic
development to occur.

Limited Agency-Based Joint Investigations Model

This basic model is the least formalized and is composed of specialized
investigative units from law enforcement that conduct joint investigations
with CPS workers using written protocols within existing agency frameworks.
This model attempts to maximize the
best use of existing agency resources.
A program coordinator is charged
with convening a steering committee,
holding case conferences, and arranging joint trainings. As the basic model
evolves, it may develop enhancements
such as the following[25]:

- Specifically designated CPS case-workers to serve as liaisons to the police department
- A police-CPS interview room with observation capabilities
- Specialized joint training opportunities
- An evaluation component that tracks cases and provides team members with case follow-up

While CPS agencies report that approximately 20% of the investigations of child maltreatment are conducted jointly, law enforcement agencies report that 80% to 95% of their investigations are conducted jointly with CPS.[25] Joint investigations often occur in the more severe cases, and approximately 42% of cases that are investigated jointly are substantiated.[25]

The greatest prevalence of joint investigations between CPS and police are noted in cases of sexual abuse.[25] This is due in part to the greater challenges and resource needs to investigate child sexual abuse compared with other forms of child maltreatment, because there is often a lack of medical findings and objective witnesses to the abuse. Physical abuse and neglect cases, on the other hand, often have obvious physical evidence, and such cases are usually seen as more straightforward by investigators.[18] Suspected sexual abuse investigations also require a number of time-consuming corroborative interviews that require a fair amount of time and experience to successfully complete. Additionally, child sexual abuse cases often require a substantial amount of judgment and expertise to

adequately interpret and make sense of all of the information available.[18]

The CPS-law enforcement collaboration is often informal, with 60% of law enforcement agencies reporting unwritten agreements and approximately 20% having signed written agreements such as interagency memorandums of understanding (MOU).[25] When formalized, the MOU contains information on the following[25]:

- Notification responsibilities
- Criteria for joint investigation
- Interviewing responsibilities during the investigation
- The jurisdiction served by the team

Figure 12.1 represents the flow of a joint investigation once the case meets the necessary criteria. In general, the CPS process consists of 6 essential stages: intake, initial assessment/investigation, family assessment, case planning, service provision, and evaluation of progress and closure.[3] Each stage in this CPS process is highlighted in Table 12.3.

The medical team at the health care facilities, as well as associated mental health providers, is often called on by CPS to help inform which steps would be in the best interests of the child and family. As the evaluation and investigation move toward the development of a treatment plan, another tier of service providers may become involved with the child and family, especially around the provision of in-home supports (eg, services in the child's own home [and wraparound mental health services]) or placement

FIGURE 12.1
Flow of a joint investigation once the case meets the necessary criteria.[a]

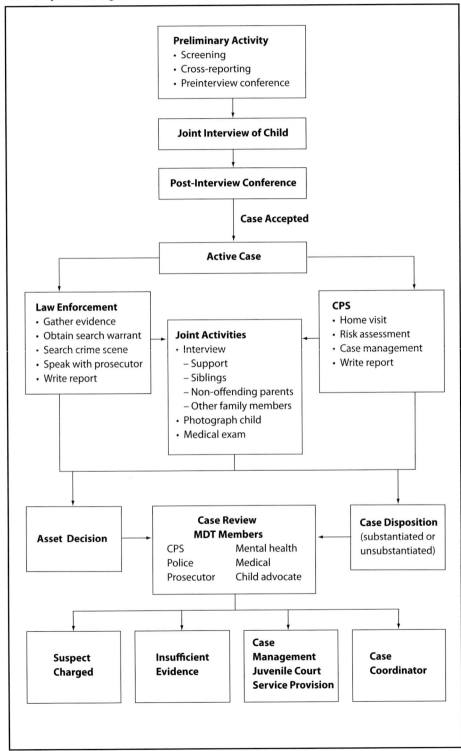

Abbreviations: CPS, child protective services; MDT, multidisciplinary team.
[a]Adapted from Sheppard DI, Zangrillo PA. Coordinating investigations of child abuse. *Public Welfare.* 1996;54:21–31.

TABLE 12.3
Child Protective Services Process[a]

Phase	Description
Intake *"getting the report"*	• Receive reports of suspected child maltreatment. • Evaluate reports against statutory and agency guidelines. • Determine urgency of response. • Educate reporters on state laws, agency guidelines, and child protective services functions.
Initial assessment/investigation *"gathering enough information and setting the tone"*	• Gather sufficient information to determine (1) whether child maltreatment has occurred, (2) risk for future maltreatment, (3) safety of the child in the home and services needed to reduce risk.
Family assessment *"building a complete picture"*	• Obtain information about nature, extent, and causes of risk. • Gain deeper understanding of how abuse occurred. • Analyze personal and environmental factors that contributed to abuse.

Case planning
"developing effective strategies"
resulted in child maltreatment
	• Determine strategies to change conditions and behaviors that
	  • Collaborate on planning when possible.
	  • Involve court when necessary.

Service provision *"implementing the plan"*	• Implement care plans. • Arrange, provide, and/or coordinate delivery of services to child and family.
Evaluation of family progress and case closure *"making sure everything is working as planned"*	• Monitor on an ongoing basis the child's safety, achievement of treatment goals, risk reduction, and success in child's and family's needs.

[a] Adapted from DePanfilis D, Salus MK. *Child Protective Services: A Guide for Caseworkers*. Washington, DC: US Department of Health and Human Services, National Center on Child Abuse and Neglect; 1992a.

in substitute care (eg, foster care and kinship care settings). Interfacing with the education system may also be an important part of the treatment plan as service plans take shape that may include early intervention, special education, and after-school and recreational enrichment activities.

Ideally, care and services are rendered in a family-centered approach that seeks to empower the family and that incorporates any strengths and abilities that the family may bring to the situation.[8] In addition, services are best delivered in a culturally competent manner that respects the cultural and ethnic diversity of the family and community.[53,54] Ideally, the perspectives of the various cultural groups that are being served in a given community should be incorporated into MDT deliberations in a substantive way, especially in the area of risk assessment.[55,56]

Creating Services Where None Exist

Some communities may not have a full range of services available to deal with all of the various aspects of cases of child maltreatment, or professionals in a given area may not be comfortable with the existing maltreatment programs. This situation, rather than engendering despair, must be seen instead as an opportunity to design and implement a set of necessary services. Inevitably, a number of challenges will arise as this effort unfolds. Each challenge will need to be faced as the community's interdisciplinary resources are identified and

marshaled to help children and families affected by sexual abuse.

A guide designed to help communities form MDTs[13] points out that the starting point should be a focus on the needs of the community's children and families. Necessary first steps to forming an MDT include the following[13]:

- Identification of members who are committed to a team approach and who are supported by their agency/employer to participate in the interdisciplinary approach to champion the effort
- Members' willingness to have an initial meeting where sharing of previous experiences with child maltreatment and teamwork occurs
- The capacity to develop a mission statement that addresses purpose, scope of activities, and agreed-on guiding principles
- The ability to create standards and written protocols that will guide practice and that specify cases to be considered, the responsibilities of each professional and agency, and agreed-on procedures for different aspects of the case

National organizations such as the National Children's Alliance (www.nca.org), the American Prosecutors Research Institute (www.apri.org), Child Welfare League of America (www.cwla.org), and others can be a resource to developing an MDT and can assist in identifying strategies to accomplish this goal. Statewide coordination of child advocacy centers also exists, and these local

TABLE 12.4
Team Composition/Membership Alternatives[a]

Organizing Alternative	Composition/Membership
Discipline	• Social worker • Physician • Psychiatrist/psychologist • Attorney • Human development specialist • Law enforcement • Nurse
Agency	• Child protective service agency • Medical center • Mental health center • Legal services • School system • Police department • Health department
Function	• Family therapist (eg, social worker, psychologist) • Community organization/social systems/resources

[a] Adapted from Kaminer BB, Crowe AH, Buddie-Giltner L. The prevalence and characteristics of multidisciplinary teams for child abuse and neglect: a national survey. In: Bross DC, Krugman RD, Lenherr MR, Rosenberg DA, Schmitt BD, eds. *The New Child Protection Team Handbook*. New York, NY: Garland; 1988:548–581.

organizations can be a tremendous resource in establishing an MDT and assisting in the identification of key stakeholders in the local community.

Especially in the initial establishment of an MDT, its success is correlated with the priority of consistently using conflict resolution practices among the participants and participating agencies. What is needed is an environment of mutual respect that recognizes both the complexity of working with child abuse cases and the valuable contribution that each professional and organization makes while serving on the MDT. Additionally, the MDT is best served by periodic evaluation, both internal and external, that serves as an ideal opportunity for self-renewal and change.[13]

When doing the initial planning for a team, several options are possible in terms of identifying who should be represented in MDTs.[57] One of 3 basic alternatives—discipline, organization, or function—can be used as a guiding principle when forming an MDT. Table 12.4 describes each composition/membership alternative. Regardless of how the membership is determined, strong community affiliations that respect the contributions of each entity and limit the barriers and turf issues common to MDTs are essential to bind the team together through the difficulties of working with child maltreatment.[5,6]

Joint training for team members has also been found to be an effective team-building strategy that creates opportunities for discussion and a sense of shared purpose among team members.[13] Some of the other benefits to joint training include common understanding of issues facing the team, practice in shared problem-solving, and the chance to openly clarify the roles and responsibilities of each team member and participating agency.

Early in the history of interdisciplinary work, the problem of tremendous physical and emotional fatigue was identified. Contributing factors such as vicarious trauma (emotional experiences of the professional as a result of repeated, chronic exposure to trauma experiences of those being served) and general work-related exhaustion can sometimes overwhelm the professionals working in direct service.[58] *Burnout,* as it is now called, is a syndrome of physical and emotional exhaustion, depersonalization, and a sense of reduced personal accomplishment that arises gradually from heavy caseloads, unrealistic expectations, increased isolation, and a social environment that fails to adequately support professionals working in a difficult area such as child maltreatment.[13,58,59] If left unattended, staff turnover, cynicism, and work-related ineffectiveness are likely results.[13,18] Preventing professional burnout remains a major challenge to teams

that provide services to children and families and that are struggling to deal with the problem of child maltreatment. A high level of compassion satisfaction (fulfillment in helping others and positive collegial relationships) and being a part of a well-functioning team can help shoulder the emotional burdens of the pressing caseloads and promote an environment that encourages team members and mitigates burnout.[58] Efforts to create organizational conditions that facilitate the processing of the negative impact of daily job stress becomes an important issue for all MDTs to ensure is addressed.[60] Many teams have used organized retreats to address this issue by creating an environment where social gatherings with team members is encouraged. This can assist in promoting a healthy work environment and reduce the risks of burnout by team members.

Directions for the Future

While there exists a rich history of MDTs over the last 4 decades, to best improve on the MDT model over the next 10 years there are many issues that still need to be addressed,[15] such as

- Consistent operational definitions of short- and long-term MDT outcomes
- Descriptive quantitative studies that evaluate the variations in MDT structure, design, and concept
- Descriptive qualitative studies of the MDT collaborative process
- Comparative quasi-experimental studies of MDT effectiveness in the relevant outcome domains (child protection, law enforcement, medical, psychological)

- Studies that provide analyses that will control for the effects of confounding issues such as differential case assignment, variations in the MDT structure, and professional composition
- Studies that are "ethnographic" in focus (ie, take into account the variations in organizational and community cultural environments)

Conclusion

Interdisciplinary approaches that foster professional collaboration in addressing child maltreatment remain the ideal in serving children and families dealing with this problem. Over the decades, professional experience has pointed consistently to the benefits of joint investigations that help coordinate community resources directed at evaluating and treating the child and family. Fostering teamwork is difficult with some readily identified barriers, but the benefits to the child, family, and professionals make the effort well worth the commitment it takes to have an effective MDT in place. Owing to the additional complexity of child sexual abuse, a variety of disciplines will need to work together to serve the child and family. This work is best done in a coordinated, collaborative manner in which the contributions of each participating discipline and agency are understood and recognized as valuable. Communities that do not have functioning teams present opportunities for committed professionals to partner around building such valuable resources to serve children and families in need.

References

1. Schmitt BD, ed. *The Child Protection Team Handbook.* New York, NY: Garland; 1978
2. Wilson EP. Multidisciplinary approach to child protection. In: Ludwig S, Kornbert AE, eds. *Child Abuse: A Medical Reference.* 2nd ed. New York, NY: Churchill Livingstone; 1992:79–84
3. DePanfilis D, Salus MK. *Child Protective Services: A Guide for Caseworkers.* Washington, DC: US Department of Health and Human Services, National Center on Child Abuse and Neglect; 1992a
4. Ludwig S. A multidisciplinary approach to child abuse. *Nurs Clin North Am.* 1981;16:161–165
5. DePanfilis D, Salus MK. *A Coordinated Response to Child Abuse and Neglect: A Basic Manual.* Washington, DC: US Department of Health and Human Services, National Center on Child Abuse and Neglect; 1992b
6. Helfer RE, Schmidt R. The community-based child abuse and neglect program. In: Helfer RE, Kempe CH, eds. *Child Abuse and Neglect: The Family and the Community.* Cambridge, MA: Ballinger; 1976:229–265
7. Siegler EL, Whitney FW, eds. *Nurse-Physician Collaboration.* New York, NY: Springer; 1994
8. Dubowitz H, DePanfilis D, eds. *Handbook for Child Protection Practice.* Thousand Oaks, CA: Sage; 2000
9. O'Neil EH. *Health Professions Education for the Future: Schools in Service to the Nations.* San Francisco, CA: Pew Health Professions Commission; 1993
10. Bassoff BZ, Ludwig S. Interdisciplinary education for health care professionals. *Health Soc Work.* 1979;4(2):58–71
11. Kindig DA. Interdisciplinary education for primary health care team delivery. *J Med Educ.* 1975;50:97–110
12. Shugars DA, O'Neill EH, Bader JD. *Healthy America: Practitioners for 2005: An Agenda for Action for U.S. Health Professional Schools.* Durham, NC: Pew Health Professions Commission; 1991

13. Ells M. *Forming a Multidisciplinary Team to Investigate Child Abuse*. Rockville, MD: Office of Juvenile Justice and Delinquency Prevention; 2000. http://www.ncjrs.org/html/ojjdp/portable_guides/forming/contents.html. Accessed March 29, 2007

14. Bross DC, Krugman RD, Lenherr MR, Rosenberg DA, Schmitt BD, eds. *The New Child Protection Team Handbook*. New York, NY: Garland; 1988

15. Lalayants M, Epstein I. Evaluating multidisciplinary child abuse and neglect teams: a research agenda. *Child Welfare League Am*. 2005;84:433–458

16. Ludwig S. Team teaching of the multidisciplinary approach. *Child Abuse Negl*. 1977;1:381–386

17. Dinsmore J. *Joint Investigations of Child Abuse: Report of a Symposium*. Washington, DC: US Department of Health and Human Services, National Center on Child Abuse and Neglect; 1993

18. Pence D, Wilson C. *Team Investigation of Child Sexual Abuse: The Uneasy Alliance*. Thousand Oaks, CA: Sage; 1994

19. Rowe DS, Leonard MF, Seashore MR, Lewiston NJ, Anderson FP. A hospital program for the detection and registration of abused and neglected children. *N Engl J Med*. 1970;282:950–952

20. Wilson EP, Hilbert D. A hospital team approach to child abuse. *Penn Med*. 1973;September:419–425

21. Jones LM, Cross, TP, Walsh WA, Simone M. Criminal investigations of child abuse. The research behind "best practices." *Trauma Violence Abuse* 2005;6:254–268

22. US Department of Health and Human Services. *Authorization for Multidisciplinary Team* (Child Abuse and Neglect State Statutes Element: No. 15). Washington, DC: Children's Bureau; 1999

23. US Department of Health and Human Services. *Reporting Laws: Cross-Reporting Among Systems* (Child Abuse and Neglect Statute Series). Washington, DC: Children's Bureau; 2002

24. Green FC. Child abuse and neglect: a priority problem for the private physician. *Pediatr Clin North Am*. 1975;22:329–339

25. Sheppard DI, Zangrillo PA. Coordinating investigations of child abuse. *Public Welfare*. 1996;54:21–31

26. Jackson SL. A USA national survey of program services provided by child advocacy centers. *Child Abuse Negl*. 2004;28:411–421

27. Faller KC, Henry J. Child sexual abuse: a case study in community collaboration. *Chlid Abuse Negl*. 2000;24:1215–1225

28. Snell L. *Child Advocacy Centers: One Stop on the Road to Performance-Based Child Protection*. Los Angeles, CA: Reason Public Policy Institute; 2003:1–25. Policy Study No.306. http://www.reason.org/ps306.pdf

29. Simone M, Cross TP, Jones LM, Walsh WA. Children's advocacy centers: understanding of a phenomenon. In: Kendall-Tackett KA, Giacomoni SM, eds. *Child Victimization*. Kingston, NJ: Civic Research Institute; 2005:22-1–22-24

30. Smith DW. Witte TH, Fricker-Elhai AE. Service outcomes in physical and sexual abuse cases: a comparison of child advocacy cener-based and standard services. *Child Maltreat*. 2006;11:354–360

31. Walsh W, Jones L, Cross T. Children's advocacy centers: one philosophy, many models. *APSAC Advisor*. 2003;15:3–7

32. Berliner L, Conte JR. The effects of disclosure and intervention on sexually abused children. *Child Abuse Negl*. 1995;19(3):371–384

33. Tedesco JF, Schnell SV. Children's reactions to sex abuse investigation and litigation. *Child Abuse Negl*. 1987;11(2):267–272

34. Henry J. System intervention trauma to child sexual abuse victims following disclosure. *J Interpers Violence*. 1997;12:499–512

35. Bruck M, Ceci SJ, Hembrooke H. Reliability and credibility of young children's reports: from research to policy and practice. *Am Psychol*. 1998;53:136–151

36. Lanning KV. Criminal investigation of sexual victimization of children. In: Myers JEB, Berliner L, Briere J, Hendrix CT, Jenny C, Reid TA, eds. *The APSAC Handbook on Child Maltreatment.* 2nd ed. Thousand Oaks, CA: Sage; 2002:329–347

37. Cross, TP, Jones LM, Walsh WA, Simone M. Multi-Site Evaluation of Children's Advocacy Centers (CACs). Crimes Against Children Research Center Web Site. www.unh.edu/ccrc/multi-site_evaluation_children.html

38. Sands RG, Stafford J, McClelland M. "I beg to differ": conflict in the interdisciplinary team. *Soc Work Health Care.* 1990;14(3):55–72

39. Baglow LJ. A multidimensional model for treatment of child abuse: a framework for cooperation. *Child Abuse Negl.* 1990;14:387–395

40. Fargason CA, Barnes D, Schneider D, Galloway BW. Enhancing multi-agency collaboration in the management of child sexual abuse. *Child Abuse Negl.* 1994;18:859–869

41. Kellogg N, Commitee on Child Abuse and Neglect. The evaluation of sexual abuse in children. *Pediatrics.* 2005;116:506–512

42. Palusci VJ, Cox EO, Cyrus TA, Heartwell SW, Vandervort FE, Pott ES. Medical assessment and legal oucome in child sexual abuse. *Arch Pediatr Adolesc Med.* 1999;153:388–392

43. Elliot NA, Carnes NC. Reactions to non-offending parents to the sexual abuse of their child: a review of the literature. *Child Maltreat.* 2001;6:314–331

44. Cohen JA, Deblinger E, Mannarino AP, Steer RA. A multisite, randomized controlled trial for children with sexual abuse-related PTSD symptoms. *J Am Acad Child Adolesc Psychiatry.* 2004;43:393–342

45. Cohen JA, Mannarino AP, Knudsen K. Treating sexually abused children: 1 year follow-up of a randomized control trial. *Child Abuse Negl.* 2005;29:135–145

46. Deblinger E, Stauffer LB, Steer RA. Comparative efficacies of supportive and cogintive behavioral group therapies for young children who have been sexually abused and their non-offending mothers. *Child Maltreat.* 2001;6:332–343

47. Spacarelli S, Kim S. Resilience criteria and factors associated with resilience in sexually abused girls. *Child Abuse Negl.* 1995;19:1171–1182

48. Morrison NC, Clavenna-Valleroy J. Perceptions of maternal support as related to self-concept and self-report of depression in sexually abused female adolescents. *J Child Sex Abuse.* 1998;7:23–40

49. Elliot DM, Briere J. Forensic sexual abuse evaluations of older children: disclosures and symptomatology. *Behav Sci Law.* 1994;12:261–277

50. Lawson L, Chaffin M. False negatives in sexual abuse dislcolsure interviews: incidence and influence of caretakers' belief in abuse in cases of accidental abuse discovery by diagnosis of STD. *J Interpers Violence.* 1992;7:532–542

51. Pence D, Everson MD, Wilson C, American Professional Society on the Abuse of Children Task Force on Investigative Interviews in Cases of Alleged Child Abuse. Investigative interviewing in cases of alleged child abuse. American Professional Society on the Abuse of Children Practice Guidelines, 2002. http://www.nca-online.org/pages/page.asp?page_id=4032

52. Sorenson E, Bottoms B, Perona A. *Handbook on Intake and Forensic Interviewing in the Children's Advocacy Center Setting.* Washington, DC: National Children's Alliance, US Department of Justice Office of Juvenile Justice and Delinquency Prevention; 1997

53. Callister LC. What the literature has taught us about culturally competent care of women and children. *MCN Am J Maternal Child Nurs.* 2005;30:380–388

54. Korbin JE. Culture and child maltreatment: cultural competence and beyond. *Child Abuse Negl.* 2002;26:637–644

55. Brissett-Chapman S. Child protection risk assessment and African American children: cultural ramifications for families and communities. *Child Welfare.* 1997a;76(1):45–63

56. Brissett-Chapman S. The culture factor in CPS: essential or elusive? In: *Decision making in Children's Protective Services: Advancing the State of the Art.* Charlotte, NC: Action for Child Protection; 1997b:75–91

57. Kaminer BB, Crowe AH, Buddie-Giltner L. The prevalence and characteristics of multidisciplinary teams for child abuse and neglect: a national survey. In: Bross DC, Krugman RD, Lenherr MR, Rosenberg DA, Schmitt BD, eds. *The New Child Protection Team Handbook.* New York, NY: Garland; 1988:548–581

58. Conrad D, Kellar-Guenther Y. Compassion fatigue, burnout, and compassion satisfaction among Colorado child protection workers. *Child Abuse Negl.* 2006;30:1071–1080

59. Lewandowski CA. Organizational factors contributing to worker frustration: the precursor to burnout. *J Soc Welfare.* 2003;30:175–185

60. DePanfilis D. Compassion fatigue, burnout, and compassion satisfaction: implication for retention of workers. *Child Abuse Negl.* 2006;30:1067–1069

Chapter 13

Legal Issues in the Medical Evaluation of Child Sexual Abuse

John E. B. Myers

Many areas of medical practice interface with the law, and this is certainly true with child sexual abuse. This chapter will discuss 4 important influences of law on medical practice with sexually abused children: the duty to report suspected child abuse to authorities, the important role that professionals play in documenting verbal evidence of abuse, the complex issue of confidentiality, and the procedures governing expert testimony.

Reporting Suspected Child Abuse

The child abuse reporting laws in every state require professionals who interact with children to report suspected child abuse. Child sexual abuse differs only from other forms of abuse by the constructs of its presentation, which are generally limited to behaviors and/or statements on the part of the child/caretaker in the absence of acute or healed injury. Without the obvious indicia of injury seen in suspected physical abuse, knowing whether a child has been sexually abused at the time of presentation may present special challenges for reporting.

The reporting obligation embraces physicians, dentists, nurses, and other medical professionals. Also included are mental health professionals, teachers, law enforcement officers, social workers, and child care professionals. Kalichman[1] wrote, "Across states, there are nearly 40 different professions specifically named in mandatory reporting laws," including animal control officers and photographic film processors.

The duty to report suspected abuse is triggered when a professional possesses the level of suspicion specified in the reporting law. Reporting laws differ slightly in the words used to describe the triggering level of suspicion. Common phrases include "cause to believe," "reasonable cause to believe," "known or suspected abuse," and "observation or examination which discloses evidence of abuse." Although the wording differs, the basic thrust of reporting laws is the same across the United States: A report is mandated when a professional has information that would lead a competent professional to believe abuse is reasonably likely. Whether the triggering level of suspicion exists depends on the facts of the case interpreted through the lens of experience and judgment.

Although it is sometimes difficult to determine when the triggering level of suspicion exists, one thing is clear: The reporting law does not require the professional to be certain that abuse occurred. Reporting is triggered by suspicion, not certainty. A professional who postpones reporting until all doubt is eliminated violates the reporting law. Moreover, a mandated reporter is required to report suspected abuse whether or not the professional believes reporting is wise. When maltreatment is suspected, reporting is mandatory, not discretionary.

The reporting law leaves final decisions about whether abuse occurred to investigating authorities, not reporters. Thus Kalichman[1] advised professionals "not to investigate the occurrence of child abuse by engaging in activities outside of ordinary professional roles." Zellman and Faller[2] added that professionals should report suspicions and leave investigation to the authorities. This is not to say that professionals ask no questions. Alternatives to abuse are considered. The point is that in-depth

investigation and decision-making about abuse is reserved for the authorities, not the reporter. Once the triggering level of suspicion is reached, the reporter turns the matter over to child protection.

Confidentiality and the Duty to Report

Professionals have ethical and legal duties to protect confidential information. Generally, a patient must consent to the release of confidential information. When the patient is a child, parents or caretakers consent to the release of confidential information. For mandated reporters, however, the child abuse reporting law supersedes confidentiality. A professional must report despite the fact that reporting requires the release of confidential information to authorities. Even so, the reporting law does not completely abrogate confidentiality. Generally, disclosure should be limited to information required by the reporting law. Confidential information that is not required by law to be disclosed should be protected.

Liability of Reporters

Liability for Failure to Report
Intentional failure to report suspected child abuse is a crime in most states. In addition to criminal liability, if a mandated reporter does not report suspected abuse and the child is further abused or killed, the professional can be sued for malpractice if reporting the original suspicion would have prevented the further abuse.[3] Several states have laws that specifically authorize lawsuits

against professionals who willfully fail to report.

Liability for Reporting

In a small number of cases, angry parents sue the professional who reported the parents to child protective services (CPS).[4] Most such lawsuits are dismissed because the child abuse reporting law gives professionals immunity from liability.

Immunity From Liability

The child abuse reporting law provides immunity from liability for professionals who report suspected child abuse, but professionals should understand what immunity does and does not do. Immunity does not prohibit an angry parent from suing. Rather, immunity gives a professional a way out of a lawsuit after the suit is filed. Immunity is like an escape hatch. If a lawsuit is filed, the judge decides whether immunity applies. If so, the professional can escape from the lawsuit at an early stage, usually long before a trial. Although immunity does not directly prohibit angry parents from suing, immunity often has the indirect effect of preventing lawsuits. The attorney working with the parents explains that immunity will probably defeat the lawsuit, and the parents decide not to sue.

If a professional testifies in court in proceedings that grow out of a report (eg, criminal or juvenile court), a different kind of immunity called *witness immunity* provides protection for what the professional says in court. Immunity is complicated, and the interested reader is referred to Myers[4] for a detailed discussion.

Guidelines Regarding Reporting

In his book on reporting, Kalichman[1] offers advice for mandated reporters.

- Knowledge of state laws regarding requirements to report suspected child maltreatment is necessary for all mandated reporters.
- Treatment and research professionals need standard informed consent procedures that detail clearly the conditions under which confidentiality is limited.
- Disclosures of child abuse can be interpreted as evidence of maltreatment and should surpass reporting thresholds.
- Suspicions of child maltreatment based on behavioral or physical indicators that do not seem to warrant reporting require close evaluation before reporting can be dismissed completely.
- Professionals operate within their areas of competence and defined professional roles and should not overstep their limitations to verify the occurrence of child abuse.
- Parents or guardians must be informed of a report before it is filed unless doing so would endanger the welfare of the child or children.
- Professionals should keep thorough and detailed records of information released in a report.
- Professionals are expected to follow up on reports to the child protection system.

- When professionals do not report suspected child maltreatment because they have caused a report to be filed by someone else, they must follow up on the case and verify that a report was filed with the child protection system.
- Cases of suspected child abuse that do not surpass reporting criteria should be discussed with a colleague to achieve some degree of objective reliability in reporting decisions.
- Training in recognizing signs of child maltreatment should be obtained by all human service professionals to the degree to which they have potential contact with abused children or abusive adults.[5]

Verbal Evidence of Abuse—Hearsay

Medical professionals are keenly aware of the forensic importance of medical and laboratory evidence of sexual abuse. Many professionals, however, are less cognizant of the forensic importance of children's words describing abuse. When a child's words are properly documented, the words may be admissible in court to prove the abuse (ie, the child's words are legal evidence). In many cases the child's statements to professionals are the most compelling evidence of maltreatment. Suppose, for example, that while 4-year-old Beth is being examined by a physician, the child points to her genital area and says, "Daddy put his pee-pee in me down there. Then he took it out and shook it up and down and white stuff came out." Beth's words are powerful evidence of abuse. In criminal

proceedings against Beth's father, the prosecutor calls the examining physician as a witness and asks the physician to repeat Beth's words and to describe her gesture. Before the doctor can speak, however, the defense attorney objects that Beth's words and gesture are hearsay. The rule in all states is that hearsay statements are inadmissible unless the statements meet the requirements of an exception to the rule against hearsay.

To determine whether Beth's words are hearsay, the judge analyzes the words according to the following definition. A child's words are hearsay when (a) the child's words were intended by the child to describe something that happened (eg, abuse), (b) the child's words were spoken before the court proceeding at which the words are repeated by someone who heard the child speak, and (c) the child's words are offered in court to prove that what the child said actually happened (ie, there is a match between the child's words and what the words are offered in court to prove).

Analysis of Beth's words reveals that they are hearsay. First, Beth intended to describe something that happened. Second, Beth made her statement before the proceeding where the prosecutor asks the physician to repeat Beth's words. Finally, the prosecutor is offering Beth's words to prove that what Beth said actually happened. Beth's words are hearsay because there is a match between her words and what the words are offered to prove. Attorneys put it this way: Beth's words are offered to prove the truth of the matter asserted by the words.

Beth's words are not the only hearsay, however. Her gesture pointing to her genital area also is hearsay. The gesture was nonverbal communication intended by Beth to describe abuse. The judge will sustain the defense attorney's hearsay objection unless the prosecutor persuades the judge that Beth's words and gesture meet the requirements of an exception to the rule against hearsay. In Beth's case, as in many other child abuse cases, the prosecutor's ability to convince the judge that Beth's hearsay statement meets the requirements of an exception to the hearsay rule depends as much on the documentation of the physician as on the legal acumen of the prosecutor. If the doctor knew what to document when Beth disclosed abuse, the prosecutor has a good chance of persuading the judge to allow the doctor to repeat Beth's words and gesture.

Exceptions to the Hearsay Rules

Although there are more than 30 exceptions to the rule against hearsay, only a few exceptions play a day-to-day role in child abuse litigation.

The Excited Utterance Exception

An excited utterance is a hearsay statement that relates to or describes a startling event. The statement must be made while the child is under the emotional stress caused by the startling event. The theory behind the excited utterance exception is that statements made under significant stress are unlikely to be lies. All states have a version of the excited utterance exception. The following factors are considered by the judge in determining whether a hearsay statement is an excited utterance.

Nature of the Event

Some events are more startling than others, and the judge considers the likely impact a particular event would have on a child of similar age and experience. In most cases, sexual or physical abuse is sufficiently startling to satisfy the excited utterance exception.

Amount of Time Elapsed Between the Startling Event and the Child's Statement Relating to the Event

The more time that passes between a startling event and a child's statement describing the event, the less likely a judge is to conclude that the statement is an excited utterance. Although passage of time is important, elapsed time is not dispositive. Judges have approved delays ranging from a few minutes to many hours. The medical professional should document as precisely as possible how much time passed between the abuse and the child's statement—minutes count.

Indications the Child Was Emotionally Upset When the Child Spoke

The judge considers whether the child was crying, frightened, or otherwise upset when the statement was made. If the child was injured or in pain, the judge is more likely to find an excited utterance.

Child's Speech Pattern

In some cases the way a child speaks, such as pressured or hurried speech, indicates excitement.

Extent to Which the Child's Statement Was Spontaneous

Spontaneity is a key factor in the excited utterance exception. The more spontaneous the statement, the more likely it meets the requirements of the exception.

Questions Used to Elicit the Child's Statement

Asking questions does not necessarily destroy the spontaneity required for the excited utterance exception. As questions become suggestive, however, spontaneity may dissipate, undermining applicability of the exception.

First Safe Opportunity

In many cases, abused children remain under the control of the abuser for hours or days after an abusive incident. When the child is finally released to a trusted adult, the child has the first safe opportunity to disclose what happened. A child's statement at the first safe opportunity may qualify as an excited utterance even though considerable time has elapsed since the abuse occurred.

Rekindled Excitement

A startling event such as abuse may be followed by a period of calm during which excitement abates. If the child is subsequently exposed to a stimulus that reminds the child of the startling event, the child's excitement may be rekindled. Rekindled excitement sometimes satisfies the excited utterance exception to the rule against hearsay.

Professionals are encouraged to document the foregoing factors and any additional evidence that a child was distraught when describing maltreatment.

Medical Diagnosis or Treatment Exception

Nearly all states have a "diagnosis or treatment" exception to the hearsay rule for certain statements to professionals providing diagnostic or treatment services. The professional to whom the child speaks may be a physician, psychiatrist, psychologist, nurse, social worker, paramedic, emergency medical technician, or technician. The diagnosis or treatment exception includes the child's statements describing medical history as well as statements describing present symptoms, pain, and other sensations. The exception also includes the child's description of the cause of illness or injury.

In many cases the child is the one who makes the hearsay statements that are admissible under the diagnosis or treatment exception. Frequently, however, an adult describes the child's history and symptoms to the professional. So long as the adult's motive is to obtain treatment for the child, the adult's statements are admissible under the exception.

The primary rationale for the diagnosis or treatment exception is that hearsay statements to professionals providing diagnostic or treatment services are reliable because the patient has an incentive to be truthful with the professional. This rationale is applicable for many older children and adolescents. Some young children, however, may not understand the need for accuracy and candor with health care providers. When a child does not understand that personal well-being may be affected by the accuracy of what is said, the rationale for the diagnosis or treatment exception evaporates, and the judge may rule that the child's hearsay statement does not satisfy the exception.

The diagnosis or treatment exception has its clearest application with children receiving traditional medical care in a hospital, clinic, or physician's office. Most children have at least some understanding of doctors and nurses, and the importance of telling the clinician "what really happened." Judges are less certain about application of the diagnosis or treatment exception to psychotherapy, where the child may not understand the importance of accuracy. Yet, when there is evidence that a child understood the need for accuracy with a mental health professional, judges generally conclude that the diagnosis or treatment exception extends to psychotherapy.

To increase the probability that a child's statement describing maltreatment satisfies the diagnosis or treatment exception to the rule against hearsay, professionals are encouraged to take the following steps:

1. Discuss with the child the clinical importance of providing accurate information and of being completely forthcoming. The physician might say, "Hello, I'm Dr Jones. I'm a doctor and I'm going to give you a checkup to make sure everything is OK. While you are here today, I'll ask you some questions so I can help you. It's important for you to listen carefully to my questions. When you answer my questions, be sure to tell me everything you know. Tell me only things that really happened. Don't pretend or make things up. Your answers to questions help me to do my job as a doctor, so it is important for you to tell me only things that really happened."

2. The diagnosis or treatment exception only applies to statements that are pertinent to the professional's ability to diagnose or treat. Thus it is important to document why information disclosed by a child is pertinent to diagnosis or treatment. For example, the professional might document that after questioning the child the professional decided to test for a sexually transmitted infection (STI).

3. If the child identifies the perpetrator, the professional should document why knowing the identity of the perpetrator is pertinent to diagnosis or treatment. For example, knowing the identity of the perpetrator is important in deciding whether it is safe to send the child home. Also, the professional needs to know the perpetrator's identity if there is a possibility the child was exposed to an STI. The decision to refer a child for mental health services is influenced in some cases by the identity of the abuser, making identity pertinent.

Residual and Child Hearsay Exceptions

Most states have a hearsay exception known as a *residual exception*, which allows use in court of reliable hearsay statements that do not meet the requirements of one of the traditional exceptions (eg, excited utterance; medical diagnosis or treatment). In addition to the residual exception, most states have a special exception for reliable hearsay statements by children in child abuse cases.

When a child's hearsay statement is offered under a residual or child hearsay exception, the most important question is whether the statement is reliable. Professionals who interview, examine, and treat children play a vital role in documenting the information judges consider to determine whether children's statements are sufficiently reliable to be admitted under residual or child hearsay exceptions. Professionals should document the following.

Spontaneity

The more spontaneous a child's statement, the more likely a judge will find it reliable.

Statements Elicited by Questioning

The reliability of a child's statement may be influenced by the type of questions asked. When questions are suggestive or leading, the possibility increases that the questioner influenced the child's statement. It should be noted, however, that suggestive questions are sometimes necessary to elicit information from children, particularly when the information is embarrassing.

The smaller the number of suggestive and leading questions, the more likely a judge is to conclude that a child's statement is reliable.

Consistent Statements

Reliability may be enhanced if the child's description of abuse is consistent over time.

Child's Affect and Emotion When Hearsay Statement Was Made

When a child's emotions are consistent with the child's statement, the reliability of the statement may be enhanced.

Play or Gestures That Corroborate the Child's Hearsay Statement

The play or gestures of a young child may strengthen confidence in the child's statement. For example, the child's use of dolls may support the reliability of the child's statement.

Developmentally Unusual Sexual Knowledge

A young child's developmentally unusual knowledge of sexual acts or anatomy supports the reliability of the child's statement.

Idiosyncratic Detail

Presence in a child's statement of idiosyncratic details of sexual acts points to reliability. Jones[6] wrote, "The interview can be examined for signs of unique or distinguishing detail. This may be found both within the account of the sexual encounter and/or in unrelated recollections. Examples include children who describe smells and tastes associated with rectal, vaginal, or oral sex."

Child's Belief That Disclosure Might Lead to Punishment of the Child

Children hesitate to make statements they believe may get them in trouble. If a child believed disclosing abuse could result in punishment, confidence in the child's statement may increase.

Child's or Adult's Motive to Fabricate

Evidence that the child or an adult had or lacked a motive to fabricate affects reliability.

Medical Evidence of Abuse

The child's statement may be corroborated by medical evidence.

Changes in Child's Behavior

When a child's behavior alters in a way that corroborates the child's description of abuse, it may be appropriate to place increased confidence in the child's statement.

None of the foregoing factors are a litmus test for reliability. Judges consider the totality of circumstances to evaluate reliability, and professionals can assist the legal system by documenting anything that indicates the child was or was not telling the truth when describing abuse.

Fresh Complaint of Sexual Assault

A child's initial disclosure of sexual abuse may be admissible in court under an ancient legal doctrine called *fresh complaint of rape or sexual assault*. In most states, a child's fresh complaint is not, technically speaking, hearsay. The law of fresh complaint varies considerably across the country. In most states, a child's initial disclosure of sexual abuse may be admissible as evidence of fresh complaint or, as it is called in some states, *outcry*.

In sum, regardless of the circumstances of the disclosure, when a child presents to the doctor's office, the responsibility of the doctor is to make a diagnosis and treat appropriately. The doctors' medical history is always the cornerstone of a diagnosis and should be obtained in a manner that furthers the understanding of what a child experienced and guides the treatment. The medical history should be documented in as precise a manner as possible, capturing the child's response to the questions asked while obtaining the medical history from the child. Although most doctors would not envision their responsibility as one of "collecting evidence," when examining children in child sexual abuse cases the medical history is frequently the most compelling "evidence" (Figure 13.1).

Limits on Admissibility of Hearsay

There are 2 sources of law that limit the admission of hearsay evidence in court. First is the rule against hearsay, discussed previously, which is part of the law of evidence. Hearsay exceptions (eg, excited utterance; medical diagnosis or treatment) are also part of evidence law. Second, in addition to the law of evidence and its hearsay rule, the US Constitution places limits on hearsay. The US Constitution's Sixth Amendment contains the so-called Confrontation Clause, which provides, "In all criminal prosecutions, the accused shall enjoy the right…to be confronted with the witnesses against

FIGURE 13.1
Verbal documentation checklist that pulls together in one location
the factors professionals should consider when obtaining a medical history

---

Child's Name: _____ Date: _____ Your Name: _____ Case No. _____

_____ Document your questions. Don't paraphrase.

_____ Document child's exact words. Don't paraphrase.

_____ Did child tell anyone else? Who? When? Why? What?

All professionals document:

_____ What happened?	According to the child, what happened?
_____ Elapsed time:	How much time elapsed between the event and the child's description? (Be precise; minutes count).
_____ Emotional condition:	Child's emotional condition when child described what happened. (crying? upset? calm? excited? traumatized?)
_____ Physical condition:	Was child hurt, injured, in pain?
_____ Spontaneous?	Was the child's description spontaneous?
_____ Consistency:	If child described the event more than once, are there consistencies across descriptions?
_____ Developmentally unusual sexual knowledge or conduct:	Document any developmentally unusual sexual knowledge or behavior, including idiosyncratic details (eg, smells or tastes).
_____ Motive to lie:	Does anyone—child or adult—have a motive to lie?
_____ Reliability:	Document anything that sheds light on the reliability of the child's statement.

Ask questions about and document:

_____ Child's memory for simple events (eg, Breakfast this morning? What was on TV today?)

_____ Child's ability to communicate.

_____ Child's understanding of the difference between the truth and lies. (Don't ask children under age 9 to define "truth" and "lie." Don't ask kids to give examples of truth or lies. Don't ask kids to explain the difference between truth and lie. Do give simple examples of something that is true and something that is a lie. Then ask the child to identify which it is (eg, hold up a blue pen and say "If someone said this is red, would that be the truth or a lie?" or "If someone said this is blue, would that be the truth or a lie?").

_____ Child's understanding of the importance of telling the truth to you.

Clinical professionals providing medical or psychological diagnosis or treatment

_____ Inform child of your clinical purpose (eg, "I'm going to give you a checkup to make sure you are healthy." "My job is talking to kids to help them with their problems.").

_____ Inform child of the clinical reasons why it is important for the child to tell the truth to you (eg, "I need you to tell me only true things, only things that really happened. I need you to tell me only true things so I can help you.").

_____ Document anything indicating the child understood your clinical role, the clinical nature of what you did or said, and why it was clinically important for the child to tell the truth to you.

_____ Document why what the child told you was pertinent to your ability to diagnose or treat the child.

_____ If child identified the perpetrator, document why knowing identity was pertinent to your ability to diagnose or treat the child.

---

him." The US Supreme Court has interpreted the Confrontation Clause to limit the types of hearsay that can be used against defendants in criminal cases. To be admissible against the defendant in a criminal trial, hearsay must satisfy *both* the Confrontation Clause and an exception to the rule against hearsay. In some situations, hearsay that fits an exception is inadmissible because it violates the Confrontation Clause.

Two decisions of the US Supreme Court—*Crawford v Washington*[7] and *Davis v Washington*[8]—define the impact of the Confrontation Clause on the admission of hearsay in criminal cases. Before discussing *Crawford* and *Davis*, however, it is important to mention 2 subsidiary principles. First, if the child who made a hearsay statement is able to testify in court and be cross-examined by the defense attorney about the hearsay, then the Confrontation Clause is satisfied and the child's hearsay can be admitted without affront to the Confrontation Clause. (Of course, the child's hearsay still has to meet the requirements of an exception to the rule against hearsay.) Second, the constitutional limits on hearsay apply only in criminal cases. Thus the Confrontation Clause is inapplicable in civil proceedings such as child protection proceedings in juvenile or family court, and in litigation to terminate parental rights.

In a criminal prosecution when the prosecutor offers hearsay against the defendant, the Confrontation Clause, as interpreted in *Crawford* and *Davis*, comes into play. As stated previously, if the child can testify and be cross-examined about the hearsay, the Confrontation Clause is satisfied. However, when the child is unable to testify in court, the question under *Crawford* and *Davis* is whether the child's hearsay statement was "testimonial" when it was made. If the child's hearsay was testimonial, then it cannot be admitted against the defendant. On the other hand, if the child's statement was non-testimonial, then the Confrontation Clause places no limit on use of the statement against the defendant.

Under *Crawford* and *Davis*, the word *testimonial* is a term of art. A hearsay statement can be testimonial even though it bears no resemblance to testimony in court. Hearsay is testimonial when a reasonable person in the position of the speaker would understand that the statement is of a type that may find its way into later court proceedings. For example, a person's answers to questions during formal police interrogation at a police station are testimonial hearsay because a reasonable person in that situation understands that the police are gathering evidence for possible use in court.

Children's hearsay statements to parents, relatives, teachers, friends, foster parents, babysitters, and other non–law enforcement individuals typically are non-testimonial. Statements to child protection social workers are sometimes testimonial, sometimes not. A statement to a social worker is testimonial if the social worker's primary purpose in questioning a child is to conduct an investigation.

Children's statements during forensic interviews at child advocacy centers are testimonial. The Minnesota Supreme Court held to the contrary in *State v Bobadilla*,[9] but the Minnesota court's ruling is out of step with other courts.

Although many statements to police officers are testimonial, some are not. The answer depends on the circumstances in which the officer questions the child. Statements to police are most likely to be non-testimonial when the police ask questions in the context of an ongoing emergency. Thus a police officer's initial questions on arriving at the scene in response to a 911 call are typically intended to assess the situation, see whether medical help is necessary, and determine whether the victim and the officer are safe. Answers to such initial questions are typically non-testimonal. As the initial emergency abates, and the officer's questions turn from securing the scene to gathering evidence, statements become testimonial. In deciding whether statements to police officers are testimonial, judges consider (1) Is there an ongoing emergency? (2) Is the child safe or in present danger? (3) Is medical assistance necessary? (4) Is the child alone or protected by others? (5) Is the child seeking help? (6) Is the child describing events that are happening as the child speaks or is the child describing past events? (7) How much time has elapsed since the events transpired? (8) What is the level of formality of the questioning?

Hearsay statements to physicians, nurses, and other medical professionals are non-testimonial when the professional's primary motive for questioning the child is clinical.[10] The fact that the professional is aware of the forensic implications of communicating with children about maltreatment does not alter this conclusion. The cases described in the remainder of this paragraph provide insight into the reasoning judges employ to determine whether hearsay statements to medical professionals are testimonial. In *State v Moses*,[11] a domestic violence victim's statements to a doctor were non-testimonial. The court wrote, "Courts that have addressed *Crawford's* impact on statements admitted under the medical diagnosis or treatment exception focus on the purpose of the [victim's] encounter with the health care provider.... In cases where courts have found such statements to health care providers are testimonial, the prosecutorial purpose of the medical examination has been clear." In *State v Griner*,[12] 4-year-old Chase made hearsay statements to a hospital admitting nurse. The court wrote, "Chase's statements to [nurse] Kaur were not testimonial. Kaur examined and questioned Chase as a routine preliminary procedure necessary prior to admitting him to the pediatrics ward. Kaur's questioning of Chase was not the equivalent of a police interrogation. Kaur was a nurse on the pediatrics ward performing her regular duties.... Chase was unafraid, smiling, wanted to play, and told Nurse Kaur that he was not in any pain. Under the standards enunciated in *Crawford*, Chase's statements to Kaur were not testimonial." In *Commonwealth v DeOliveria*,[13] the court considered a 6-year-old's hearsay statements to a pediatrician in the emergency department. Concluding that the child's statements were non-testimonial, the court wrote, "Patricia's statements cannot persuasively be said to have been made in response to police interrogation. Although police officers were present at the hospital, there is no indication in the record that they were present during the doctor's examination of Patricia, or that they had instructed the doctor on the manner in which his examination should proceed. Nothing in the record would support a determination that the doctor acted as an agent of law enforcement. Indeed, the doctor's testimony as to his role as a physician entirely independent from law enforcement, and the judge's findings in connection with his medical evaluation of Patricia, are all to the contrary. Police presence at a hospital cannot turn questioning of a patient by a physician during a medical examination into interrogation by law enforcement." In *State v Wyble*,[14] a 3-year-old made hearsay statements while in the emergency department. Concluding that the child's statements were non-testimonial, the court wrote, "The child's statements in the emergency room, to the effect that she did not want anyone to touch her private areas, as reported by the nurse, were made in connection with the diagnosis and treatment of the redness and discomfort she was experiencing. They were related to the child's then present experience, not to past events. The child was not calm, but was distressed. While medical personnel are, of course, required to report

indications of child abuse, there were no statements made by the child about past events.... Here, [the medical professionals], according to their own testimony, stated they were not driven by the purpose of prosecution." In *Hobgood v State*,[15] a 5-year-old's statements to a therapist and a physician were non-testimonial. The court wrote, "These individuals were not working in connection with the police.... Had the police directed the victim to seek treatment from a doctor and a therapist for the purpose of discovering evidence to aid in the investigation then it might be possible for the statement to implicate the Confrontation Clause." In *Hernandez v State*,[16] the child was taken by a deputy sheriff to the child protection center at a hospital, where the child was interviewed and examined by a nurse practitioner for medical and forensic purposes. The court concluded that the child's statements to the nurse were testimonial "because the nurse was acting in concert with law enforcement in questioning the child and her parents to gather information for a potential criminal prosecution, we conclude that their statements to the nurse were testimonial." In *People v Cage*,[17] the court ruled that the fact that physicians are required to report suspected child abuse does not render statements to physicians testimonial. In sum, hearsay statements to medical providers are non-testimonial when the provider's primary purpose in questioning the child is provision of medical care.

Importance of Documentation

Medical professionals are in an excellent position to document children's hearsay statements as part and parcel of the medical history. Without careful documentation of exactly what questions are asked and exactly what children say, the professional will not likely remember months or years later when the professional is called as a witness and asked to repeat what the child said. Documentation is needed not only to preserve the child's words, but also to preserve a record of the factors indicating whether the child's hearsay statements meet the requirements of an exception to the hearsay rule and whether the statements are non-testimonial.

Confidential Records and Privileged Communications

Abused and neglected children interact with many professionals. Each professional who comes in contact with the child documents the interaction. Much of this information is confidential and must be protected from inappropriate disclosure. Confidentiality arises from 3 sources: (a) the broad ethical duty to protect confidential information, (b) laws that make certain records confidential, and (c) privileges that apply in legal proceedings.

Ethical Duty to Safeguard Confidential Information

The ethical principles of medicine, nursing, and other professions require professionals to safeguard confidential information revealed by patients.

The principles of medical ethics of the American Medical Association require physicians to "safeguard patient confidences within the constraints of the law."[18] The Hippocratic oath states, "whatsoever I shall see or hear in the course of my profession…if it be what should not be published abroad, I will never divulge, holding such things to be holy secrets." The Code of Ethics of the American Nurses Association states that nurses safeguard the patient's right to privacy by carefully protecting information of a confidential nature.[19]

Laws That Make Patient Records Confidential

Every state has laws that make certain records confidential. Some of the laws pertain to records compiled by government agencies such as CPS, public hospitals, and courts. Other laws govern records created by professionals and institutions in the private sector such as physicians, psychotherapists, and private hospitals. The federal Health Insurance Portability and Accountability Act (HIPAA) also governs the confidentiality of records.

Privileged Communications

The ethical duty to protect confidential information applies in all settings: in the clinic, the cafeteria, the courtroom—everywhere. In the narrow context of legal proceedings, however, certain professionals have an additional duty to protect confidential information. In legal proceedings the law prohibits disclosure of confidential communications between certain professionals and their patients. These laws are called *privileges.*

Unlike the expansive ethical obligation to protect confidential patient information, privileges apply only in legal proceedings. Privileges clearly apply when professionals testify in court and are asked to reveal privileged information. Privileges also apply during legal proceedings outside the courtroom. For example, in most civil cases and in some criminal cases, attorneys take pretrial depositions of potential witnesses. During a deposition, questions may be asked that call for disclosure of privileged information. If this occurs, the professional or one of the attorneys should raise the privilege issue.

Communication between a patient and a professional is privileged when 3 requirements are fulfilled. First, the communication (oral or written) must be between a patient and a professional with whom privileged communication is possible. All states have some form of physician-patient and psychotherapist-patient privilege. Not all professionals are covered by privilege statutes, however. For example, if a patient communicates with a psychotherapist who is not covered by privilege law, no privilege applies. (A privilege may apply if a therapist who is not covered by a privilege is working under the supervision of a therapist who is covered by a privilege.) Of course, the fact that a privilege does not apply does nothing to undermine the therapist's ethical duty to protect confidential information.

The second requirement for a privilege to apply is that the patient must seek professional services. The patient must consult the professional to obtain diagnosis or treatment.

The third requirement of privilege law is that the patient must intend to communicate in confidence with the professional. Privileges only cover communications that the patient intends to be confidential. The privilege covers confidential statements from the patient to the professional as well as statements by the professional to the patient. Thus privilege is a 2-way street. Privilege generally does not attach to communications the patient intends to be released to other people.

In legal proceedings the presence or absence of a privilege is important. In court, a professional may have to answer questions that require disclosure of information the professional is ethically bound to protect. By contrast, the professional generally does not have to answer questions that require disclosure of privileged information. Thus in legal proceedings, a privilege gives protection to confidentiality that is not available under the ethical duty to protect confidential information.

The fact that a third person is present when a patient discloses information may or may not eliminate the confidentiality required for privilege. The deciding factor usually is whether the third person is needed to assist the professional. For example, suppose a physician is conducting a physical examination and obtaining a medical history from a child. The presence of a nurse during the examination does not undermine the confidentiality of information revealed to the doctor. Furthermore, presence of a child's parents need not defeat privilege. Again, the important factor is whether the third person is needed to assist the professional. A privilege is not destroyed when colleagues consult about cases.

Privileged communications remain privileged when the relationship with the patient ends. In most situations, the patient's death does not end the privilege.

The privilege belongs to the patient, not the professional. In legal parlance, the patient is the "holder" of the privilege. As the privilege holder, the patient can prevent the professional from disclosing privileged information in legal proceedings. For example, suppose a treating physician is subpoenaed to testify about a patient. While the physician is on the witness stand, an attorney asks a question that calls for privileged information. At that point, the patient's attorney should object. The patient's attorney asserts the privilege on behalf of the privilege holder—the patient. The judge then decides whether a privilege applies. If the patient's attorney fails to object to a question calling for privileged information, or if the patient is not represented by an attorney, the professional may assert the privilege on behalf of the patient. Indeed, the professional has an ethical duty to assert the privilege if no one else does. The professional might address the judge, "Your Honor, I would rather not answer that question because answering would require disclosure of information I believe is privileged." When the judge learns that a privilege may exist, the judge decides whether the question should be answered.

Disclosure of Confidential and Privileged Information

This section discusses disclosure of confidential and privileged information.

Patient Consent

Patient consent plays the central role in release of confidential or privileged information. Gutheil and Appelbaum[20] observed, "With rare exceptions, identifiable data can be transmitted to third parties only with the patient's explicit consent." A competent adult may consent to release of privileged or confidential information to attorneys, courts, or anyone else. The patient's consent should be informed and voluntary. The professional should explain any disadvantages of disclosing confidential or privileged information. For example, the patient may be told that release to third persons may waive privileges that would otherwise apply.

A professional who discloses confidential or privileged information without patient consent can be sued. With an eye toward such lawsuits, Gutheil and Appelbaum[20] wrote, "It is probably wise for therapists always to require the written consent of their patients before releasing information to third parties. Written consent is advisable for at least two reasons: (1) it makes clear to both parties involved that consent has, in fact, been given; (2) if the fact, nature or timing of the consent should ever be challenged, a documentary record exists. The consent should be made a part of the patient's permanent chart."

When the patient is a child, parents normally have authority to make decisions about release of confidential and privileged information. When a parent is accused of abusing or neglecting a child, however, it may not be appropriate for the parent to make decisions regarding the child's confidential or privileged information. In the event of a conflict between the interests of the child and a parent, a judge may appoint someone else, such as a guardian ad litem, to make decisions about confidential and privileged information.

Limitations of the Physician-Patient Privilege

Privileges are not absolute. In many states, for example, the physician-patient privilege applies only in civil cases and is not applicable in criminal trials. Thus in a criminal trial confidential communications between patient and doctor that would normally be privileged may have to be revealed. The psychotherapist-client privilege generally applies in civil and criminal cases, making the psychotherapist-client broader than the physician-patient privilege.

Subpoenas

A subpoena is issued by a court, typically at the request of an attorney. A subpoena is a court order and cannot be ignored. Disobedience of a subpoena can be punished as contempt of court. The 2 types of subpoenas are a subpoena requiring an individual to appear at a designated time and place to provide testimony, called a *subpoena ad testificandum,* and a subpoena requiring a person to produce records or documents, called a *subpoena duces tecum.*

A subpoena does not override the physician-patient and psychotherapist-patient privileges. A subpoena for testimony requires the professional to appear, but the subpoena does not mean the professional has to disclose privileged information. A judge decides whether a privilege applies and whether a professional has to answer questions or release records.

Before responding to a subpoena, the professional should contact the patient or, in the case of a child, a responsible adult. The patient may desire to release confidential or privileged information.

It is often useful, with the patient's permission of course, to communicate with the attorney issuing the subpoena. In some cases, the conversation lets the attorney know the professional has nothing that can assist the attorney, and the attorney withdraws the subpoena. Even if the attorney insists on compliance with the subpoena, the conversation may clarify the limits of relevant information in the professional's possession. Care should be taken during such conversations to avoid disclosing confidential or privileged information.

If doubts exist concerning how to respond to a subpoena, consult an attorney. Legal advice should not be obtained from the attorney who issued the subpoena.

Reviewing Patient Records Before or During Testimony

When a professional is asked to testify, relevant records are reviewed to refresh the professional's memory. In some cases, the professional leaves the record at the office. In other cases the record is taken to court. Generally, it is entirely appropriate to review pertinent records before testifying. Indeed, such review is often essential for accurate and detailed testimony. Professionals should be aware, however, that reviewing records before or during testimony may compromise the confidentiality or privileged status of the records.

While a professional is on the witness stand, the attorney for the alleged perpetrator may ask whether the professional reviewed the child's record prior to coming to court. If the answer is yes, the attorney may ask the judge to order the record produced for the attorney's inspection. In most states, the judge has authority to order the record produced.

When records are reviewed *before* testifying, the judge has considerable discretion to decide whether to order disclosure of the records to the attorney for the alleged perpetrator. If the professional takes the record to court and refers to it while testifying, however, the judge is very likely to order the record disclosed.

Whether a professional reviews a child's record before or during testimony, a judge is more likely to require disclosure of non-privileged records than records that are protected by a privilege. Unfortunately, in most states, the law is unsettled regarding the impact of record review on privileged communications. With the law unsettled, steps can be taken to reduce the likelihood that reviewing records will jeopardize confidentiality or privilege.

1. It is often advisable to determine what information has already been released to the parties as part of the legal process. If the parties already have access to the entire record as part of the discovery process, then there is less reason for the professional to be concerned that their review of the record will implicate concerns about privileged or confidential records.

2. When reviewing a child's record before going to court, consider limiting review to portions of the record that are needed to prepare for testifying. Document the parts of the record reviewed and not reviewed. In this way if a judge orders the record disclosed to the attorney for the alleged perpetrator, an argument can be made that disclosure should be limited to portions of the record actually used to prepare for testifying.

3. Recall that records containing privileged communications probably have greater protection from disclosure than non-privileged records. With this distinction in mind, professionals may wish to organize records so that privileged information is maintained separately from non-privileged information. When a record that is arranged in this manner is reviewed before testifying, it is sometimes possible to avoid reviewing privileged

communications. This done, if a judge orders the record disclosed, the judge may be willing to limit disclosure to non-privileged portions of the record. Although this approach entails the burden of separating records into privileged and non-privileged sections, and may not persuade all judges, the technique is worth considering.

4. If it is necessary to take the record to court, consider taking only the portions of the record that will be useful during testimony and leaving the remainder at the office.

5. If the record is taken to court, the record can remain in the briefcase rather than be taken to the witness stand. Make no mention of the record unless it becomes necessary to refer to it while testifying. Once the record is used during testimony, the attorney for the alleged perpetrator probably has a right to inspect it.

6. If the record is taken to court and to the witness stand it may be possible to testify without referring to the record.

Legal advice should be obtained before implementing any of the foregoing suggestions. Some of the recommendations may not be permitted in some states.

Child Abuse Reporting Laws Override Confidentiality and Privilege

Child abuse reporting laws require professionals to report suspected child abuse and neglect to designated authorities. The reporting laws override the ethical duty to protect confidential client information. Additionally, the reporting requirement overrides privileges.

Although reporting laws abrogate confidentiality and privilege, abrogation usually is not complete. In many states, professionals may limit the information they report to the information required by law. Information that is not required to be reported remains confidential and/or privileged.

Psychotherapist's Duty to Warn Potential Victims About Dangerous Clients

In 1974, the California Supreme Court ruled in *Tarasoff v Regents of the University of California*[21] that a psychotherapist has a legal duty to warn the potential victim of a psychiatric patient who threatens the victim. The duty to warn overcomes both the ethical duty to protect confidential information and the psychotherapist-patient privilege. If the therapist fails to take reasonable steps to warn the victim and the patient carries out the threat, the therapist can be sued.

Emergencies

In emergencies, a professional may have little choice but to release confidential information without prior authorization from the patient. The law allows release of confidential information in genuine emergencies.

Court-Ordered Medical and Psychological Examinations

A judge may order an individual to submit to a medical or psychological evaluation to help the judge decide the

case. Because everyone knows from
the outset that the professional's report
will be shared with the judge and the
attorneys, the obligation to protect confidential information is limited, and
privileges generally do not attach.

Expert Testimony in Child Sexual Abuse Litigation

Expert testimony in child sexual abuse
litigation is provided by physicians,
nurses, psychologists, social workers,
and other professionals.

Who Qualifies as an Expert Witness

Before a professional may testify as
an expert witness, the judge must
be persuaded that the professional
possesses sufficient knowledge, skill,
experience, training, and education to
qualify as an expert. To provide the
judge information on the professional's
qualifications, the professional takes
the witness stand and answers questions about the professional's education, specialized training, and relevant
experience. Typically, the attorney who
offers a professional's testimony asks all
the questions related to qualifications.
Occasionally the judge asks questions.
The opposing attorney has the right to
question the professional in an effort to
convince the judge that the professional
should not be allowed to testify as an
expert. Such questioning by opposing
counsel is called *voir dire*. When the
professional's qualifications are
obvious, there usually is no voir dire.

Preparation for Expert Testimony

When a professional prepares to testify,
it is important to meet with the attorney

for whom the expert will testify. Pretrial conferences are ethically and
legally proper. Chadwick[22] observed,
"Face-to-face conferences between…
attorneys and [expert witnesses] are
always desirable, and rarely impossible."
During preparation the expert and the
attorney discuss questions the attorney
plans to ask as well as likely areas of
cross-examination.

Preparation includes review of relevant
records, although professionals should
keep in mind that reviewing records
can compromise confidentiality (see
previous discussion). Preparation
includes creation and discussion of any
exhibits, charts, or demonstrative aids
that will be used during testimony.

Forms of Expert Testimony

Expert testimony usually takes 1 of
3 forms: (1) an opinion, (2) a lecture
providing technical or clinical information for the judge or jury, or (3) an
answer to a hypothetical question. It is
not uncommon for expert testimony
to take more than one form.

Opinion Testimony

The most common form of expert
testimony is an opinion. Thus a
physician might opine that a child's
history and the findings of a physical
examination are consistent with sexual
abuse. An expert may offer an opinion
that a child was penetrated.

An expert must be reasonably confident
of the opinion that is offered in court.
Lawyers use the term *reasonable
certainty* to describe the necessary
degree of confidence. Unfortunately,
reasonable certainty is not well defined

in law. It is clear that experts may not speculate or guess. It is equally clear that experts do not have to be 100% certain their opinion is correct. Thus reasonable certainty lies somewhere between speculation and certainty—closer to the latter than the former.

A helpful way to assess the degree of certainty supporting expert opinion is to equate reasonable certainty with the scientific concepts of validity and reliability. Ask the following questions: In formulating my opinion did I consider all the relevant facts? Do I have a thorough understanding of the pertinent clinical and scientific principles? Did I use methods of diagnosis and assessment that are appropriate, reliable, and valid? Are my assumptions, inferences, and conclusions reasonable and supported by the data? The California Supreme Court reminds us, "Like a house built on sand, the expert's opinion is no better than the facts on which it is based."[23]

A Lecture to Educate the Jury

Experts may testify in the form of a lecture that provides the jury with information on technical, clinical, or scientific issues. This form of expert testimony is offered in sexual abuse cases when the defense attorney asserts that a child's delayed reporting, inconsistent disclosure, or recantation means the child cannot be believed. When the defense attacks a child's credibility this way, judges typically allow an expert witness to inform the jury that it is not uncommon for sexually abused children to delay reporting, provide partial or piecemeal disclosures, and recant. Equipped with this information, the jury is in a better position to evaluate the child's credibility.

The Hypothetical Question

In some cases expert testimony is elicited in response to a hypothetical question. The hypothetical question asks the expert to assume that certain facts have been established. Consider, for example, a physical abuse case in which the expert was the child's treating physician in the hospital. The attorney says, "Now doctor, let me ask you to assume that all of the following facts are true." The attorney then describes testimony by earlier witnesses regarding the child's condition and symptoms prior to hospitalization, including the child's eating, feeding, and sleeping patterns, the time when the 911 call was placed, the child's condition when the paramedics arrived, and observations made by emergency department doctors on admission. The attorney then asks the expert to consider the child's injuries and condition when the expert examined the child at the hospital. The attorney ends by asking, "Doctor, based on these facts, do you have an opinion, based on a reasonable degree of medical certainty, when the child was injured in relation to the 911 call?" Alternatively, the hypothetical question might be, "Doctor, assuming that the child had been injured by a mechanism involving violent shaking, how soon after the shaking episode would you expect the child to exhibit symptoms and what would those symptoms look like?"

Attorneys cross-examining expert witnesses often ask hypothetical questions. The cross-examiner may try to undermine the expert's opinion by presenting a hypothetical set of facts that differs from the facts described by the expert. The cross-examiner then asks, "Now doctor, if the hypothetical facts I have suggested to you turn out to be true, would that change your opinion?" Chadwick[22] observed that it is "common to encounter hypothetical questions based on hypotheses that are extremely unlikely, and the witness may need to point out the unlikelihood." When asked about a hypothetical set of facts, be reasonable, but stick to your opinion and do not commit to an answer when the facts suggested by the attorney are not accurate.

Daubert and *Frye* Hearings

Professionals have heard of *Daubert* and *Frye* hearings, but most clinicians have little idea what the terms mean. Basically, *Daubert* and *Frye* are short-hand terms for the procedure judges use to determine whether expert testimony is sufficiently valid and reliable to be used in court.

The judge presiding over a trial is re-sponsible for ensuring that expert tes-timony is sufficiently valid and reliable to warrant consideration. Judges realize that although most expert testimony is based on well-accepted science, occasions arise when novel and un-tested scientific principles underlie expert testimony or, worse, when junk science is passed off as legitimate. In trials where there is a jury, judges worry

that jurors will be over-impressed—swept away, if you will—by highly polished expert testimony that stands on shaky scientific ground. Jurors are not in a good position to critically evaluate the scientific foundation for expert testimony. Moreover, attorneys are often little better than jurors at separating scientific wheat from chaff, with the result that attorneys too often fail to expose unreliable expert testimony.

With these concerns in mind, in a 1923 case called *Frye v Unites States,*[24] the Court of Appeals for the District of Columbia fashioned a procedure to evaluate the validity and reliability of expert testimony based on novel scientific principles. In *Frye* the court ruled that expert testimony based on novel scientific principles cannot be used in court until the principles are generally accepted as valid and reliable by the scientific community. *Frye* is known as the "general acceptance" test for novel scientific evidence. When questions are raised about the validity or reliability of scientifically based expert testimony, the judge holds a hearing—a *Frye* hearing—to determine whether the principles underlying the testimony have achieved general acceptance in the scientific community.

For most of the 20th century, *Frye* was the dominant procedure in the United States for evaluating novel scientific evidence. Over the years, however, *Frye* was criticized because *Frye's* requirement of general acceptance occasionally led to the exclusion of scientific evidence that had yet to achieve general acceptance but that was nevertheless sufficiently valid and reliable for use in court. Criticism of *Frye* culminated in the United States Supreme Court's 1993 decision in *Daubert v Merrell Dow Pharaceuticals, Inc.*[25] In *Daubert,* the Supreme Court rejected *Frye* and replaced it with an expanded procedure to evaluate the validity and reliability of scientific evidence.

Under *Daubert,* the trial judge is the gatekeeper for all scientific evidence. As with *Frye,* an attorney under *Daubert* may object that expert testimony is based on invalid and unreliable scientific principles and request a hearing—now called a *Daubert* hearing. Unlike *Frye*, however, where the only issue was general acceptance, the judge conducting a *Daubert* hearing considers *all* evidence shedding light on validity and reliability.

In a *Daubert* hearing the judge considers whether the scientific principle in question has been subjected to testing for accuracy. The judge asks whether the principle has been published in peer-reviewed journals and whether the principle has a measurable error rate. Are there standards governing proper use of the principle? Finally, and borrowing from *Frye,* the judge asks whether the principle has gained general acceptance in the scientific community. A scientific principle that has yet to achieve general acceptance may never the less be sufficiently trustworthy to be used in court, but general acceptance remains an important factor in assessing validity and reliability.

The *Daubert* decision dealt with expert testimony based on science. Following *Daubert,* judges and attorneys were uncertain whether *Daubert* applied to expert testimony that combines science, clinical judgment, and subjective interpretation. In 1999 the US Supreme Court removed the uncertainty by ruling in *Kumho Tire Company, Ltd. v Carmichael*[26] that "*Daubert*'s general holding—setting forth the trial judge's 'gatekeeping' obligation—applies not only to testimony based on 'scientific' knowledge, but also to testimony based on 'technical' and 'other specialized' knowledge." In *Kumho,* the Supreme Court reiterated that the trial judge should consider all evidence shedding light on the validity and reliability of expert testimony.

The Supreme Court's rulings in *Daubert* and *Kumho* are only binding on federal courts and do not compel individual states to abandon *Frye*. As of 2008, most states had jettisoned *Frye* in favor of *Daubert.*

In most child sexual abuse cases there is no request for a *Frye* or *Daubert* hearing. The expert testifies and is cross-examined, and that is the end of it. *Frye* and *Daubert* do not come up. *Frye* or *Daubert* only arise when serious questions arise about the validity or reliability of expert testimony. A few states (eg, California and Florida) have a rule that *Frye/Daubert* do not apply to opinion testimony.

Cross-Examination and Impeachment of Expert Witnesses

Testifying begins with direct examination. During direct examination, the expert witness answers questions from the attorney who asked the expert to testify. After direct examination, the opposing attorney has the right to cross-examine the expert. Cross-examination is sometimes followed by redirect examination. Redirect examination affords the attorney who asked the expert to testify an opportunity to clarify issues that were raised on cross-examination.[27,28]

Positive and Negative Cross-Examination

Cross-examination can be broken down into 2 types: positive and negative. With positive cross-examination, the cross-examining attorney does not attack the expert. Rather, the attorney questions the expert in a positive—even friendly—way, seeking agreement from the expert on certain facts or inferences that may be helpful to the attorney's client. With negative cross-examination, by contrast, the attorney seeks to undermine (impeach) the expert's testimony.

A cross-examining attorney who plans to use negative as well as positive cross-examination typically begins with positive questioning in the hope of eliciting favorable testimony from the expert. Negative cross-examination is postponed until positive cross-examination pans out.

Master the Facts of the Case

The skilled cross-examiner masters the facts of the case and shapes questions to manipulate the witness into providing answers that favor the cross-examiner's client. To avoid being manipulated, the expert must know the facts as well as the cross-examiner.

Maintain a Calm, Professional Demeanor

The experienced expert refuses to be cajoled, dragged, or tricked into verbal sparring with the cross-examiner. The professional is at all times just that—professional. Given the aggression of some cross-examiners, it can be a challenge to maintain a calm, professional demeanor on the witness stand. Remember, however, that the jury is looking to you for guidance and wisdom. The jury wants a strong expert, but not someone who takes off the gloves and fights it out with the cross-examiner. This does not mean, of course, that the expert cannot employ pointed responses during cross-examination. The expert should express confidence when challenged and should not vacillate or equivocate in the face of attack. On the other hand, the expert should concede weak points and acknowledge conflicting evidence.

Ask for Clarification

Do not answer a question unless you fully understand it. When in doubt, ask the attorney to clarify. Such a request does not show weakness. After all, if you do not understand a question, you can bet the jury doesn't either. When a cross-examiner's question is 2 or 3 questions in one, the other attorney may object that the question is "compound." Absent an objection, it is proper for the expert to respond to the question by asking the cross-examiner which of the several questions the attorney would like answered.

Leading Questions During Cross-Examination

From the lawyer's perspective, the key to successful cross-examination is controlling what the witness says in response to the cross-examiner's questions. With the goal of "witness control" in mind, the cross-examiner asks leading—often highly leading—questions. Unlike the attorney conducting direct examination, who is not supposed to ask leading questions, the cross-examiner has free reign to ask all the leading questions the examiner desires. Indeed, some cross-examiners almost never ask non-leading questions during cross-examination.

The cross-examiner seeks to control the expert with leading questions that require short, specific answers, preferably limited to "yes" or "no." The cross-examiner keeps the witness hemmed in with leading questions, and seldom asks "why" or "how" something happened. "Why" and "how" questions relinquish control to the expert, the relinquishing of control is precisely what the cross-examiner does not want.

When an expert attempts to explain an answer to a leading question, the cross-examiner may interrupt and say, "Please just answer yes or no." If the expert persists, the cross-examiner may ask the judge to admonish the expert

to limit answers to the questions asked. Experts are understandably frustrated when an attorney thwarts efforts at clarification. It is sometimes proper to say, "Counsel, it is not possible for me to answer with a simple yes or no. May I explain myself?" Chadwick[22] advised, "When a question is posed in a strictly 'yes or no' fashion, but the correct answer is 'maybe,' the witness should find a way to express the true answer. A direct appeal to the judge may be helpful in some cases." Judges sometimes permit witnesses to amplify their opinion during cross-examination. Finally, remember that after cross-examination there is redirect examination, during which the attorney who asked you to testify is allowed to ask further questions. During redirect examination you have an opportunity to clarify matters that were left unclear during cross-examination.

Undermine the Expert's Facts, Inferences, or Conclusions

One of the most effective cross-examination techniques with expert witnesses is to get the expert to agree to the facts, inferences, and conclusions that support the expert's opinion, and then to dispute or undermine one or more of those facts, inferences, or conclusions. Consider a case where a physician testifies a child experienced vaginal penetration. The cross-examiner begins by committing the doctor to the facts and assumptions underlying the opinion. The attorney says, "So doctor, your opinion is based exclusively on the history, the physical examination, and on what the child told you. Is that correct? And there is nothing else you relied on to form your opinion. Is that correct?" The cross-examiner commits the doctor to a specific set of facts and assumptions so that when the cross-examiner disputes those facts or assumptions, the doctor's opinion cannot be justified on some other basis.

Once the cross-examiner pins down the basis of the doctor's opinion, the cross-examiner attacks the opinion by disputing one or more of the facts, inferences, or conclusions that support it. The attorney might ask whether the doctor's opinion would change if certain facts were different (a hypothetical question). The attorney might press the doctor to acknowledge alternative explanations for the doctor's conclusion. The attorney might ask the doctor whether experts could come to different conclusions based on the same facts.

Rather than attack the doctor's facts, inferences, or conclusions during cross-examination, the attorney may limit cross-examination to pinning the doctor down to a limited set of facts, inferences, and conclusions and then, when the doctor has left the witness stand, offer another expert to contradict the doctor's testimony.

Learned Treatises

The cross-examiner may seek to undermine the expert's testimony by confronting the expert with books or articles (called *learned treatises*) that contradict the expert. The rules on impeachment with learned treatises vary from state to state. There is agreement on one thing, however. When an expert is confronted with a sentence or a paragraph selected by an attorney from an article or chapter, the expert has the right to put the selected passage in context by reading surrounding material. The expert might say to the cross-examiner, "Counsel, I cannot comment on the sentence you have selected unless I first read the entire article. If you will permit me to read the article, I'll be happy to comment on the sentence that interests you."

Bias

The cross-examiner may raise the possibility that the expert is biased. For example, if the expert is part of a multidisciplinary child abuse team, the cross-examiner might proceed as follows:

Q: Now doctor, you are employed by Children's Hospital, isn't that correct?

A: Right.

Q: At the hospital, are you a member of the multidisciplinary team that investigates allegations of child abuse?

A: As a doctor I obtain the medical history and conduct the medical examination. I do not investigate. The police investigate. But yes, I am a member of the hospital's multidisciplinary child abuse team.

Q: You regularly perform examinations and interviews at the request of the prosecuting attorney's office, isn't that correct?

A: No. At the request of the prosecutor I examine children to diagnose and treat any effect of the alleged abuse and in that context I obtain a medical history.

Q: When you complete your examination for the prosecutor, you prepare a report for the prosecutor, don't you?

A: A medical report and recommendation are prepared and placed in the child's medical record. On request, the team provides a copy of the report to the prosecutor and, I might add, to the defense.

Q: After your team prepares its report and provides a copy to the prosecutor, you often come to court to testify as an expert witness for the prosecution in child abuse cases, isn't that right, doctor?

A: Yes.

Q: Do you usually testify for the prosecution rather than the defense?

A: Correct.

Q: In fact, would I be correct in saying that you always testify for the prosecution and never for the defense?

A: I am willing to testify for the defense, but so far I have always testified for the prosecution.

Q: Thank you, doctor. I have no further questions.

The cross-examiner seeks to portray the doctor as biased in favor of the prosecution, but the cross-examiner does not ask, "Well then, doctor, isn't it a fact that because of your close working relationship with the prosecution, you are biased in favor of the prosecution?" The cross-examiner knows the answer is no, so the cross-examiner simply plants seeds of doubt in the jurors' minds and then, when it is time for closing argument, the cross-examiner reminds the jury of the doctor's close working relationship with the prosecution.

Recall that cross-examination is followed by redirect examination. During redirect, the prosecutor might ask, "Doctor, in light of the defense attorney's questions about your responsibilities with the multidisciplinary team, are you biased in favor of the prosecution?" The doctor can then set the record straight.

In conclusion preparation for court testimony is grounded in sound medical practice. The legal concepts presented in this chapter provide a foundation for understanding basic legal issues as they relate to child abuse. An understanding of legal concepts is no substitute for enhancing one's professional expertise. Expertise is reflected in the medical record as demonstrated by excellent documentation; thoroughness of a medical assessment; appropriate testing; a differential diagnosis; and an objective, well-balanced, and defensible formulation of a medical opinion.

References

1. Kalichman SC. *Mandated Reporting of Suspected Child Abuse: Ethics, Law & Policy.* Washington, DC: American Psychological Association; 1993

2. Zellman GL, Faller KC. Reporting of child maltreatment. In: Briere J, Berliner L, Buckley JA, et al, eds. *The APSAC Handbook on Child Maltreatment.* Thousand Oaks, CA: Sage; 1996

3. *Landeros v Flood,* 551 P2d 389 (Cal 1976)

4. Myers JEB. *Legal Issues in Child Abuse and Neglect Practice.* 2nd ed. Thousand Oaks, CA: Sage; 1998

5. Kalichman SC. *Mandated Reporting of Suspected Child Abuse: Ethics, Law & Policy*. Washington, DC: American Psychological Association; 1999

6. Jones DPH. *Interviewing the Sexually Abused Child: Investigation of Suspected Abuse*. Great Britain: Gaskell—Royal College of Psychiatrists; 1992

7. *Crawford v Washington,* 541 US 36 (2004)

8. *Davis v Washington,* 126 S Ct 2266 (2006)

9. *State v Bobadilla,* 709 NW2d 243 (Minn 2006)

10. *State v Blue,* 717 NW2d 558 (ND 2006)

11. *State v Moses,* 119 P3d 906 (Wash Ct App 2005)

12. *State v Griner,* 899 A2d 189 (Md Ct App 2006)

13. *Commonwealth v DeOliveria,* 849 NE2d 243 (Mass 2006)

14. *State v Wyble,* 2007 WL 43612 (Mo Ct App 2007)

15. *Hobgood v State,* 926 So2d 847 (Miss 2006)

16. *Hernandez v State,* 2007 WL 188417 (Fla Ct App 2007)

17. *People v Cage* Apr 09 SC S127344 (2007)

18. American Medical Association. *Code of Ethics*. American Medical Association Web site. http://www.ama-assn.org/ama/pub/category/2498.html. Accessed April 22, 2008

19. American Nurses Association. *Code of Ethics for Nurses*. American Nurses Association Web site. http://nursingworld.org/ethics/. Accessed April 22, 2008

20. Gutheil TG, Appelbaum PS. *Clinical Handbook of Psychiatry and the Law*. New York, NY: McGraw-Hill; 1982

21. *Tarasoff v Regents of the University of California,* 551 P2d 334 (Cal 1976)

22. Chadwick DL. Preparation for court testimony in child abuse cases. *Pediatr Clin North Am.* 1990;37:955–970

23. *People v Gardeley,* 927 P2d 713 (Cal 1997)

24. *Frye v United States,* 293 F 1013 (DC 1923)

25. *Daubert v Merrell Dow Pharmaceuticals, Inc.,* 509 US 579 (1993)

26. *Kumho Tire Co., Ltd. v Carmichael,* 526 US 137 (1999)

27. Brodsky SL. *Coping with Cross-Examination*. Washington, DC: American Psychological Association; 2004

28. Stern P. *Preparing and Presenting Expert Testimony in Child Abuse Litigation: A Guide for Expert Witnesses and Attorneys*. Thousand Oaks, CA: Sage; 1997

Chapter 14

Child Sexual Exploitation: Recognition and Prevention Considerations

Sharon W. Cooper

The 21st century has brought with it great strides in technology. Health care, communication, and business have gained significantly from these strides. However, there is another aspect of society that has grown over the past 10 years because of technology—that of the sexual abuse and exploitation of children and youths. The combination of sexual abuse with an unjust use of the victim for an offender's financial profit or social networking advantage is sexual exploitation. Prior to the advent of the Internet, such exploitation was often secretive and when pornography production was a component, limited to the photography of young victims often sold via a black market for distribution via print magazines. There is an emerging sobering realization among professionals that a significant number of child sexual abuse cases that have been investigated and adjudicated have been incompletely evaluated in that victim pornography production

was never known at the time of a trial. Sexual exploitation prior to the Internet included human traffickers who sold youths for sex in hidden places both in urban and rural America as well as often through the importation of children from foreign countries. Sexual exploitation has expanded significantly since the advent of the World Wide Web, and no discussion of child abuse and sexual violence can be complete without addressing a phenomenon that has caused the most significant change in society today—information and communication technology.[1]

The sexual exploitation of children is a complex issue that has both global and political perspectives. This form of child abuse not only involves impoverished families, but multibillion dollar financial institutions. It may involve online networking of families who sexually abuse their own children live, with Web cam transmissions throughout the world via highly secure venues.[2] It often involves commercial exploitation of children sexually abused for money and marketed from within their families or by brutal offenders who recruit youths who have run away or have become "throw away" children.[3] There are 5 types of child sexual exploitation: child pornography; the prostitution of children and youths; the cyber-enticement of children and youths by Internet initiation or facilitation; child sex tourism; and the domestic or international trafficking of children and youths for pros-titution, illegal labor, sexual slavery, and/or civil rights violations (Table 14.1).

Each of these forms of abuse has specific dynamics with respect to victimology and offender characteristics. For example, recent research has revealed that more than one-third of convicted child pornography producers had multiple victims, and often these children were victimized simultaneously in groups. These groups of child victims were often siblings, or if the multiple victims were unrelated, one was usually used to recruit other children.[4]

TABLE 14.1
Types of Child Sexual Exploitation

Type	Definition
Child pornography	The photographic record of child sexual abuse, which may reveal lascivious images of the genitals or pubic area or sexual acts between an adult and a child or between 2 or more children who are younger than 18 years.[1]
Prostitution of children and youths	The sexual exploitation of children or youths almost entirely for financial or economic reasons, which may be monetary but may also be for food, shelter, or drugs, and that universally benefits the exploiter with complete disregard to the rights and well-being of the child.
Cyber-enticement	Grooming or luring a minor either initiated or facilitated by a computer or communication device for the end result of a sexual abuse encounter between an adult and a minor. Consent cannot be given in this context.
Child sex tourism	A form of child sexual abuse associated with travel of the offender from one country to another to achieve this end.
Human trafficking	The movement of men, women, or children from one country to another or from one part of a country to another for the purpose of commercial sexual exploitation, sexual slavery, or labor law violations.

Consideration of prevention in this area of sexual exploitation consequently does require a complete understanding of the nature of grooming, luring, and factors that contribute to compliant victimization.

Sexual exploitation is perhaps the worst form of sexual abuse because it removes a child's right to the privacy of their victimization and can multiply offenders with just the click of a mouse. Child sexual exploitation affects every aspect of the victim impact of sexual abuse as never before imagined.

Stages of Sexual Abuse Adjudication

- Disclosure or outcry: The presence of exploitation is a deterrent to disclosure in part because of increased feelings on the part of children of guilt, self-blame, and shame.
- Investigation: If images are discovered before a child discloses abuse, or if a child is rescued from prostitution, feelings of self-blame or collusion often resort in victim denial that the contraband are self-images, or that a trafficker is exploiting a youth through prostitution compared with the youth committing the offense on his or her own.
- Prosecution (civil and/or criminal): Civil prosecution is still met with disbelief and poor understanding of grooming in Internet crimes—particularly in the circumstances of cyber-enticement. In the criminal prosecution areas, victims who have been poorly prepared may deny their abuse or minimize the role of the offenders, particularly inintrafamilial cases.

- Treatment: If child sexual images are part of the victimization, therapists have had poor training in the reality of the extent of the abuse that children have experienced. Cognitive-behavioral therapy may not be the ideal means of treatment. Additional problems of sexualized behaviors in this form of child abuse resulting in online sexual role-playing via social networking sites and Internet dating can present as additional problems seen in this form of abuse.

It is very important to understand that child sexual abuse is usually disclosed by a victim who has come to the point of feeling a need to tell. The spontaneous disclosure, whether it occurs during a fit of anger, as a desire to protect another potential victim, because of painful physical symptoms or behavioral concerns, or on the chance that there was an eyewitness, is almost always delayed in nature. On the other hand, sexual exploitation may often become known because others have witnessed the abuse of the child without the victim even being aware. This difference is very relevant to therapists, investigators, prosecutors, the victim, and families who are seeking to learn the truth and move on. Defense mechanisms that many children have when confronted with a charge of participating in acts that they perceive to be wrong and their fault often result in denial of the presence of pornographic images, even if the victim is able to acknowledge the sexual abuse. Because of the nature of this form of child abuse, continuous or recurrent victimization is very likely.

There is a close relationship between each of these forms of sexual exploitation and pornography. At times pornography (either of children or adults) is used to normalize and desensitize victims to the acceptability of a sexual encounter between an adult and a child. At other times, child pornography is used to educate children regarding the sexual wishes of the offender. In addition, child pornography is used to extort victims into silence with the threat of exposure of their willing participation of this form of child sexual abuse. Exposure to child pornography is also used to groom and convince children that a sexual assault will not be painful and that many children experience sexual satisfaction with adults or other children through these behaviors.

The final role of child pornography in sexual exploitation is that its continued production, possession, and distribution increases demand for the contraband and has given birth to a market for more graphic and violent images as well as sexual abuse images of younger and younger victims.

Child Pornography

The problem of sexual abuse associated with memorialization through photography or videography has been a difficult concept to accept. For some time it was assumed that a significant amount of computer-based images of children were technologically derived or virtual in nature. This theory led many professionals to believe that the ever-increasing number of images on the Internet actually were either adults

who were shaved and made to look as if they were under-aged minors, or that the images had all been "morphed," a graphics skill that allowed placing body images together like the pieces of a puzzle. For this reason, the United States Supreme Court decision of *Ashcroft v Free Speech Coalition*[5] in 2002 led many in the field of child abuse to ignore the warning smoke of an ever-increasing firestorm of victimization. This ruling required that the government prove that at least one image in a collection was that of a real child, as opposed to one that was completely computer-generated, and that the offender knew that the image was real. The overwhelming numbers of images on the Internet are of unidentified victims. This ruling led to the immense cost of bringing in foreign investigators who had identified children depicted in well-known series of images, often included in an offender's collection, to verify that the victims were known to be children at the time of the pornography production. For more than a year, the criminal acts of possession and distribution of sexual abuse images increased with minimal investigations and prosecutions. Fortunately, the PROTECT Act of 2003[6] provided a remedy such that prevention could be reinstituted through prosecution and community education.

From the standpoint of prevention involving the individual victim, child pornography constitutes insult to injury. The injury is that of child sexual abuse—an adverse childhood experience known to have a high association with delayed disclosure and long-term impact on an individual's physical and mental health.[7] One aspect of prevention for child sexual abuse is the encouragement of disclosure to hopefully bring an end to the recurrent nature of this form of child abuse. The insult is that of memorialization of the abuse through computer or communication technology images, videotapes, or photographs. A dynamic that has emerged when this insult is in place is that of "double silencing."[8] This refers to a phenomenon about sexual abuse and pornography that contributes to a victim's denial that the images are actually his or her own. They are silenced because of the sexual abuse and silenced because of incriminating pictures available for all to see. This added dimension of victim impact requires that professionals in the field of child sexual abuse understand and communicate to others the differences in evaluation and treatment of exploitation victims.[9] Protocols should be in place for these special situations to prevent further victimization by the system. From a prevention perspective, pointed efforts must promote the understanding of professionals in the field and a proactive protocol should be implemented to provide subsequent protection of these children from further exploitation—through the investigation, the courtroom process, media coverage, and in therapy (Table 14.2).

It is imperative to prevent further harm to victims, as can occur in the media, in the courtroom, and as reports on the Internet. Recommendations for the prevention of further exploitation of victims would include courtroom protocols that would easily allow a closed courtroom in such cases, viewing of images only by the judge and jury, and clear guidance that victims should not necessarily be shown images of their own abuse in court preparation. Another method of prevention of further harm to victims is to file both federal and state charges against an offender for different aspects of his criminal sexual behavior, which might lead the offender to plead guilty. Offenders might particularly prefer to plead guilty to federal charges to avoid state prison systems. Federal agencies, such as the Office of Victims of Crime, as well as state victims' advocate academies, should include in their training best practices in the cases of children who have been exploited through child pornography production.

When a child decides to disclose sexual abuse, she has often mentally struggled and determined that telling might be the best way to make the abuse stop. Sometimes young victims disclose to protect other children in the family, or if there is parental estrangement, they disclose because they feel safe enough to do so and desire not to have visitation with a parent who is abusing them. On the other hand, in cases of sexual exploitation associated with child pornography production, the images are often discovered before the victim is ready to tell.

Instead of an experienced child protective services professional as the first point of contact, these children are often identified at their schools or

TABLE 14.2
Prevention of Revictimization in Child Pornography

Prevention Needs	Actions
Pornographic images discovered without victim disclosure	Perform careful victim interview avoiding efforts to "force" a confession by the child victim of the presence of methods of abuse.
Victim discloses presence of pornographic images	Manage case empathetically with careful protection of contraband availability and facilitation of therapeutic interventions.
Impact of exploitation on family support systems	Provide family support and counseling to prevent further emotional victimization.
Court preparations of victims	Avoid exposing the child victim to images of his or her own sexual abuse.
Courtroom protections	Strongly advocate for closed court setting during victim testimony; careful management of contraband images with access only to judge and/or jury members.
Child pornography community education	Provide information through media regarding compliant victimization, online grooming, alcohol and drug impact on adolescent brain development and function, as well as long-term victim impact of pornography.
Communication technology child pornography prevention	Educate parents and adolescents regarding the use of cell phone cameras in the production or distribution of child pornography.
Bullying through online or communication technology pornographic exploitation	Educate schools, families, and youths regarding victimization of this nature with establishment of appropriate consequences.

homes by an expert in Internet crimes against children, who may not have forensic interviewing skills. This may lead to a delay in the child and family accessing services because of continued denial. In a multiple victim case from Sweden, researchers noted how hard it was for the children to either acknowledge the abuse or reveal that they knew pictures were being taken.[2] The reasons for this include

- The children feel that they are being seen to let the abuse happen.
- They might, quite frequently, be smiling and therefore appear to be "enjoying" the activity (in reality they are forced to do so by the perpetrator).
- They may have been encouraged to introduce other children to the perpetrator and thus feel responsible for letting it happen to others.

- They may have been encouraged to be proactive in either their own sexual abuse or that of other children.
- They may have been shown their own abuse images by the perpetrator with threats that he will tell of, or even show, the pictures to their parents or caregivers or other significant people in their lives if they do not cooperate, and they may carry the shame of not stopping the abuse.

The greatest inhibitor to disclosing what has happened to these victims is the humiliation that the children feel regarding who may have seen their images and their fear of being recognized. They feel they have been literally "caught in the act."[10]

A good prevention strategy in the case of child pornography should include multidisciplinary team education regarding the special circumstances of failure to disclose in child sexual abuse with pornographic exploitation. Another aspect of prevention of this form of sexual abuse includes recognizing the modus operandi of offenders that have been demonstrated in child sexual abuse images. The differences that are more common in Internet images include simultaneous multiple victims, who are particularly encouraged to sexually interact with each other. Many times, these children are of similar ages compared with the more familiar youth sex offender scenario where age differences are obvious.

Programs that encourage would-be offender self-regulation such as Stop It Now! are also important prevention models that would discourage the learned skills of predators such as how they lure children, gain their trust as well as their family members, groom the children into compliance in the sexually abusive behaviors, and maintain their silence. Recognition of these dynamics provides a platform for the development of prevention efforts for non-offending parents and family members, specialists in child protection and investigation, as well as court systems and the community at large.[11]

Two successful prevention strategies to diminish the availability of child pornography images exist presently because of a law that requires Internet service providers to (1) shut down any known child pornography sites and (2) transfer information regarding images in the United States to the National Center for Missing and Exploited Children for further efforts to identify victims. Failure to comply brings with it a very stiff financial penalty.

Child pornography is one of the most common threads in all aspects of child sexual exploitation. Pornography is used to educate and extort youths into prostitution in association with romance grooming and often intimate partner violence. Threats of distribution of pornographic videos or photographs to the families of runaway or throwaway youths provide enough impetus for their cooperation with offenders who then frequently traffick these juveniles to various parts of the country away from their home of record so as to further isolate them and ensure their dependence on the exploiter.

Child Sex Tourism

Child sex tourism is frequently associated with a "travel keepsake" (eg, photos or videos of a sexual encounter with minor children). Because Americans comprise the largest number of sex tourists, prevention efforts continue by the World Travel Organization and advocacy groups such as ECPAT (End Child Prostitution, Child Pornography and Trafficking of Children for Sexual Purposes) as well as the United Nations as they work hard with local countries to discourage the marketing of children for sex.

The various types of cases and offender behaviors as described by Sullivan[12] include

- Those who take the opportunity such as a holiday environment to abuse children
- Those who travel abroad in the company of intended child victims
- Those who speculatively explore traveling to locate where children are apt to be available for sex
- Those who arrange through others to meet and abuse children at a specific location
- Those who are resident foreigners who reside in countries where primarily due to poverty, children are vulnerable to abuse
- Those who abuse in the course of their voluntary nongovernmental work in a foreign country

Prevention in each of these scenarios will be case specific, but should at least include careful screening at the disembarkation border for sex offender registration for those traveling to high-risk destinations. On return, a careful customs check for possession of child pornography is indicated because of the high risk of recidivism in this kind of sexual offending. Education of non-profit outreach programs regarding sex tourism and the stiff penalties associated with conviction of such criminal activities is another measure that may deter otherwise opportunistic offenders.

Cyber-enticement

In cases of computer-initiated crimes, as is typically seen in cyber-enticement, offenders will often send by e-mail images of themselves, clothed and then nude, as well as participate in explicit autoerotic behaviors both to normalize such online exposure to the youth and to encourage reciprocation. Gifts that make it easier for a teen to self-exploit such as Web cams, digital cameras, and cell phones with cameras are tools of the trade for these types of offenders. Prevention in this area would obviously include increasing public awareness of the immense potential for exploitation and extortion when an adult and a child embark on an illicit romantic online relationship. Parents should be provided anticipatory guidance from health care providers, school personnel, and their faith community supports as well as through public service announcements of the immense patience found in individuals who commit this type of crime.

Information as is noted in a study
of 129 victims of cyber-enticement
(Table 14.3) reveals numerous details
that attest to the tenacity in online
grooming, such as the fact that 48% of
offenders communicated online with
children more 1 to 6 months before
arranging a meeting.[13]

Recent reports of cases of cyber-
enticement from social networking
sites such as MySpace.com, Facebook.
com, Bebo.com, and others require
further considerations in prevention.
Social networking sites provide the
ability to upload information about
oneself and interact with others

through online blogging (Web logs)
and information exchange. Prevention
recommendations in these areas, which
are often referred to as Web 2.0, include
frequent communication between
parents and their children on how
many social networking sites they use;
the importance of avoiding personal
information such as full name, school,
home address, or phone number; and
continued encouragement to maintain
a sense of skepticism regarding those
who visit online. Many of these sites
require a minimum age of 14 to have an
account. Communities are beginning to
practice prevention of cyber-enticement
or cyber-bullying by removing social

TABLE 14.3
Characteristics of Victims and Offender Dynamics in Cyber-enticement[a]

Victim Age, y	n=129		Gender	Victim	Offender
12	1%		Female	75%	1%
13	26%		Male	25%	99%
14	22%				
15	28%				
16	14%				
17	8%				

Offender communicated online with victim for
1 month or less............ 27%
More than 1 to 6 months...... 48%
More than 6 months........ 16%
Missing values............ 9%

Distance offender traveled to initial meeting
10 miles or less........... 8%
More than 10 to 50 miles...... 32%
More than 50 miles 41%

Offender or victim traveled more than 50 miles to initial meeting 50%

Victim was in love with or felt close to offender.......... 50%

Sexual offense was committed at face-to-face meeting...... 93%

Victim spent the night with the offender......... 41%

Offender and victim met more than once 73%

Most serious sexual offense committed
Oral sex 18%
Intercourse or other penetration 71%

[a]Adapted with permission from Wolak J, Finkelhor D, Mitchell K. Internet-initiated sex crimes against minors: implications for prevention based on findings from a national study. *J Adolesc Health.* 2004;35(5):e11–e20.

networking sites from the computers in public middle schools and high schools. Other school districts are beginning to forbid camera phones on the school campus. An excellent resource for parents with a multitude of prevention parenting points, *MySpace Unraveled: A Parent's Guide to Teen Social Networking from the Directors of BlogSafety.com*[14] was recently written in response to public concerns about sexual exploitation through the medium of MySpace.com, the most popular of social networking sites, hosting more than 180 million members.

Prostitution and Human Trafficking

Exploitation through prostitution is likely one of the worst forms of human rights violations of children and youths. This aspect of child sexual abuse has been thought in the past to be self-promotion and entrepreneurial. Victims even as young as 10 and 11 years of age had been incarcerated in juvenile detention centers criminally charged for solicitation without strong efforts being made to define the modus operandi of their exploitation.

Fortunately, in the past several years the Office of Juvenile Justice and Delinquency Prevention of the US Department of Justice has begun taking proactive measures to rescue these youths from some of the most vicious and organized criminals set on marketing sex for money.

Children who have been sexually abused are 28 times more likely to be arrested for prostitution compared with children who have not been sexual abuse victims. This statistic compels the field of counseling to address the sexual self-objectification that can occur in victims of sexual abuse. In addition, child placement in numerous foster care settings places children at increased risk for the run away behaviors, which so often results in what is euphemistically referred to as "survival sex" on the streets. Prevention should begin with child sexual abuse prevention strategies, but if children are nevertheless victimized, safe and consistent after care is essential.

Intrafamilial prostitution is another poorly recognized phenomenon that often precedes runaway behaviors, subsequently leading to commercial sexual exploitation through prostitution. Prevention of this form of abuse requires CPS training so that investigators will recognize that children who have made disclosures of sexual abuse and who are repeatedly ignored by caregivers might actually represent a victim whose sexuality is traded for the financial support of a spouse or paramour.

When underaged minors are foreign nationals, a consideration for organized crime has become a very real issue, and the US Department of State has assisted in defining those countries in the world that are referred to as *third tier* (ie, having no significant proactive or reactive laws to protect children from being trafficked or prostituted). Part of prevention of international human trafficking includes financial support of the countries of origin who are taking proactive measures to diminish the abduction and transport of their children and youths for labor law violations, prostitution, and sexual slavery. In 2005, 82 million dollars in anti-trafficking assistance was provided to foreign governments in an effort to diminish the flow of this form of exploitation.[15]

In the United States, prevention of prostitution of children and youths has in the past been focused on prevention of recidivism. Victims are often trafficked across the country and, under the guise of romance with the exploiter or pimp, are exposed to immense physical and mental health risks. The most common cause of death for a person who is being prostituted is murder and the second most common cause of death is HIV/AIDS.[16] Prevention strategies presently rest on enhancing child protection measures for victims in intrafamilial cases, as well as improving the investigative skills in rescuing children and youths marketed on the streets and via the Internet. Further prevention, however, should be modeled after landmark programs for children exploited through prostitution, such as the Los Angeles, CA, Children of the Night; the Minneapolis, MN, Breaking Free program, which has a preferential service delivery to minority populations; and the New York City outreach program the Girls Education and Mentoring Services, Inc. (GEMS) Program.

These outreach programs provide safety, vocational rehabilitation,

medical and substance abuse treatment, education, and support for prosecution issues to youths rescued from streets and brothels. Treatment of addictions, the immense degree of mental impact, social deprivation, and the medical results of physical and sexual violence are all parts of the necessary interventions for youths in this tragic predicament. It is also very important to understand the link between child sexual abuse and prostitution. Victims of child sexual abuse were 28 times more likely to be arrested for prostitution in their lifetimes than children who had not been sexually abused.[17]

Attention to the plight of the gay, lesbian, bisexual, transgender, and questioning (GLBTQ) youths is essential because many may be at risk for commercial sexual exploitation. The dynamics of victimization are different for these adolescents and include the important problems of running away or being thrown out of their homes. Self-exploitation can at times be additional behaviors that youths will use to meet potential partners. This strategy often results in youths loitering near gay bars, placing them at much higher risk for sexual assault and physical violence as well as commercial sexual exploitation.

Prevention of victimization of the GLBTQ youths should include clinical guidelines for primary caregivers to recognize youth sexual orientation and gender identity differences. School counselors and teachers who recognize any problems that such youths are exhibiting should be provided a toolbox for social, educational, and family interventions. Policy changes regarding homeless youth shelters and the existing restrictions to admitting GLBTQ youths for overnight stays should take place. Prevention should also include education of all service delivery agencies that will interact with such youths. Support for such organizational practices must be victim driven, because at-risk youths remain despite a political climate.

An Emerging Culture of Sexploitation: An Impetus for Compliant Victimization

Of concern today is the increasing emphasis in media, entertainment, music, fashion, and advertising of the glorification of pimping and a glamorization of prostitution as pervasive images of acceptability of a most heinous form of exploitation. Frequently referred to as the *normalization of sexual harm,* this campaign has already begun to demonstrate a degree of compliant victimization among teens that must be addressed at all levels of youth culture. There is a dual representation of exploitation and violence in many of the music videos that are shown repetitively on numerous cable television channels. Youths who listen to and watch videos of sexually explicit music with degrading lyrics typical of the prostitution genre have an earlier onset of sexual intercourse and participation in more advanced levels of noncoital sexual activity (eg, oral sex) than those youths who experience equally sexually explicit music without degrading lyrics.[18] The rap and present-day hip hop musical genres provide in some cases the most explicit examples

of what the entertainment industry calls *sexploitation.* From a prevention perspective, this form of imagery in so many venues normalizes sexual harm and promotes unhealthy beliefs about gender roles and sexual relationships to youths who are still in the developmental stages of their psychosexual values.

The toxicity of these sexploitation messages promotes misogyny, mutual intimate partner violence, disrespect, bullying, and exploitation. It also provides very negative role models for males, encouraging dominance and violence in relationships with females and encouraging males to treat females as sexual commodities. These behavioral tenets form the basis of the messages promoted in prostitution. In addition, power and control themes are particularly constant in many music videos, which continuously denigrate women and girls. Adulation of extravagant expenditures on champagne; cars; and bejeweled drug, alcohol, and pimp paraphernalia are almost always seen in many of these productions.

There seems to be a link between the amount of exposure youths have to these constant negative messages and delinquency outcomes. A public health study of African American adolescent females who were prospectively exposed to an increased amount of derogatory and sexually explicit music videos resulted in significantly negative behaviors. They were 3 times more likely to assault a teacher, twice as likely to be arrested and have multiple sexual partners, and 1½ times more likely to use drugs and alcohol and acquire a sexually transmitted infection.[19]

The concern for compliant victimization of exploitation through prostitu-tion is underscored by a study sponsored by the National Institute on Drug Abuse in conjunction with data from the National Longitudinal Study of Adolescent Health. This research revealed that in a national representative study of 7th- to 12th-grade students, 3.5% (650,000) of youths had exchanged sex for money or drugs. Two-thirds of these youths were boys, and the median number of sex exchanges was one, suggesting that the motivation for the sex exchange was other than that of survival on the streets. The study also noted that the likelihood of sex exchange is elevated for youths who are involved in drug use in general, have run away from home, are depressed, and have engaged in various high-risk sexual behaviors.[20] These data were collected between 1995 and 1996, which continued to be a period of popular "gangsta rap" and music symbolic of the "pimp and ho culture."

In response to these and other studies regarding the constant messages that are resulting in an increase in dating violence among teens and a concern for earlier sexually risky behaviors, the Centers for Disease Control and Prevention has launched a Web-based prevention initiative called Choose Respect to encourage youths to choose respect in their interpersonal relationships. This model allows interaction and discussion and has the potential

for use in youth groups, schools, and other venues where youths gather.[21]

Additional campaigns such as My Strength Is Not for Hurting by the organization Men Can Stop Rape and the help line available from Stop It Now!, which encourages adults to identify problematic sexual behavior and to take appropriate action even when the one who may need intervention is someone they know and love. The establishment of a new national hotline for adolescent intimate partner violence is another means to add to the emerging and promising measures to promote healthy relationships, protect and prevent child sexual exploitation as part of a community, and societal response.

It is essential to recognize that sexual exploitation is often linked with violence. When this problem becomes evident in a school setting, careful consultation and analysis may be necessary to include focus groups and mediation. Providing a common language for students and parents is important when discussing sexual problems in a school setting. Prevention is typically enhanced when education is included for all parties. Education helps bystanders and reluctant participants to take a stand on behalf of what is right and in defense of a potential victim.[22]

Prevention and intervention in school sexual behavior problems such as was noted in 2006, when a group of 6- to 8-year-old boys attacked a similar-aged girl in a school bathroom in what appeared to be an attempt to gang rape her, becomes an imperative skill in communities.[23] Such frightful occurrences demand a careful consideration of the sexually intolerant and toxic environment that children are living in. In addition, open communication within the home, schools, and youth groups about youth sexuality in the Web 2.0 age is essential to assist youth in making wise decisions.[23] Newly emerging terms such as *self-exploitation* require anticipatory guidance by parents regarding online behaviors that might actually represent illegal child pornography production. When teen boys sexually assault a girl and end the crime by taking several cell phone camera pictures of the wounded victim with the threat of exposure on the Internet or to others should she report the crime, professionals must understand the milieu of sexual exploitation and the associated victim impact.

The role of industry is an important component of prevention, and appealing to responsible marketing must be an ongoing dialogue. Parent support groups who lobby on behalf of a safe childhood directly with lawmakers or watchdog agencies should be given direction and strategies on the most successful means of eradicating any and all factors that contribute to the sexual exploitation of children and youths.

Child sexual abuse continues to be the basis of maltreatment in child sexual exploitation. Prevention strategies will likely require numerous types of approaches because of the diverse presentations of this form of child abuse. More than an individual's awareness or skills and more than an individual parent's actions must be in place for the various psychological and technological dynamics of this form of abuse. In addition, an ever-present realization of grooming to compliance has never been more important in an area of child abuse. Countering social norms, the role of the Internet and other emerging technologies, and a need to ensure the safety of children and families are essential pieces of the puzzle that will continue to require multimodal interventions and prevention.

References

1. ECPAT International. *Violence Against Children in Cyberspace: A Contribution to the United Nations Study on Violence against Children.* Bangkok, Thailand: ECPAT International; 2005. http://www.ecpat.net/eng/publications/Cyberspace/PDF/ECPAT_Cyberspace_2005-ENG.pdf. Accessed April 21, 2008

2. Remarks of US Customs Commissioner Robert C. Bonner: Press Conference on Operation Hamlet. August 9, 2002. http://www.cbp.gov/xp/cgov/newsroom/commissioner/speeches_statements/archives/2002/aug092002.xml. Accessed April 21, 2008

3. Estes RJ, Weiner NA. The commercial sexual exploitation of children in the United States. In: Cooper SW, Estes RJ, Giardino AP, Kellogg ND, Vieth VI, eds. *Medical, Legal & Social Science Aspects of Child Sexual Exploitation: A Comprehensive Review of Pornography, Prostitution and Internet Crimes.* St Louis, MO: GW Medical Publishers; 2005:95–128

4. Wolak J, Finkelhor D, Mitchell K. The varieties of child pornography production. In: *Viewing Child Pornography on the Internet: Understanding the Offense, Managing the Offender, Helping the Victims.* Dorset, England: Russell House Publishing; 2005:31–48

5. *Ashcroft v Free Speech Coalition*, 535 US 234 (9th Cir 2002)

6. Prosecutorial Remedies and Other Tools to end the Exploitation of Children Today Act (PROTECT Act), 2003

7. Edwards VJ, Anda RF, Dube SR, Dong M, Chapman DP, Felitti VJ. The wide-ranging health outcomes of adverse childhood experiences In: Kendall-Tackett K, Giacomoni S, eds. *Child Victimization, Maltreatment, Bullying, and Dating Violence Prevention and Intervention.* Kingston, NJ: Civic Research Institute; 2005:8.1–8.13

8. Children and Young Persons with Abusive and Violent Experiences Connected to Cyberspace Challenges for Research, Rehabilitation, Prevention and Protection. Report from: Expert Meeting of Swedish Child Welfare Foundation; May 29–31, 2006; Sutra Bruk, Sweden

9. Svedin CG, Black K. *Children Who Don't Speak Out.* Stockholm, Sweden: Radda Barnen (Save the Children, Sweden); 1996

10. Palmer T. Behind the screen: children who are the subjects of abusive images. In: Quayle E, Taylor M, eds. *Viewing Child Pornography on the Internet: Understanding the Offence, Managing the Offender, Helping the Victims.* Lyme Regis Dorset, England: Russell House Publishing; 2005:61–65

11. Kaufman KL, Mosher H, Carter M, Estes L. An empirically based situational prevention model for child sexual abuse. In: Wortley R, Smallbone S, eds. *Situational Prevention of Child Sexual Abuse. Crime Prevention Studies.* Vol. 19. Monsey, NY: Criminal Justice Press; 2006

12. Sullivan J. Presentation at: International Online Child Sexual Victimization Symposium sponsored by the Federal Bureau of Investigation Critical Incident Response Group's National Center for the Analysis of Violent Crimes; 2001; Leesburg, VA

13. Wolak J, Finkelhor D, Mitchell K. Internet-initiated sex crimes against minors: implications for prevention based on findings from a national study. *J Adolesc Health* 2004;35(5):e11–e20

14. Magid L, Collier A. *MySpace Unraveled: A Parent's Guide to Teen Social Networking from the Directors of BlogSafety.com.* Berkeley, CA: Peachpit Press; 2006

15. US Department of State (USDOS). *Trafficking in Persons Report, 2006.* Washington, DC: USDOS, Office to Monitor and Combat Trafficking in Persons; 2006

16. Sheridan DJ, Van Pelt D. Intimate partner violence in the lives of prostituted adolescents. In: Cooper SW, Estes RJ, Giardino AP, Kellogg ND, Vieth VI, eds. *Medical, Legal & Social Science Aspects of Child Sexual Exploitation: A Comprehensive Review of Pornography, Prostitution and Internet Crimes.* St Louis, MO: GW Medical Publishers; 2005:423–435

17. Widom CS. *Victims of Childhood Sexual Abuse—Later Criminal Consequences.* Washington, DC: US Department of Justice, National Institute of Justice; 1995. NCJ151525

18. Martino SC, Collins RL, Elliott MN, Strachman A, Kanouse DE, Berry SH. Exposure to degrading versus nondegrading music lyrics and sexual behavior among youth. *Pediatrics.* 2006;118:430–441

19. Wingood GM, DiClemente RJ, Cosby R, et al. A prospective study of exposure to rap music videos and African American female adolescents' health. *Am J Public Health.* 2003;93(3):437–439

20. Edwards JM, Iritani BJ, Hallfors DD. Prevalence and correlates of exchanging sex for drugs or money among adolescents in the United States. *Sex Transm Infect.* 2006;82:354–358

21. Department of Health and Human Services, Centers for Disease Control and Prevention and the National Center for Injury Prevention and Control. Choose Respect Web site. http://www.chooserespect.org/scripts/aboutus.asp. Accessed April 21, 2008

22. Anderson C. *Prevention and Intervention of Sexual Violence in Schools Talking About "It."* St Paul, MN: Sensibilities, Inc.; 2005. http://www.co.ramsey.mn.us/NR/rdonlyres/AD200AC3-F5D9-4AD8-B47B-9B90CB84FAEE/811/Talkingaboutit.pdf

23. Montgomery R, Adler E. Sexual assaults by children set off experts' alarms. *The Kansas City Star.* May 11, 2006

Chapter 15

Documentation, Report Formulation, and Conclusions

Martin A. Finkel

Detail of the Medical Record

The clinician should assume that every medical record of a child examined for the purpose of diagnosis and treatment of residua to alleged abuse will potentially undergo legal scrutiny. Thus the medical record must be constructed with exacting attention to detail in anticipation of critical and adversarial review. The medical record must be legible, well-constructed, and educational, and the conclusions must be defensible.[1,2] A medical record that memorializes carefully and objectively the verbal and visual findings can be a powerful instrument to articulate the physician's diagnosis and treatment recommendations.[3] An incomplete and poorly formulated record suggests lack of attention to detail and sloppy medical practice, and it undermines the credibility of the diagnostic assessment.[4–7]

The medical record provides valuable information for caseworkers, for case management discussions in the context of a multidisciplinary team review, for court proceedings, or for future reference should there be a new allegation of abuse. This chapter describes the essential components of the documen-tation of the medical history, physical examination, and diagnostic assessment. Examples are provided to illustrate how a diagnosis can be formulated.

Stating the Purpose of the Medical Examination

The medical examination is an essential component of the complete assessment of any child suspected of being sexually abused. The evaluation of a child suspected of being abused dictates the need for clinicians to work in a collaborative fashion with professionals from child protection, mental health, and law enforcement. The clinician must make it clear to child protection and law enforcement that the purpose of examining a child suspected of being abused is to diagnose and treat any residua to the alleged sexual contact. Medical professionals' primary concern is the patient's well-being; thus, all aspects of the examination are conducted in a manner that should be therapeutic to the child, whether the result is that of reassurance or of treatment for acute injuries or sexually transmitted infections (STIs).

Granted, a comprehensive medical evaluation may have value to child protection and law enforcement as they investigate allegations of abuse, but that is not the purpose of such an examination. The clinician's diagnosis and recommendations not only serve the needs of the child directly but also help nonmedical colleagues understand and facilitate the child's specific treatment needs.

Physicians address patients needs by providing treatment or, simply, the time-honored method of reassuring the patient that he or she is going to be fine. Although some children will require treatment for an STI or for acute injuries, most children will be "treated" by the reassurance that follows a complete examination. The health benefit of reassurance by a clinician that the child's body is OK and that there will be no long-term adverse health consequences can be enormously therapeutic.

Every allegation of abuse can be thought of as a diagnostic puzzle, and medicine is a critical and sometimes ordinal piece of it. As with any puzzle, the more pieces that are available, the greater the potential to appreciate fully the complete picture. The medical evaluation and the accompanying record can provide important insight into what a child may have experienced and the treatment he or she requires.

Every patient who presents for medical care should be told, in a developmentally appropriate way, that he or she is being seen for the purpose of diagnosis and treatment. The failure to explain

the purpose of the examination and to document the child's understanding that he or she is being seen for diagnosis and treatment may result in the child's medical history being inadmissible under the diagnosing and treating physician's exception to hearsay.

Although the manner of relaying the purpose of the examination will be accomplished in varying ways depending on the child's age, the following serves as an example of how this issue can be addressed with most children. The clinician might begin with an introductory comment such as, "When you have gone to the doctor in the past and not felt well, what does the doctor do? They ask you all kinds of questions, like does your tummy hurt? Do you have a headache, or have you had a fever? The reason the doctor asks those questions is simply to understand what's been bothering you, so the doctor can decide what to take a look at and whether you will need any special tests or medicines to get you better. I am going to ask you some questions about what happened. The questions I am going to ask are not to embarrass you or make you uncomfortable, but simply to understand what happened." Ask the child if he or she understands and has any questions. Continue by asking, "Is it important to tell the doctor the truth?" The child usually answers yes. Then ask the child to explain why it is important to tell the truth. The child might respond by saying, "Because the doctor can help me get better." Continue with, "It is always important to tell the truth, but particularly important to tell the doctor the truth. If you told me that your toe hurt and it was really your thumb that hurt, would that make it harder or easier for the doctor to help?" The child responds "harder." Then say, "You can tell doctors anything the worries you, upsets you, or confuses you. The more you tell the doctor the better the doctor can understand and help. Doctors and kids work together to solve problems."

The medical history obtained from the child should be recorded in writing as a part of the medical record and included in the consultative report. In the case of very young children, or children who are emotionally unavailable to provide a history of the concern, other sources are relied on and must be assessed as best as possible for their reliability. Pediatricians, of course, rely on this approach routinely for the care of infants and young children.

Although it seems obvious that the purpose of seeking medical care is to get better, children are rarely in a position to seek medical care on their own and are thus dependent on others to recognize the need. Children may appreciate the need to see a doctor if they have been injured, but they would not be expected to fully understand the potential consequences of sexual interactions. Even parents may not fully appreciate the potential consequences of the sexual interactions and should receive guidance in seeking diagnostic and treatment services. Thus it is incumbent on medical professionals to educate parents, as well as colleagues in child protection, mental health, and law enforcement, regarding the potential medical consequences of sexual abuse and the need to make referrals for diagnostic and treatment services for children who are suspected of being sexually abused.

Medical History Documentation

The medical record is a reflection of the sum and substance of an evaluation of a child suspected of being sexually abused. The record must speak to the thoroughness with which the clinician obtained the medical history, conducted the examination, and formulated a diagnosis.

The source of all information obtained and used to formulate a diagnosis must be noted. Information provided by individuals other than the child is generally considered hearsay and should not be used in formulating a diagnosis but may be included in the report. The clinician's diagnosis will be a marriage of 3 components: medical history, physical examination findings, and laboratory test results. When obtaining a medical history from the child and/or caretaker, it is not sufficient to record a summary note of the information provided. All information must be recorded verbatim—all introductory comments, the exact questions asked, and the child's exact responses. The health care professional should never rely on memory to reconstruct the details of the medical record. The handwritten notes serve to refresh the physician's memory when constructing the medical report.

Background information provided by child protection, law enforcement, or a non-offending parent is important but should not be relied on as the sole source of information when formulating a diagnosis. Information obtained from the above sources does not negate the need to speak to the child independently to obtain the medical history of the alleged interactions.

In some communities, clinicians have been discouraged from speaking to the child about the alleged experience, presumably so the child does not have to experience the trauma of retelling his or her experience. However, children can find retelling to be therapeutic, especially when they talk to a medical professional who understands and can help them express their worries or concerns. As one child said, "I can tell you because you're a doctor." Many of the questions asked by the clinician for medical diagnostic purposes would not be expected to have been addressed by nonmedical professionals.

Components of the Medical Record

The child's medical history and review of systems (ROS) should be obtained from the non-offending parent/caretaker. If the child is present in the room, it is best not to discuss any of the details of the child's alleged experiences. Reassure the child that he or she will be spoken to independently and will have an opportunity to share any worries or concerns during the examination. The non-offending parent/caretaker should provide his or her understanding of the concerns

as he or she heard or observed either firsthand or through a third party. The caretaker's information is important to frame the issue, but generally it should not be used in formulating a diagnosis. If hearsay is used in formulating a diagnosis, then the use of such information should be qualified and noted appropriately. Whenever possible, the "chief complaint" or history of the alleged contact should be obtained from the child when he or she is not in the presence of the caretaker.

The medical history should include the following components:

1. Birth history
2. Family history
3. Social history
4. Developmental history
5. Hospitalizations/emergency department visits
6. Surgery
7. Medications/allergies
8. Review of body systems, with particular attention to the genitourinary and gastrointestinal systems
9. History regarding presenting concern obtained from caretaker
10. History obtained from child

If the child's caretaker is unavailable to provide the medical history, then try to obtain medical records for review. When obtaining details of the caretaker's observations and concerns, structure the questioning in such a way to obtain the best possible chronology of events and/or observations. Questions that enable the child to provide contextual detail to observations and statements result in greater insight. For example, if the child made a statement to a caretaker in a manner that was spontaneous and idiosyncratic, it would be important to understand the circumstances under which the statement occurred. Inquire as to the caretaker's exact response to the child's disclosure or observed behavior and the child's reaction to that response.

Review of Systems

Although each of the body systems should be included in the medical history, the genitourinary (GU) and gastrointestinal (GI) ROS obtained from the caretaker is one of the most important aspects of the child's history that can be relevant to issues of sexual contact. The importance of the ROS originates from the need to identify any current or preexisting medical conditions that should be considered when assessing any GU or GI complaints that may have been associated with the alleged sexual contact. The clinician must consider the differential diagnosis of GU or GI complaints and take into account alternative explanations for the child's symptoms. If the child has had either GI or GU symptomatology for reasons unrelated to the alleged sexual contact, preexisting knowledge of such symptoms will be used to undermine the presence of the same symptoms when the result is from sexual contact.

One of the most important medical history details that can be obtained from a child and can confirm with medical certainty that he or she has experienced genital trauma is a history

of dysuria, which commonly follows either genital fondling, vulvar coitus, or coitus. Dysuria results from rubbing and resultant superficial trauma to the periurethral and/or vestibular structures. Because most of the injuries that result from genital fondling, vulvar coitus, or coitus will be superficial, they heal very quickly without demonstrative residual or nonspecific signs.

A history of urinary tract infections (UTIs) with associated dysuria in a child's ROS may help to rule out inappropriate contact. The clinician can best anticipate these challenges by conducting a thorough ROS. When preexisting conditions must be considered, the clinician carefully evaluates the temporal relationship between symptoms associated with that condition and the child's complaint(s) referable to the contact. Genitourinary questions should include history of UTIs, vaginal discharges, vaginal odor, vaginal bleeding, diaper dermatitis, urinary incontinence, use of bubble baths, treatment for any STIs, menstrual history, use of tampons, abortions, accidental genital injuries, vaginal foreign bodies, prior examinations of the genitalia for any reason other than routine health care, and self-exploratory activities/masturbation. It should be determined whether the child requires any anogenital care and if so by whom.

The GI ROS should include age of toilet training; use of rectal suppositories, enemas, or medications for stooling; history of constipation; painful bowel movements; frequency/character of stools; history of recurrent vomiting; diarrhea; hematochezia; hemorrhoids; fecal incontinence; rectal itching; and pinworms.

Myers[1,2] has identified some essential elements from a legal perspective that clinicians should be aware of and when addressed contribute to creating a more complete and defensible medical record.

1. Document the child's age at the time of the statement.
2. Note the length of time that elapsed between the suspected abuse and the child's statements.
3. Specify who was present when the child made the statement, where the statement was made, and to whom it was made.
4. Document whether specific statements are made in response to questions or are spontaneous.
5. Note whether the child's responses are made to leading or non-leading questions.
6. Note if the child's statement was made at the first opportunity that the child felt safe to talk.
7. Document the emotional state of the child. Note if the child was excited or distressed at the time of the statement and, if so, what signs or symptoms of excitement or distress were observed.
8. Document whether the child was calm, placid, or sleeping prior to making the statement, or soon thereafter.
9. Use the exact words that the child used to describe the characteristics of the event.
10. Document the child's physical condition at the time of the statement.
11. Note any suspected incentives for the child to fabricate or distort the truth.

Recording the Physical Examination Findings

The medical record should reflect that the physical examination was thorough, and the documentation should support it. The record should include the overall medical condition of the child and the general physical examination findings, and it should describe in meticulous detail the appearance of all genital and anal structures and appropriate extragenital findings. A detailed report goes a long way toward demonstrating that the examiner understands the importance of being thorough and has recorded the examination findings in as precise a manner as possible.

To augment the medical record's written description of physical findings, it is equally important that there be visual documentation of any physical findings interpreted to be either diagnostic or supportive of the diagnosis. The availability of photographic and/or video documentation should eliminate the potential for an adversary to request that a child undergo a repeat examination for a second opinion. If a physical finding is diagnostic, then objective visual documentation of that finding should be available for a second opinion. The benefit of obtaining visual documentation for all examinations, whether diagnostic findings are present or not, is justifiable if there is reason to believe the child remains at risk for abuse in the future. If further abuse occurs, then the baseline documentation of the initial examination may serve as a useful comparative reference. The need for baseline documentation is particularly evident when a child presents in the context of a custody dispute, or the allegations are unsubstantiated but are of concern. Chapter 4 details the process by which images are obtained, processed, and stored.

Describing the Physical Examination

The physical examination is a head-to-toe examination. All aspects of the general medical examination should be described appropriately. Children who experience sexual abuse may also experience physical abuse and neglect, and thus the examination should record any findings supportive of that abuse. The genital and anal examinations, as well as any extragenital findings, need to be described in detail and supplemented by photographs.

When no acute or chronic signs of trauma are found on examination, it is inadequate to simply state that no evidence of sexual abuse exists or that the examination is "normal." More appropriately, clear descriptions of examination findings are recorded in the medical chart, and an explanation for the lack of acute or chronic residua is given. Conclusions such as "the examination neither confirms nor denies the history provided" or "an examination without diagnostic residua is consistent with the history" are inadequate as well. Ambiguous conclusions should be avoided. The best diagnostic assessment integrates

the physical examination findings, laboratory results, and medical history in a manner that is clear and educative.

The recording of the physical examination should be descriptive. Rather than using a preformed checklist that designates findings as either normal or abnormal, the following example illustrates an alternative way to describe the genital and anal examination. The example provided represents excerpts from the complete report and illustrate the description of only the anogenital aspects of the physical examination.

Example Description of an Anogenital Examination

The child was examined in both the supine frog-leg and knee-chest positions. The examination was conducted and recorded with the use of video colposcopy at ×4, ×6, ×10, and ×16 magnifications with white- and red-free light. The child's sexual maturity rating (Tanner stage) is 1 for both breast and pubic hair development and Huffman stage 1 for estrogenization of external genitalia. The clitoral hood and labia majora and minora are well-formed without acute or chronic signs of trauma. The structures of the vaginal vestibule were examined first in the supine frog-leg position with the use of labial separation and traction. Examination of the vestibular structures demonstrated no abnormal degree of redness, vaginal discharge, or malodor. There was redundant tissue surrounding the urethral meatus. The hymenal membrane had a crescentic-shaped orifice, with an uninterrupted thin and translucent border along its edge from 2 to 10 o'clock with the child supine. The transverse hymenal orifice diameter measured between 3 to 5 mm depending on the degree of labial separation, traction, and relaxation. The external surface of the hymenal membrane, fossa navicularis, and posterior fourchette did not demonstrate any acute or chronic signs of injury. There was a fine lacy vascular pattern to vestibular mucosa. The child was placed in the knee-chest position. The appearance of the hymenal membrane orifice edge in this position was unchanged. There were no stigmata of STI. The external anal verge tissues and perineum were examined in the supine knee-chest position with the legs flexed onto the abdomen. There was a sym-metrical rugal pattern, normal sphincter tone, a constrictive response to separation of the buttocks, no post-inflammatory pigmentary changes, and slight venous pooling during the later part of the examination, which disappeared with anal constriction. There were no acute or chronic signs of trauma to the external anal verge tissues, the distal portion of the anal rectal canal, or the perineum.

Putting It All Together: Formulating a Diagnosis

The medical diagnosis is the cornerstone of the final assessment. As such, the diagnosis must be formulated in a manner that is clear and educative. When formulating the diagnostic assessment, the clinician must consider and incorporate salient aspects of each of the following:

- Historical details and behavioral indicators reflective of the contact
- Symptoms that result from the contact
- Acute genital/anal injuries and/or chronic residua
- Forensic evidence
- STIs

When discrepancies exist between the child's perception of what he or she experienced and the examination findings, the reasons should be explained. Throughout all aspects of the diagnostic and treatment process, the clinician must be objective, know the limitations of clinical observations, and formulate the diagnosis in a neutral manner.

The following are examples of common case scenarios, each of which requires a different diagnostic assessment.

1. Medical history/behaviors are clear and descriptive of inappropriate sexual contact but no physical diagnostic residua are present.
2. Medical history/behaviors are clear and descriptive of inappropriate sexual contact with symptom-specific complaints reflective of genital and/or anal trauma.
3. Medical history/behaviors are clear and descriptive of inappropriate sexual contact and physical diagnostic residua are present (ie, acute/healed injuries, STI, other physical forensic evidence).
4. Medical history/behaviors are suspicious and/or concerning that child either experienced something inappropriate and/or was exposed to something inappropriate and the examination is without physical diagnostic residua.

Although the constellation of historical, behavioral, and examination findings will vary from case to case, the following serve as examples of how the concluding component of the diagnostic assessment could be formulated in each of the following common scenarios:

- Medical history/behaviors are clear and descriptive of inappropriate sexual contact but no physical diagnostic residua are present.

The medical history presented by this 8-year-old female reflects progression of a variety of inappropriate sexual activities over time initially represented to her in a caring and loving context. Although the initial interactions were described as playful, the activities progressed with correspondingly escalating threats to maintain secrecy. The young girl did not complain of experiencing any physical discomfort following the genital fondling or the stroking of her uncle's genitalia. During the medical history, she described icky stuff that came out of his "pee pee" and explained that she had to wipe it from her "peach" using a tissue. In addition, she said that she was worried that people could tell just by the way that they looked at her that she had to do those disgusting things. In light of the history regarding contact with genital secretions, she is at risk for contracting an STI. I have evaluated this young lady for STIs. Treatment and follow-up will be initiated should any of the test results be positive. Her physical examination does not demonstrate any acute or chronic residua to the sexual contact, nor would be anticipated to in light of

her denial of discomfort associated with the contact. Her body image concern is common among children who experience sexual abuse. There isn't any alternative explanation for this child's history of progressive engagement in sexual activities, threats to maintain secrecy, detailed description of a variety of sexually explicit interactions, and concerns about body image other than from experiencing such. The most signifi-cant impact of her inappropriate sexual experiences is psychological. She needs to undergo a pretreatment evaluation by a clinical child psychologist to assess the impact of her inappropriate experiences, develop a therapeutic plan for trauma-focused cognitive-behavioral therapy, and the provision of anticipatory guidance regarding personal body safety.

- Medical history/behaviors are clear and descriptive of inappropriate sexual contact and physical diagnostic residua are present (ie, acute/healed injuries, STI, other physical forensic evidence).

This 9-year-old female provided a clear and detailed medical history reflecting her experiencing genital-to-genital contact and being coerced into placing her mouth on her father's genitalia. Her perception was that the genital-to-genital contact involved penetration into her vagina. She provided a history of bleeding, genital pain, and dysuria following the genital-to-genital contact although she never disclosed such to her mother because of threats to maintain secrecy. Her initial disclosure occurred 2 months following the last contact. Her physical examination demonstrates diagnostic residua to the contact as evidenced by a well-defined healed transection of the posterior portion of her hymen extending to the base of its attachment on the posterior vaginal wall. This finding is diagnostic of blunt force penetrating trauma and reflects the introduction of a foreign body through the structures of the vaginal vestibule, the hymenal orifice, and into the vagina. She did not complain of physical discomfort associated with the history of oral-genital contact, although she stated that her father peed in her mouth, placing her at additional risk for an STI.

- Medical history/behaviors are clear and descriptive of inappropriate sexual contact with symptom-specific complaints reflective of genital and/or anal trauma.

This 8-year-old female provided a detailed history of a variety of sexually inappropriate interactions with her uncle spanning a 6-month time frame. The initial activities involved exposure to child pornography as a way to represent the activities and create the impression for the child that the interactions were acceptable. The most recent event, 10 days prior to disclosure, involved her uncle touching her genitalia and placing his "stuff" into her coochie. When asked to explain what she meant by "inside" her coochie, with the use of an anatomical model of the female genitalia, she demonstrated that she thought his "stuff" went inside in the adult sense of penetration. However, on physical examination there were no acute or

chronic signs of trauma to her perceived vaginal penetration. The hymenal membrane edge was without interruption, and the orifice diameter of 5 mm was insufficient to have allowed introduction of a foreign body, such as a penis. The genital-to-genital contact that she described was limited to penetration of the vaginal vestibule. When asked what the genital-to-genital touching felt like, she provided a history of discomfort that followed the rubbing of his genitalia on hers. She denied seeing anything following the contact that made her know she had discomfort. When asked to explain what she meant by the genital-to-genital contact causing her discomfort, she stated that it hurt her after he stopped when she went to go "pee pee." When asked to describe the discomfort when peeing, she stated that it stung. When asked how long the discomfort lasted she responded "only a day." She denied ever having felt anything like that before and only had that feeling when he did it again. Her ROS to address differential considerations for dysuria was negative. The symptom of dysuria temporally related to the genital-to-genital contact with no alternative explanation reflects trauma to the periurethral area as a result of rubbing. The only way this young girl could know about the symptom of dysuria temporally related to the genital-to-genital contact is by experiencing such contact. This confirms with medical certainty that she experienced penetration into the structures of the vaginal vestibule. The trauma incurred to the distal urethra/vestibular mucosa was superficial and has since healed without residua as anticipated. Her physical examination does not demonstrate any acute or chronic residua and testing for STIs was negative.

- Insufficient historical, behavioral, or physical examination findings to support referents concern that child experienced anything of a sexually inappropriate nature.

A 2½-year-old male was examined to diagnose and treat any residua to the concern that he may have been touched in a sexually inappropriate manner. This concern arose because of a diaper rash, intermittent self-stimulatory behaviors, and some resistance to having his diaper changed. The mother raised the question as to whether her son may have been touched in a sexually inappropriate manner to account for the genital irritation, increased genital touching, and resistance to have his diaper changed. The mother stated that she had been sexually abused by her father as a child and wanted to protect her son from the same. The maternal grandparents occasionally baby-sit for her son. His physical examination is positive for diaper dermatitis due to *Candida albicans*. The historical and behavioral details that have been provided are insufficient to confirm with medical certainty that this young man has experienced anything of a sexually inappropriate nature. The constellation of behavioral changes are best attributed to his diaper dermatitis and not sexually inappropriate contact. The mother was advised that she should provide to her son anticipatory guidance regarding body safety in a developmentally appropriate manner when

he has the language to communicate. Baseline documentation of the appearance of his anogenital anatomy was obtained should there be any concern in the future. If so, this will serve as a useful reference. The mother will need to address some unresolved issues concerning her own experience and exercise caution in leaving her child in the care of any individual for whom she has concern.

The following are examples of less common presenting scenarios:

- On examination, the clinician identifies a healed injury with no prior suspicion of abuse and for which no historical or behavioral indicators are presented.
- A child presents with a concern by a caretaker without historical or behavioral details to support the concern.
- An STI is diagnosed in a young child, and no explanation for how the child contracted the infection is evident following a complete investigation.
- A child presents with fabricated or misinterpreted behaviors and/or a history alleging sexual abuse.
- Concerns arise in a family with custody/visitation arrangements in a young child requiring genital care.
- Medical findings that mimic sexual abuse on evaluation are found to be associated with medical conditions and not the result of abuse.
- Witnessed inappropriate sexual interactions without physical diagnostic residua.

In circumstances in which the history and examination findings do not support each other, a statement that the examination is inconsistent with the history and that an alternative explanation should be sought is most appropriate.

The examples of diagnostic assessments presented in this chapter serve to illustrate components of a diagnostic assessment and how a physician might clearly articulate findings and their significance. A detailed medical record that is clear in its conclusions reduces the likelihood that the clinician will need to appear in court. Conclusion options should include a recommendation that the child have a complete mental health assessment of the impact of the experience, as well as indicate the need to develop a treatment plan.

Conclusion

The sexual abuse of children is a complex form of victimization that requires a multidisciplinary approach during initial evaluation and treatment. The goal of any intervention is to protect the child and, if possible, correct the environment that allowed the abuse to occur or continue. The health care professional is called on to provide medical diagnostic and treatment services. The clinician's assessment should serve the purpose of bringing a more complete understanding of a child's experience when sexual abuse is suspected to assist colleagues in child protection and law enforcement in meeting the child's therapeutic needs when abuse is substantiated. For the

child and caretaker the medical assessment serves to both diagnose and treat any physical consequences of the sexual contact as well as address any concerns the child might have regarding their sense of "body intactness."

For health care professionals to serve the needs of children alleged to have been sexually abused, they need to avail themselves of relevant information on patterns of victimization, the medical and mental health consequences of sexual abuse, and therapeutic approaches to meet both short- and long-term needs of the child and family. Health care professionals should seek active involvement with multidisciplinary teams in their communities.

We anticipate that health care professionals, after reading this text, will be more comfortable evaluating children suspected of being sexually abused. We believe that they will understand the importance of a thorough evaluation and the "how-tos" of interpreting, documenting, and formulating a defensible medical diagnosis. If health care professionals view their role as advocating for children who experience abuse, the only way this can be achieved is by developing the clinical skills to conduct examinations with knowledge, skill, and sensitivity that forms the foundation for the articulation of diagnostic opinions that are balanced and objective.

Summary

Dos

- Describe findings simply and clearly.
- Be aware of the child's developmental status and the expressive limitations associated with it.
- Use exacting words in the documentation.
- Use non-leading but focused questions throughout the medical history.
- Record both questions asked of the child/caretaker and the specific answers given.
- Use diagrams, videotapes, or photographs to supplement the written documentation.
- Obtain visual documentation of all physical findings that are considered diagnostic.

Don'ts

- Don't use leading questions if at all possible.
- Don't rely on memory; rather, create a well-documented chart that can be consulted later for details.
- Don't use imprecise terms such as "virginal" or "intact" hymen.
- Don't use diagnostic conclusions such as "examination neither confirms or denies," "examination consistent with history," or "no evidence of abuse."

References

1. Myers JEB. *Evidence in Child Abuse and Neglect Cases.* 3rd ed. New York, NY: John Wiley; 1997
2. Myers JEB. Investigative interviewing regarding child maltreatment. In: *Legal Issues in Child Abuse and Neglect Practice.* 2nd ed. Thousand Oaks, CA: Sage Publications; 1998:102–152
3. Finkel MA, Ricci LR. Documentation and preservation of visual evidence in child abuse. *Child Maltreat.* 1997;2(4):322–330
4. Boyce MC, Melhorn KJ, Vargo G. Pediatric trauma documentation. Adequacy for assessment of child abuse. *Arch Pediatr Adolesc Med.* 1996;150(7):730–732
5. Parra JM, Huston RL, Foulds DM. Resident documentation of diagnostic impression in sexual abuse evaluations. *Clin Pediatr.* 1997;36(12):691–694
6. Socolar RR, Champion M, Green C. Physicians' documentation of sexual abuse of children. *Arch Pediatr Adolesc Med.* 1996;150(2):191–196
7. Socolar RR, Raines B, Chen-Mok M, Runyan DK, Green C, Paterno S. Intervention to improve physician documentation and knowledge of child sexual abuse: a randomized, controlled trial. *Pediatrics.* 1998;101(5):817–824

Index